Global Health, Humanity and the COVID-19 Pandemic

Francis Egbokhare • Adeshina Afolayan
Editors

Global Health, Humanity and the COVID-19 Pandemic

Philosophical and Sociological Challenges and Imperatives

palgrave
macmillan

Editors
Francis Egbokhare
Linguistics and African Languages
University of Ibadan
Ibadan, Nigeria

Adeshina Afolayan
Department of Philosophy
University of Ibadan
Ibadan, Nigeria

ISBN 978-3-031-17428-5 ISBN 978-3-031-17429-2 (eBook)
https://doi.org/10.1007/978-3-031-17429-2

Cover illustration: Jasmina007 Getty Images

This Palgrave Macmillan imprint is published by the registered company Springer Nature Switzerland AG.
The registered company address is: Gewerbestrasse 11, 6330 Cham, Switzerland

Preface and Acknowledgements

Pandemics have always been a part of the world's historical heritage. From the first series of plague pandemic—or the Justinian plague—of 541 to c. 767 down to the second plague pandemic—or the Black Death—of the fourteenth century that killed between 75 and 200 million people, to the Spanish Flu of the twentieth century (that decimated over a hundred million) and the HIV/AIDS pandemic that started in 1981 (that has so far killed over thirty seven million), humanity has always battled unknown pathogens that were unleashed, sometimes as the consequences of human activities under the auspice of the march of civilization. Since the dawn of the twenty-first century, scientists have identified a new species of virus—severe acute respiratory syndrome-related coronavirus (SARSr-CoV)—with the capacity to infect humans. Two strains of the virus have been responsible for millions of deaths. The first one, SARS-CoV-1, manifested between 2002 and 2004, across about 29 countries, and led to over 800 deaths. The second strain, SARS-CoV-2 (also referred to as COVID-19), has had a worse impact than the first strain. Both strains were first discovered in China from where they became worldwide pandemics.

The emergence of pathogens has been simultaneous with the inexorable civilizational progress of humans. And science and technology have played the most fundamental role in the defining of the human world as we have come to know it. Both have been borne by the epistemological legitimacy that science constructed for itself as the template for human knowledge, especially about the universe and its dynamics. And that template has been consistently applied to societal understanding of human activities, all to the deliberate sidelining of the humanities themselves. In other words, the sciences have attempted to be humanitarian without any consideration for the humanistic values and sensibility that derives from the humanities. And from that disregard has emerged the horrors of the atomic bomb, climate change and the tragedy of pandemics that have transformed the human world.

Global health denotes the cumulative health profile of the entire global population. It refers to the complex of not only the framework of researches and practices that investigates and improves the health of all people on the globe, but also the range of humanistic issues—economic, cultural, social, ideological—that constitute the sources of inequities and threat to the achievement of a positive global health profile. Pandemics of all sorts in human history, including the recent COVID-19, have constituted the major threat to the framework of global health. Science can no longer be scientistic in its explanation of the universe. And that depends a lot on the humanities jettisoning its besieged mentality in order to be able to take its pace besides science and technology in the understanding of the world, and the appropriate monitoring of the progress of civilization. It is the hope that this volume will serve as a space-clearing gesture that will outline an interrogation of science through a humanistic analysis of the COVID-19 pandemic and how a post-pandemic world would be better with science walking side by side with the humanities in the reconstruction of a new world order where dangerous pathogens are kept at bay.

In putting together this volume, we would like to first appreciate all the contributors who are united in their collective belief in the values of the humanities and how they could be deployed to make the world better. They have patiently and assiduously committed themselves to making this volume a reality.

Ibadan, Nigeria

Francis Egbokhare
Adeshina Afolayan

Contents

1 **Introduction: Humanity and Disease Discourse** 1
Francis Egbokhare and Adeshina Afolayan

Part I Humanistic Understanding of Disease 13

2 **Toward a Fuller Understanding of the Enigma of Health** 15
Peter Amato

3 **Ubuntu and COVID-19: A Philosophical Reflection** 33
M. S. C. Okolo

4 **Limits of Science-Based Approaches in Global Health: Sociocultural and Moral Lessons from Ebola and COVID-19** 51
Samuel J. Ujewe

5 **The Vaccination Mandate Debate Revisited** 75
Peter Aloysius Ikhane

Part II Critical Framing of the Pandemic in Africa 95

6 An African Perspective on the Ethics and Politics of Foreign Medical Aid in a Pandemic 97
Adeolu Oluwaseyi Oyekan and Ademola Kazeem Fayemi

7 Disease Discourses, African Knowledge Systems, and COVID-19 in Senegal 123
Karen S. Barton, Jieun Lee, and Ivan J. Ramírez

8 *Ẹnulẹbọ*: Ethical Imperative of Yorùbá Thought on Eating for COVID-19-Related Crises 151
Adewale O. Owoseni

9 Epidemiology and an Epistemic Evaluation of the Management of COVID-19 in Nigeria 171
Anselm K. Jimoh and Francis Ikhianosime

10 Borders, Boundaries, and Identities: Navigating the Barriers to Solidarity and Cohesion in a Pandemic 197
Adeolu Oluwaseyi Oyekan and Wasiu Abiodun Balogun

11 Discourses of the Wandering Almajiri Child as Representation of the (Post-)COVID Generation 223
Malami Buba and Mika'ilu Ibrahim

12 Quarantining the Holy Spirit: Africa and the Pentecostal Economy of COVID-19 Pandemic 247
Asonzeh Ukah

13 On Pandemic Planning and the Frontline Workers in Nigeria 283
Damilola Victoria Oduola

14 **Dialogism and Polyphony in the Interpretations of COVID-19 Discourse in Zimbabwe** 303
Tobias Marevesa and Esther Mavengano

Part III Representing COVID-19 327

15 **Cartooning COVID-19 on Facebook** 329
James Yékú

16 **"It's in Your Hands": Communicating a Pandemic to a Disengaged Public** 353
Eyitayo Aloh

17 **Musical Representations of COVID-19 on Social Media Among Young People in Nigeria** 373
Toyin Samuel Ajose and Jeremiah Oluwadara Omotayo

18 **COVID-19, Food and Freedom to Worship: An Analytic Approach to Nigeria's Religioscape** 401
Benson Ohihon Igboin

19 **Analysis of COVID-19 Risk Communication and Community Engagement on Social Media in Nigeria** 427
Abiola I. Odejide and Olayinka A. Egbokhare

20 **COVID-19 (Post)Proverbials: Twisting the Word Against the Virus** 461
Aderemi Raji-Oyelade

Index 483

Notes on Contributors

Adeshina Afolayan teaches philosophy at the University of Ibadan, Nigeria. His areas of specialization include philosophy of politics, African cultural studies and African philosophy. He is the author of *Philosophy and National Development in Nigeria* (2018), a coeditor of the *Palgrave Handbook of African Philosophy* (2017), *Pentecostalism and Politics in Africa* (2018), *Pathways to Alternative Epistemologies in Africa* (2021), the editor of *Identities, Histories and Values in Postcolonial Nigeria* (2021) and the co-author of *Fela Anikulapo-Kuti: Afrobeat, Rebellion, and Philosophy* (2022).

Toyin Samuel Ajose is an ethnomusicologist with broad research interest in Christian/gospel music in Nigeria/African Pentecostalism. His research focuses on musical expressions in Prayer Mountain Spirituality among Yoruba Pentecostals in Southwestern Nigeria, and Christian music and social engagements in contemporary Nigeria. He holds a doctorate degree from the University of Ibadan, Nigeria. He currently serves as the Ag. Head of Department of Music, University of Ibadan, and also the Director of Music at the Chapel of the Resurrection, University of Ibadan. He is also the Public Relation Officer of the Association of Nigerian Musicologists (ANIM).

Eyitayo Aloh is currently an assistant professor (limited term) at Trent University, Peterborough. His research focuses on the representation and portrayal of Black/African Canadian Identity in Literature and Popular Culture, and how immigration plays a role in shaping this representation. He is particularly interested in how such representations are problematized in humour and comedy productions in the mainstream Canadian media. Aloh has authored four children's books, contributed to poetry and prose anthologies, and is a regular writer and columnist for *New Telegraph* newspaper, Nigeria. His research interest includes cultural studies (broadly defined but with a particular focus on Yoruba oral culture), postcolonial studies and its cultural interpretations, masculinity, media and communication studies and interdisciplinary studies.

Peter Amato teaches philosophy, politics and economics in the Department of English and Philosophy at Drexel University in Philadelphia, PA, USA. His areas of specialization include political philosophy, ethics, phenomenology and Marxism. He also researches in the history of Western philosophy and African philosophies.

Wasiu Abiodun Balogun is a scholar of history, diplomacy, global energy developments and maritime affairs. His current research focuses on energy and maritime security challenges in West and Central Africa. Balogun had his bachelor's degree in History and Diplomatic Studies from Ogun State University and a Masters in International Relations from Obafemi Awolowo University, Ile-Ife, Nigeria. He then moved to the Centre for Energy Petroleum Mineral Law and Policy (CEPMLP), University of Dundee, Scotland, where he obtained a Master of Science degree in Energy Studies, specializing in Energy and the Environment. Balogun had his doctoral degree in Energy and Maritime Security from the Department of International Relations, Lancaster University, Lancaster, England.

Karen S. Barton is Professor of Geography, GIS and Sustainability at the University of Northern Colorado. Her work focuses on Africa, community resilience and adaptation in marine and agricultural communities, and global environmental change. With support from Fulbright and the National Endowment for the Humanities, she recently published *Africa's Joola Shipwreck: Causes and Consequences of a Humanitarian Disaster* (2020). Barton has led numerous expeditions abroad focused on conservation and local communities, including Iceland, Peru, Nicaragua, Nepal and Guyana. In 2022, she was selected as a fellow for Cohort 7 of

Homeward Bound, a global leadership initiative for women in science. She currently serves as a fellow of the Explorers Club, the Royal Geographical Society, and is the Co-President of the Fulbright Colorado. She is also the president of the Society of Women Geographers, a group formed in 1925 when women were denied entry into most professional organizations. In September 2022, she carried the SWG's expedition flag to the oceanic site of the Joola disaster in memory of the 1863 individuals who lost their lives.

Malami Buba has been a professor in the Division of African Studies, Hankuk University of Foreign Studies, Korea, since 2016. Before then, he was a professor in the Department of English Language and Linguistics, Sokoto State University (Nigeria) as well as the Deputy Vice-Chancellor, Administration, in the same university. He was also a professor in the Department of Modern European Languages and Linguistics, Usmanu Ɗanfodiyo University, Sokoto (Nigeria). He has held visiting scholar positions in the USA (Indiana University, Bloomington), Germany (University of Potsdam) and the Netherlands (Leiden University). His recent publications include: "Hausa 'Native' Speakers and the Racialisation of Knowledge Production" (2021) and "Look East" and Look Back: Lessons for Africa in the Changing Global Order (2022)

Francis Egbokhare is Professor of Linguistics at the University of Ibadan, a public intellectual and a former president of the Nigerian Academy of Letters (NAL). His areas of specialization include ethics, linguistics and syntax. He is the coeditor (with R. P. Schaefer) of *A Dictionary of Emai* (2007), *A Grammar of Emai* (2016) and *Class Marking in Emai* (2019). He is currently working on a dictionary of Nigerian Pidgin.

Olayinka Egbokhare is a senior lecturer in the Department of Communication and Language Arts, University of Ibadan. She is also a Commonwealth Rutherford Fellow. Her research interests cover media effects, marketing communications, creative writing, literacy, gender and health advocacy.

Ademola Kazeem Fayemi is a senior lecturer in the Department of Philosophy, University of Lagos, Nigeria. He is a principal investigator at the African Cluster Centre of the Africa Multiple Cluster of Excellence,

University of Lagos. He writes and lectures widely in African philosophy, African Bioethics and African environmental ethics. Fayemi received Global Excellence Postdoctoral Fellowship Award from the University of Johannesburg in 2017 where he interrogated beauty by surgical and non-surgical designs in sub-Sahara Africa through an Afro-bioethical lens. He won the 2020 Mark S. Ehrenreich Prize in Healthcare Ethics Research for the African region, awarded by the Pacific Center for Health Policy and Ethics, University of Southern California at the 15th World Congress of Bioethics Virtual Conference for being the best paper from Africa presented at the Congress. Until recently, he was a research fellow, Moi University African Cluster Centre of the Africa Multiple Cluster of Excellence, Kenya. Fayemi's current research is on developing a relational framework for research ethics in African Studies.

Mika'ilu Ibrahim is a specialist in applied linguistics with interest in discourse studies and early grade reading instruction in education systems. He coordinated international reading projects in Nigeria and is currently the Education Adviser for Foreign Commonwealth and Development Office (FCDO). He was a technical advisor and lead on Reading and Numeracy Activity (RANA) which aims at ensuring sustainable reading practices and policies in Nigeria. In the academics, he taught and conducted research on English language and reading instruction at Usmanu Danfodiyo University, Sokoto and Zamfara State College of Education Maru, Nigeria.

Benson Ohihon Igboin is Professor of Philosophy of Religion, Adekunle Ajasin University, Nigeria. He is also an academic associate in the Research Institute of Theology and Religion, University of South Africa. His areas of interest include philosophy of religion, African cultural values, African Pentecostalism, among others. He is the editor of *Corruption: A New Thinking in the Reverse Order* (2018), coeditor, *African Pentecostalism: Probity and Accountability* (2019), *The Mighty Temple of the Gods: A Festschrift for Professor (Bishop Theologian) Dapo F. Asaju* (2021), *Nigerian Pentecostalism and COVID-19: Dynamics, Worship, and Creativities* (2022) and "I am an African" (2021).

Peter Aloysius Ikhane holds a PhD in Philosophy from the University of Ibadan, Nigeria, where he also lectures. He is presently completing an

MSc degree in Bioethics in the Department of Bioethics and Medical Humanities from the same university. His areas of research interest include rationality and multilateral trade relations, rational choice theory, decision theory, global health discourse, applied epistemology and African epistemology. He is a co-editor of *African Epistemology: Essays on Being and Knowledge* (2023).

Francis Ikhianosime teaches philosophy in the Department of Philosophy, Seminary of All Saints, Uhiele-Ekpoma, Nigeria, with research interests in social epistemology, contemporary philosophy and metaphysics. Some of his publications in peer-reviewed books and journals include: "Levinas' Theory of Alterity and the Sketching of an Epistemology of Otherness" (2018), "Prejudicial Dysfunctions, Epistemic Practices and Priestly Formation: Anselm Jimoh and the Pursuit of Genuine Knowledge" (2019), "The Metaphysics of Empiricism: Two Dogmas of Empiricism Reexamined" (2021), "What Can a Woman Know? Epistemic Bias as Depersonalization" (2021).

Anselm K. Jimoh is Professor of Philosophy with specialization in epistemology and a special interest in African epistemology. He is currently the Head of Department of Philosophy, SS. Peter and Paul Catholic Major Seminary, Bodija, Ibadan, Nigeria. He is the author of *Certitude and Doubt: A Study Guide in Epistemology* (2017); *Philosophy: A Guide for Beginners* (2021); *Introduction to Existentialism, Phenomenology and Hermeneutics* (2014); "Reconstructing a Fractured Indigenous Knowledge System" (2018); and many other papers in local and international peer-reviewed journals. He is currently working on the prospect of a decolonized African epistemology and African philosophy curriculum in African universities.

Jieun Lee is a professional geographer and a faculty member in the Geography, GIS and Sustainability Department at University of Northern Colorado. Her research focuses on the intersection of urban environments, travel behaviour and community health. Her search focuses on disparities in accessibility and health through the lens of social equity for marginalized populations due to their income, race and ethnicity and gender using various Geographic Information Systems and Sciences (GIS) applications and geospatial analysis. Specifically, her recent studies explore interconnectedness between housing affordability and public health crises such as mental health and COVID-19 in Colorado. She has published in journals such as *Urban Studies*, *Journal of Urban Design*, the *Journal of Urban Affairs*, *International Journal of Environmental Research and Public Health International Journal of Disaster Risk Science*, *Spatial and Spatio-temporal Epidemiology* and *Behavioral Medicine*. She has also authored several book chapters—including in the *Handbook for Teaching and Learning in Geography* and the *Handbook of Global Urban Health*—and has published in the London School of Economics Urban Centre's Politics and Policy blog.

Tobias Marevesa is New Testament Lecturer in the Department of Philosophy and Religious Studies, under the Joshua Nkomo School of Arts and Humanities at the Great Zimbabwe University where he teaches New Testament Studies and New Testament Greek. He is a research fellow at the Research Institute for Theology and Religion, College of Human Sciences, South Africa. He holds a PhD from the University of Pretoria in South Africa. His areas of interest are New Testament studies and politics, Pentecostal expressions in Zimbabwean Christianity, culture, human rights and gender-based violence. He has also published in the area of New Testament studies and conflict-resolution in the Zimbabwean political landscape. He has attended and presented a number of papers in both regional and international conferences and has published articles in reputable international journals.

Esther Mavengano is Lecturer in areas of Linguistics and Literature in the Department of English and Media Studies at Great Zimbabwe University. She is also a research fellow at the Research Institute for Theology and Religion, College of Human Sciences, UNISA, South Africa. She holds a PhD in Linguistics and Literary studies from the University of North West in South Africa. Her areas of interests are applied linguistics, discourse analysis, poetics and English as a Second Language. She has published in these areas.

Abiola Odejide is Emeritus Professor of Communication and Language Arts, University of Ibadan, Nigeria. Her research interests are in communication skills development, gender issues in higher education, women in the media and institutional cultures of higher educational institutions.

Damilola Victoria Oduola is a graduate student in the Department of Philosophy, University of Ibadan, Nigeria. Her areas of interest include applied ethics, social and political philosophy and African philosophy.

M. S. C. Okolo is a lecturer at the Federal University of Agriculture, Abeokuta, Nigeria. She studied Philosophy at the Universities of Calabar and Ibadan. A Civitella Ranieri Fellow, she is the author of *African Literature as Political Philosophy*, *Philosophy: Contemporary Concerns in Africa, and, Contesting the African Public Sphere*. She also has several published novels, and has contributed to many short story and poetry anthologies. Okolo's research interests include philosophy and African literature, political philosophy, and African identity. She is the recipient of CODESRIA Doctoral Prize for Africa in 2005.

Jeremiah Oluwadara Omotayo is a junior research fellow in the Political and Governance Policy Department, Nigerian Institute of Social and Economic Research (NISER). He is currently a PhD student of Political Sociology, Department of Political Science, University of Ibadan. Omotayo has engaged in several political and social research studies across Nigeria. As a public policy practitioner, he has engaged in the consultancy and training of civil servants. He has contributed to scholarly articles on youth politics, federalism, security studies and peace and conflict.

Adewale O. Owoseni holds a doctoral degree in philosophy from the University of Ibadan, Nigeria. His research interests include African philosophy, Animal and Environmental Ethics, Philosophy of Culture and Development. He recently published a co-authored article titled "A Complementarity Reflection on Human Interest and Common Good in Africa."

Adeolu Oluwaseyi Oyekan holds a Bachelor's and Master's degree in Philosophy from the Olabisi Onabanjo University, Ago-Iwoye, and a PhD in Philosophy from the University of Lagos. He has taught at undergraduate and postgraduate levels in the Department of Philosophy, Lagos

State University, Ojo, Nigeria, and published peer-reviewed articles in political philosophy, ethics and gender theory. He is currently a research fellow of Identities and Social Cohesion in Africa (ISCIA) at the Nelson Mandela University, Port Elizabeth, South Africa.

Aderemi Raji-Oyelade teaches Literature of the African Diaspora, Literary Theory, Creative Writing and New Media in the Department of English, University of Ibadan, Nigeria. His scholarly essays have appeared in journals including *Research in African Literatures*, *ARIEL*, *Wasafiri*, *Matatu* and *African Literature Today*. His book *Playful Blasphemies: Postproverbials as Archetypes of Modernity in Yoruba Culture* (2012) has received acclaim as a seminal work in contemporary African studies. Raji-Oyelade has won multiple literary and academic prizes, including the ANA/Cadbury Prize (Nigeria), the Ford Foundation Research Grant (USA), the West African Research Council Prize (West Africa) and the Harry Oppenheimer Award (South Africa). He is the coordinator of the multi-site, pan-African research project on the theory and practices of postproverbials in seven African countries.

Ivan J. Ramírez is a geographer whose research focuses on the intersections of climate change, urban health, disasters and environmental justice. Using geospatial and community-based approaches, he seeks to address health and social inequities across and between communities in the USA and internationally. Current projects include El Niño-Southern Oscillation impacts on malaria, ecosyndemics and syndemic vulnerability in Colorado. His work is published in interdisciplinary journals such as *Weather, Climate, and Society*, *EcoHealth*, *International Journal of Disaster Risk Science*, *Behavioral Medicine* and *Spatial & Spatio-temporal Epidemiology*. As a teacher, he is committed to diversity, equity and inclusion, and cross-disciplinary environmental and public health education. Ivan is a faculty member in the Department of Health and Behavioral Sciences at University of Colorado (CU), Denver. He is also an affiliate at the Consortium for Capacity Building (CCB), INSTAAR at CU Boulder. Ivan has a PhD in Geography from Michigan State University with specializations in Ethics, Development, and Community Engagement, and an MA in Climate and Society from Columbia University.

Samuel J. Ujewe is a researcher and expert in Bioethics and Health Policy, especially global health ethics and policy, health research ethics, healthcare ethics, ethics of clinical trials, ethics of infectious diseases and international bioethics—with vast international experience in leading ethics research teams and delivering on several ethics projects. He obtained a First Class BA Hons in Philosophy from the University of Zimbabwe; a Master of Health Sciences (MHSc) in Bioethics from the University of Otago, New Zealand; and a PhD in Bioethics and Health Policy from the University of Central Lancashire, United Kingdom. He is the coeditor of *Socio-cultural Dimensions of Emerging Infectious Diseases in Africa: An Indigenous Response to Deadly Epidemics* (2019). Ujewe is a fellow and sub-faculty chair at the Global Emerging Pathogens Treatment Consortium (GET-Africa), leading projects and research within the Cultural, Anthropological, Social, and Economic Impact (CASE) Work Group.

Asonzeh Ukah is Professor of Christianity and African Religions in the Department for the Study of Religions, University of Cape Town. He is also the chair of Religious Studies and the director of a newly created research unit, African Centre for Religion, Ethics and Society (ACRES) at the same institution. He trained as a sociologist of religion and a historian of religion, and has taught in several universities in Africa and Europe. With fieldwork experience in west, east and southern Africa, his research interests include Religious Urbanism, New Religious Movements, Sociology of Pentecostalism and the Media. From 2014 till January 2022, he was the director of the Research Institute for Christianity and Society in Africa (RICSA); since 2019, he has been the Head of Department for the Study of Religions, University of Cape Town, South Africa. He has published extensively in internationally reputable journals in English, German and Spanish.

James Yékú is Assistant Professor of African and African American studies at the University of Kansas, where he leads the African digital humanities program. He is the author of *Cultural Netizenship: Social Media, Popular Culture, and Performance in Nigeria* (Indiana University Press), and a book of poetry, *Where the Baedeke*r *Leads* (Toronto). Yékú is a 2022 fellow at the Center for Advanced Internet Studies (CAIS) in Bochum, Germany.

List of Figures

Fig. 7.1	Senegal's COVID-19 cases by regions; COVID incidence per 1000	127
Fig. 7.2	Map of Senegal and The Gambia. (Source: Jieun Lee)	130
Fig. 7.3	Percentage of elderly per region (>60)	135
Fig. 7.4	Sleeve Your Sneeze Graffiti	137
Fig. 7.5	Combat coronavirus postage stamp. (*Le Poste* 2020)	138
Fig. 7.6	October new case counts for Senegal post-Magal. (Source: JHU CSSE COVID-19)	140
Fig. 7.7	Urbanization rates in Senegal	142
Fig. 12.1	A public message about COVID-19 (Photo: author 2021)	253
Fig. 12.2	A Public Service advertisement to curb religion-induced vaccine hesitancy in South Africa (Photo: author)	264
Fig. 15.1	The Death Trap (*Facebook*)	337
Fig. 15.2	Flattening The Curve in Kano (*Facebook*)	339
Fig. 15.3	Masks of The Beast (*Facebook*)	341
Fig. 15.4	When Equity Forgets To Wash Its Hands (Facebook. https://www.facebook.com/photo.php?fbid=10222867151567898 &set=a.2058448341395&type=3&theater)	347
Fig. 19.1	Video types	436
Fig. 19.2	Type of message	437
Fig. 19.3	Identified sponsors	437

Fig. 19.4 Languages used 438
Fig. 19.5 Types of appeal 439
Fig. 19.6 Cultural resonance 439

1

Introduction: Humanity and Disease Discourse

Francis Egbokhare and Adeshina Afolayan

It was the best of times, it was the worst of times, it was the age of wisdom, it was the age of foolishness, it was the epoch of belief, it was the epoch of incredulity, it was the season of light, it was the season of darkness, it was the spring of hope, it was the winter of despair.
—Charles Dickens, *A Tale of Two Cities* (1859)

When Charles Dickens penned this famous opening statement of his iconic novel, England was in the grip of a world-historic event. Industrialization, as well as the impending revolutions in America and France, was already fundamentally restructuring the social fabric of

F. Egbokhare (✉)
Department of Linguistics and African Languages, University of Ibadan, Ibadan, Nigeria
e-mail: fo.egbokhare@ui.edu.ng

A. Afolayan
Department of Philosophy, University of Ibadan, Ibadan, Nigeria
e-mail: a.afolayan@ui.edu.ng

F. Egbokhare, A. Afolayan (eds.), *Global Health, Humanity and the COVID-19 Pandemic*, https://doi.org/10.1007/978-3-031-17429-2_1

Victorian England, and it had become so terrible that there was a serious concern with the threat of gradual dehumanization. *A Tale of Two Cities* therefore is a historical novel concerned with the problem of historical dehumanization (Marcus 1976: 57). Dickens' understanding of history was catastrophic. Thus, the "haunted and contradictory" quality of the opening paragraph attests to both the vision of that historical continuum and the possibility of liberation from it. According to J. M. Rignall, Dickens' distinctive vision of history:

> is a peculiarly grim one. As oppression is shown to breed oppression, violence to beget violence, evil to provoke evil, a pattern emerges that is too deterministic to owe much to Carlyle and profoundly at odds with the conventional complacencies of Whig history. Instead of progress there is something more like the catastrophic continuum that is Walter Benjamin's description of the historical process: the single catastrophe, piling wreckage upon wreckage. (1984: 575)

The London that is depicted in most of Dickens' novels, and in *A Tale of Two Cities*, is one that is already in deep misery, not only from what has been called the "mysterious circulation of capital" (Robinson 2004: 76) but also from the terrible spread of diseases that claim thousands of lives. With capitalism and diseases, we arrive at the intention of Dickens through the passage: a deep confusion about the inability to achieve a neat certainty about one's era. The contrastive literary framework deployed in the famous paragraph also speaks to the contemporary period caught in the awful grip of the coronavirus pandemic.

In terms of the urgency of finding a solution to the scourge of the COVID-19, we can also reiterate that it is the best and the worst of times for all of humanity. When an epidemic or a pandemic breaks out, it affects not only the physical/biological configurations of humanity but also its infrastructural fabric—social, economic, religious, financial, moral, relational, and developmental. The COVID-19, like all other pandemics in the history of humankind, has not only invaded the human physiognomy and wrecked mortal and fatal havoc, but it has also brought the global economies to the point of recession, transformed social thinking, initiated political maneuvers, generated mental health issues, forced a rethinking of governance measures, and excavated the best and the worst in the human relational dynamics. In essence, this pandemic had practically stopped humanity dead in its track. With global statistics of over 636 million cases, number of deaths at 6.61 million, and still counting, and new variants of the coronavirus still threatening and killing, the last two years, from 2020, has been humanity's *annus horribilis*.

As has usually been the case with all the disease outbreaks in history, the response to the COVID-19 pandemic has been largely reckoned with in scientific terms. The World Health Organization (WHO), together with global pharmaceutical giants and other health consortiums, has been at the forefront of the massive and concerted global efforts to arrest the tragic decimation of human populations by the virus. The search for vaccines that will undermine the deadly drift of the virus began immediately. And success has been recorded in terms of the AstraZeneca, Moderna, Pfizer, Johnson & Johnson, as well as many other vaccines that have been developed in record times to battle the scourge. These vaccines preceded other scientific infrastructures that led to the mapping of the virus' structure, the epidemiological understanding of its behavior, and the containment of its spread. Indeed, it was so easy for science to step into the breach of the pandemic scourge. Since the beginning of the seventeenth century and the Enlightenment, the scientific worldview has gradually evolved to the point of defining and determining the architecture of the universe and all its components, including humans. With the collective efforts of the Vienna Circle of logical positivists, the scientific conception of the world gained a clearer and firmer foothold on the world's imagination. According to Otto Neurath, one of the most formidable members of the Vienna Circle, the scientific world-conception is characterized by two fundamental features: "*First* it is *empiricist and positivist*: there is knowledge only from experience, which rests on what is immediately given. This sets the limits for the content of legitimate science. *Second*, the scientific world-conception is marked by application of a certain method, namely *logical analysis*. The aim of scientific effort is to reach the goal, unified science, by applying logical analysis to the empirical material" (1973: 309). In other words, this scientific worldview, the search for a unified science, springs from:

> the search for a neutral system of formulae, for a symbolism freed from the slag of historical languages; and also the search for a total system of

> concepts. Neatness and clarity are striven for, and dark distances and unfathomable depths rejected. In science there are no "depths"; there is surface everywhere: all experience forms a complex network, which cannot always be surveyed and can often be grasped only in parts. Everything is accessible to man; and man is the measure of all things. Here is an affinity with the Sophists, not with the Platonists; with the Epicureans, not with the Pythagoreans; with all those who stand for earthly being and the here and now. The scientific world-conception knows *no unsolvable riddle.* Clarification of the traditional philosophical problems leads us partly to unmask them as pseudo-problems, and partly to transform them into empirical problems and thereby subject them to the judgment of experimental science. (ibid.: 306. Emphasis in original)

This scientific world-conception also offers what Wilfred Sellars regards as the "scientific image of man-in-the-world." And this image of humans is constructed by science to overshadow what anyone would have mistaken for a naïve understanding of humans. Sellars contrasts between the "manifest" and "scientific" images of man (both derived from an "original" image of man-in-the-world).[1] While the manifest conception of man-in-the-world is "the framework in terms of which man encountered himself" (2001: 476), it is different from the scientific image essentially on the basis of deploying different scientific methodologies for understanding human. In other words, Sellars warns that in juxtaposing the manifest image to the scientific, we should not make the mistake of thinking we are comparing a pre-scientific understanding of man with a more scientific understanding. On the contrary, according to him:

> ...what I mean by the manifest image is a refinement or sophistication of what might be called the "original" image.... Thus the conceptual framework which I am calling the manifest image is, in an appropriate sense, itself a scientific image. It is not only disciplined and critical; it also make use of those aspects of the scientific method which might be lumped

[1] By the "original" image, Sellars means a framework of reckoning, before the gradual unfolding of civilization, within which all objects are perceived as persons and all kinds of objects constitute ways of being persons. "This means that the sort of things that are said of objects in this framework are the sort of things that are said of persons" (ibid.: 478). However, the refinement of this original image, which Sellars calls the "manifest" image, is characterized, with the advancement of civilization, by the "de-personalization" of all objects other than persons.

> together under the heading "correlational induction." There is however one type of scientific reasoning which it by stipulation does *not* include, namely, that which involves the postulation of imperceptible entities, and principles pertaining to them, to explain the behavior of perceptible things. (ibid.: 476)

What is then called the scientific image of humans emerged from many integrated images deriving from several sciences which then determines itself to be "a *complete* image, i.e., to define a framework which could be the *whole truth* about that which belong to the image" (ibid.: 484). It is therefore just a little step from this conception of the scientific image as a complete image to its understanding as a *rival* to the manifest image. And the logic becomes almost unassailable: if the scientific image constitutes a complete image of man-in-the-world, then the manifest image must be, by that fact, "an 'inadequate' but pragmatically useful likeness of a reality which first finds its adequate…likeness in the scientific image" (ibid.: 484). Unfortunately, to reject the manifest image, argues Sellars, is for the scientific image to reject its own foundation since the postulational idealization of the scientific image of man-in-the-world is constructed on a foundation taken from the manifest image itself. In other words, for Sellars, we can assume that "the categories of a theoretical science are logically dependent on categories pertaining to its methodological foundation in the manifest world of sophisticated common sense in such a way that there would be an absurdity in the notion of a world which illustrated it theoretical principles *without also illustrating the categories and principles of the manifest world*" (ibid. Emphasis in original).

But then, it is not just the grounding of the positivistic understanding of science in the methodological omnipotence of the scientific method but most importantly the epistemological arrogance of science being the only mode of genuine knowledge that facilitates the construction of the scientific image of the world and of humans. Scientism speaks to the assumption that science is the best and even the *only* legitimate means by which knowledge could be deployed for material and social progress. In Jurgen Habermas' words, scientism constitutes "science's belief in itself: that is, the conviction that we can no longer understand science as one form of possible knowledge, but rather must identify knowledge with science" (1971: 4). The fundamental questions faced by scientism and the scientific image of humans, which underlies this entire volume and its adjudication of the rift between science and the humanities in the understanding of global health and the COVID-19, are as follows: can humans be scientifically conceived in strictly neurophysiological terms? Or is there an irreducible core to the understanding of *human* that goes beyond its description as a mere scientific specimen? Wilfred Sellars provides a fundamental and even transcendental argument that takes humans away from the descriptive specimen-tation of the scientific image into the intentional framework of being in community of meaningful discourse. According to him, "To say that a certain person desired to do A, thought it his duty to do B but was forced to do C is not to *describe* him as one might describe a scientific specimen. One does, indeed, describe him, but one does something more. And it is this something more which is the irreducible core of the framework of persons" (ibid.: 495). To be a person, that is, is to be construed as being within the communal context with other persons, a context of a "we" that imbues the person's actions and deeds with intentions and meanings.

However, such a proper specification of persons within the scientific image seems out of sync with what that image demands. The epistemic arrogance underlying scientism is founded on the disdain for what Hans Radder sees as "the reflexive Kantian question of the general conditions of the possibility of scientific knowledge" (2009: 62). For positivism to have arrived at science's self-appraisal of its own epistemic significance, it needed to circumvent the possibility of an external reflexivity. This made it impossible to interrogate science "within the horizon of possible and a priori reflected knowledge" (1971: 71). Positivism's understanding of the supremacy of science arose out of the funeral pyre of the "perceiving and judging subject" (ibid.: 73). Essentially, however, it is human actions that constitute the condition that makes scientific knowledge possible. Habermas argues that,

> Science can only be comprehended epistemologically, which means as one category of possible knowledge, as long as knowledge is not equated either effusively with the absolute knowledge of a great philosophy or blindly with the scientistic self-understanding of the actual business of research

> (*Forschung*). Both equations close off the dimension in which an epistemological concept of science can be formed—in which, therefore, science can be made comprehensible within the horizon of possible knowledge and legitimated. Compared with "absolute knowledge" scientific knowledge necessarily appears narrow-minded, and the only task remaining is then the critical dissolution of the boundaries of positive knowledge. (ibid.: 4)

Indeed, for Habermas, communicative action—the condition for the possibility of the humanities—serve ultimately as the platform from which scientific knowledge can be critically interrogated. It therefore takes little reflection to see how the scientism that rejects the self-reflexivity demanded by philosophy[2] will equally reject the imperatives of the humanities. It is this rejection of reflection and the conditions that make it possible that create the epistemic dissonance between science as scientism and the humanities. With this seemingly unassailable scientific conception of the world, and the epistemological strength of scientism that flows from it, humanities seems to go deeper into crisis. And that crisis seems accentuated by the near invisibility of the humanities in any consideration of the search for a cure for the COVID-19 pandemic.

The crisis of the humanities today, accentuated by capitalism's redefinition of pedagogical relevance for worldly progress through the emergence of the STEM—science, technology, engineering, and mathematics—curriculum, is deepened by the scientized understanding of higher education across the globe. And this has severely undermined the significance of humanistic values in contributing to the conversation of humankind. Eric Adler makes a convincing argument:

> The triumph of the sciences would spell serious trouble for humanism. The latter, after all, foregrounds the wisdom of the past as the means to shape a student's character. The sciences, by contrast, promote the creation of new knowledge. And the dominance of the scientific outlook in higher education has turned the modern humanities distinctly un-humanistic.... Our scientized universities focus almost exclusively on what the great humanist

[2] Indeed, Habermas argues that scientism makes possible the effacement of epistemology for the emergence of scientific knowledge. In other words, "Positivism is philosophical only insofar as is necessary for the immunization of the sciences against philosophy" (ibid.: 67).

> Irving Babbitt called humanitarianism: the drive to improve the material conditions of the world. They desperately require a balancing emphasis on humanism: the drive to improve the self. Bereft of the humanities, education only accomplishes half of what it should. We cannot, of course, improve the world if we cannot improve ourselves. And the humanities cannot thrive without the spirit of humanism. (2020)

Unfortunately, the humanitarianism-without-humanism template of the scientized response to the coronavirus pandemic has definitely not attenuated the numerous consequences of the pandemic, from vaccine nationalism to the anti-vaxxers, and from the accentuation of racial inequalities to the relationship between the pandemic and underdevelopment. We cannot even begin to talk about a search for a universal scientific panacea that overlooks the contextual reactions to the coronavirus. And this becomes a critical issue in the face of the underlying ideological dynamics that already divides the world along several doctrines and ideologies. Indeed, the COVID-19 was initially recognized in racial terms as the "Wuhan" or "Chinese" virus. And Africa, as the famous "diseased" continent, has had its fair share of innuendos and references in relations to this virus and with diseases in general.[3] Even though the World Health Organization has spearheaded the scientific response to the resolution of this crisis, it is already clear that a universal vaccine will get bogged down in ideological and pecuniary warfare fought on several fronts. Essentially, COVID-19 instigated an all-encompassing human development catastrophe that magnified horizontal inequalities across and within countries. Gender, income, class, and racial dynamics became very significant in mapping the unequal power relations that the pandemic exhumed.[4] Populations groups and their unique physiological configurations, for

[3] In April 2020, two French doctors, Dr Jean-Paul Mira and Camille Locht, the research director for France's National Institute of Health and Medical Research, stirred ideological controversy when they suggested that the BCG tuberculosis vaccine that was about to enter into trials as a potential treatment for COVID-19 be tested in Africa, "where there are no [face] masks, no treatments and no ICUs." Even though the suggestion was met with a swift and angry global reaction (the director-general of WHO saw it as "a hangover from a colonial mentality"), the doctors' suggestion coheres with a historical trajectory that takes Africa and the rest of the developing third world as an experimentation laboratory.

[4] See Carolina Rivera et al. (2020), William Mude et al. (2021), and Maitrayee Chaudhuri (2021).

instance, have demonstrated why the deployment of universal vaccines is ill-thought-out. The gender, structural, and health inequalities that the pandemic reinforced attest to this.

There is also the significant issue of how vaccination infringes personal freedoms. The anti-vaccine activism suggests the reaction against vaccination is not just an issue of ignorance about the dynamics of vaccination or the efficacy of vaccines. On the contrary, the twenty-first century vaccine resistance has a deeper root. According to Kenneth Rochel de Camargo, Jr., we can track this resistance at three levels. Two are significant here. The first has to do with the "misapprehensions of the risks of both vaccinating, which are overestimated, and not vaccinating, which are underestimated" (2020: 2). But the second reason is even more fundamental in the age of the Internet. And this has to do with the anti-establishment sensibility of anti-vaccine activism, tied to a deep distrust of traditional science and medicine, and especially the big connection between big pharma and big business (or big pharma *as* big business). Thus, "Distrust of everything that concerns medicine is often associated with the idea that only economic interests, often undisclosed, are the sole determinants of the decisions of health specialists" (ibid.). Vaccine resistance, in this sense, therefore takes on a postmodern ideology—"hostility towards singular truths; aversion to scientific objectivity; and decreased trust in expertise" (ibid.). To put in a broader perspective, a significant part of vaccine hesitation and resistance has a lot to do with an argument about whether the state has any right to intervene in the health profile of her citizens.

Thus, as the entire world continue to grapple with the pandemic, new issues are beginning to emerge, while old ones are becoming more accentuated and aggravated. What is the relationship between science and non-science? How do the humanities feature in the search for a global health profile for humanity? What is the nature of scientific truth? How are such truths to be effectively communicated to the general populace? What is the role of faith and hope in health crisis? What is the relationship between scientific engagement and political negotiations? And how do the humanities mediate the two? How does the world handle the consequences of what has been called "vaccine nationalism" as well as the ideological modulation of causes, consequences, and resolution of health crises? The COVID-19 pandemic has, for instance, given the fake news phenomenon (i.e., infodemic) a new and even more critical and dangerous dimension. It has not only exacerbated the distinction between what is fake and real; it has also brought to stark perception the possible effects of an incomplete understanding of the pandemic situation by the scientific community itself. The profusion of the various conspiracy theories thus critically undermines the legitimacy of scientific truth, as well as generating new challenges for an effective communication management. In other words, the separation between science and the cost of information gaps in engaging with the populace leads to the deep crisis of managing the crucial information flow within the acceptable ambit of censor and control.

The humanities have therefore been challenged to play a fundamental role in looking for an all-encompassing "vaccine" for curbing and eliminating a virus that has invaded the physiognomy of humanity and has endangered global health and the future *of* human well-being. The humanities are concerned with humanity in all its manifestations. They study human frailties and human achievements. They also investigate the nature of the human spirit as well as its capacity and elasticity in the face of existential difficulties. For the humanities, a pandemic becomes a measure of the human spirit in the face of an existential challenge. It therefore stands to reason that not only this pandemic but also a post-COVID-19 human society cannot be imagined outside of the prism provided by the humanities. Scientism's false hope of being the only legitimate epistemic prism into the human world has been belied by its struggle to adequately contain the myriads of consequences, both scientific and non-scientific, that pandemics, and especially the COVID-19, have offloaded on humanity.

This volume explores the possible responses of the humanities to the challenges posed specifically by the COVID-19 pandemic and generally by global health crises. Its twofold objective is to interrogate (a) the neglect of the humanities in the overreliance on epidemiological models (often situated within the cultural dynamics of a supposed center) in the search for an amelioration of the effects and consequences of the COVID-19 pandemic and (b) the reluctance of the humanities themselves to weigh in on the behavioral and attitudinal prescriptions that could lead to the understanding and evaluations of global health issues. The volume samples analyses from humanities scholars and disciplines that enunciate models, strategies, insights, methodologies, and discourses that can enlighten our understanding of pandemics, the ongoing search for a resolution of this crisis and the prevention of others, as well as other issues involved in the management of global health.

References

Adler, Eric. 2020. Scientism, the Coronavirus, and the Death of the Humanities. OUPblog, October 30. https://blog.oup.com/2020/10/scientism-the-coronavirus-and-the-death-of-the-humanities/.

Camargo, Kenneth Rochel, Jr. 2020. Here We Go Again: The Reemergence of Anti-vaccine Activism on the Internet. *Cadernos de Saude Publica* (Reports in Public Health) 36 (2): 1–8.

Chaudhuri, Maitrayee. 2021. COVID-19 and Structural Inequalities: Some Reflections on the Practice of Sociology. *Sociological Bulletin* 70 (2): 252–258.

Habermas, Jurgen. 1971. *Knowledge and Human Interests*. Translated by Jeremy J. Shapiro. Boston: Beacon Press.

Marcus, David D. 1976. The Carlylean Vision of 'A Tale of Two Cities'. *Studies in the Novel* 8 (1, Spring): 56–68.

Mude, William, Victor M. Oguoma, Lillian Mwanri TafadzwaNyanhanda, and Carolyne Njue. 2021. Racial Disparities in COVID-19 Pandemic Cases, Hospitalisations, and Deaths: A Systematic Review and Meta-analysis. *Journal of Global Health* 11. https://doi.org/10.7189/jogh.11.05015.

Neurath, Otto. 1973. *Empiricism and Sociology*. Edited by Marie Neurath and Robert C. Cohen. Dordrecht: D. Reidel Publishing Co.

Radder, Hans. 2009. Science and Technology: Positivism and Critique. In *A Companion to the Philosophy of Technology*, ed. Jan Kyrre Berg Olsen, Stig Andur Pedersen, and Vincent F. Hendricks, 61–65. Malden, MA: Blackwell Publishing.

Rignall, J.M. 1984. Dickens and the Catastrophic Continuum of History in A Tale of Two Cities. *ELH* 51 (3, Autumn): 575–587.

Rivera, Carolina, Yu-Chieh Hsu, Fernanda Pavez Esbry, and Esuna Dugarova. 2020. Gender Inequality and the COVID-19 Crisis: A Human Development Perspective. Human Development working paper. http://hdr.undp.org/sites/default/files/gendercovid_final.xlsx.

Robinson, Alan. 2004. *Imagining London, 1770–1900*. London: Palgrave Macmillan.

Sellars, Wilfred. 2001. Philosophy and the Scientific Image of Man. In *Analytic Philosophy: An Anthology*, ed. A.P. Martinich and David Sosa, 473–496. Malden, MA: Blackwell Publisher.

Part I

Humanistic Understanding of Disease

2

Toward a Fuller Understanding of the Enigma of Health

Peter Amato

It has been frequently observed of the Great Irish Famine of 1845–1852 that "a mold caused the blight, but political-economy caused the famine."[1] At least a million people died, and perhaps an equal number emigrated as a result of the famine according to some estimates (Woodham-Smith 1962; Bloy 2015). Although the tiny mold *Phytophthora infestans* directly killed potato plants, not humans, the tragedy of the famine illustrates how social institutions and political-economic relations may greatly mag-

[1] I paraphrase the oft-quoted statement of John Mitchel, a contemporary observer of the famine that, "The Almighty, indeed, sent the potato blight, but the English created the Famine" (Daly 1997: 596). According to Daly, Mitchel is regarded by historians as linking the famine directly with British political-economic policies in Ireland (595). Bloy (2015) endorses Mitchel's remark insofar as successive British governments "did little to help the Irish population." In her now classic study, Cecil Woodham-Smith is more direct: "All this wretchedness and misery could, almost without exception, be traced to a single source—the system under which land had come to be occupied and owned in Ireland, a system produced by centuries of successive conquests, rebellions, confiscations and punitive legislation" (1962: 20).

P. Amato (✉)
Drexel University, Philadelphia, PA, USA
e-mail: peterama@drexel.edu

F. Egbokhare, A. Afolayan (eds.), *Global Health, Humanity and the COVID-19 Pandemic*, https://doi.org/10.1007/978-3-031-17429-2_2

nify a biological hazard. There are many lessons of the COVID-19 pandemic, many related to this general truth we have always known—*that no person's health or illness is ever just a biological issue*. The major theme I take up here is how, despite knowing this, it nevertheless often appears from how we talk about, think about, and act toward the pandemic and other public health issues that we nevertheless believe *that it is*. In the theory and practice of medicine in the pursuit of health, we seem convinced that the institutional conditions and relations that structure the world we share with viruses, bacteria, and each other play only a minor role in our actual experience and knowledge of health and illness. And this is despite the fact that we know, and have perhaps always known, that their role is quite large. The pandemic has forced this paradox upon us with new urgency the world round—we kinda know but are unwilling or afraid to face up to the implications of the ways individual and social health are not merely interwoven but mutually determining. We keep being shown signs of how deeply everyone yearns for and deserves a return to normalcy, despite the exposure of its mortal dysfunction.

The idea that "medicine isn't just biology" is not new, particularly from the standpoint of the discipline of public health, and especially with reference to the limits at which a rigorously scientific approach to health must give way to "softer," "alternative," or "humanistic" approaches. But if, on the most general level, medicine is the promotion of individual bodily or spiritual health, simply pursuing that aim with determination leads sooner or later to the threshold of public health whether one is ready to cross into it or not. Yet even where the social dimensions of individual health are forced into view, deeper-lying problems in thinking about ourselves and how we "know" anything that characterize modern science remain. The health sciences as a whole are responsible for an enormous amount of lifesaving work, and many lives depend directly on the expertise and energetic work of public health professionals. Nevertheless, to a significant degree, the public health perspective responds to some of the biggest gaps in modern health science without challenging its underlying assumptions, which has the effect of deferring rather than improving our understanding of health.

The occasion for this reminder is the current global calamity the human race finds itself in the midst of even after at least a million deaths—about half in my country, the USA. Although much smaller than the mold spores that spread the potato blight, the COVID-19 novel coronavirus has attacked our entire species directly. Like the mold, it found humans woefully unprepared. From my vantage point, the public discussion and international debate about fighting the pandemic have mostly been about logistics and math. How distant should people remain in enclosed spaces? How fast can we vaccinate people? Who should be first? How do we measure the effectiveness of the vaccines? When will the risk be low enough that we can open up restaurants and stop wearing masks? When can the children go back to school? *When can we get back to normal?* It is common for the news in the USA to cite the grim statistics showing how poverty, racism, sexism, and inequality are manifest in the COVID-19 death and illness reports. It is quite rare however for them to facilitate any discussion of these conditions themselves as part of the "health" equation, as fundamental to what is undermining "health."

I am interested here in why there isn't a lot more to talk about concerning the pandemic than math and how we are even able to think about health—in this case public health—without following to the next logical set of concerns that are essential to it, which are broadly of a political-economic, ethical, and humanistic nature. Why isn't a health crisis of these proportions as such a *moral* and *humanitarian* crisis—not simply a matter of logistics to master *via* technology but a matter that makes a claim upon us as persons to restore our own and others' wholeness or integrity? I am focused here on the health sciences as an institution and the ways of thinking about health that dominate it. I want to discuss and illuminate something about what it means to be "scientific" about human health right now because, following Hans-Georg Gadamer's critique, I think there is a way we have become blind to dimensions of "health" that we know are there, that are in plain sight, but that we refuse to recognize and acknowledge the implications of.

Although countless physicians, nurses, healthcare workers, caregivers, and public health authorities in municipalities, states, and countries around the world have been truly heroic in this time of calamity, the issues raised here help to account for some of the institutional obstacles that have arisen to undermine their intentions and effectiveness in saving lives and giving comfort. Many became patients and casualties of

COVID-19 themselves in part as the result of institutional obstacles rooted in the historical reality of modern science and its distorted thinking about health and medicine. I believe the pandemic has shown how unclear thinking and bad ideas sometimes have swift and deadly repercussions. Again, this is not something we did not know, but it is the kind of truth it takes a certain kind of care and careful work to remind ourselves is true—and to fully work out the implications of.

With more than three million dead and counting, after one year of the COVID-19 pandemic, and the effects of global warming making themselves increasingly felt worldwide, it may be more obvious than ever in human history that a thorough-going, far-ranging critical rethinking of major global institutions is necessary if humans are to flourish and perhaps if we are even to survive on the planet much longer. Gadamer does not call for such a response to "the enigma of health," but I believe he illuminates compellingly how modern science distorts our thinking and confounds our hopes related to "health" and "illness." In what follows, I develop some themes from Gadamer's *The Enigma of Health: The Art of Healing in a Scientific Age* in order to show how his thinking can help us emerge from the crisis and trauma the world is presently enduring with a fuller understanding of what "health" is and greater prospects for more people to live healthier lives in the future.

In the preface which begins Gadamer's collection of essays entitled *The Enigma of Health: The Art of Healing in a Scientific Age*, he emphasizes the limits of science and its role in the larger whole of society. At the close of the twentieth century, science and technology have developed "astounding" technical capacities that have not been "integrate[d] into the social and political order as a whole," leaving the "humanitarian optimism which animated the eighteenth century" unfulfilled (Gadamer 1996: viii). We have learned from physics of limits to what can be measured in the physical universe. In the case of health, an object whose study is inseparable from the conditions experienced by human subjects, more caution would seem warranted, yet science and technology have reinterpreted the experience of health for modern humanity in ways that distort and undermine it.

Some of the warranted caution we nevertheless hear in the way we still talk about medical treatment. Despite the overwhelming influence of the modern scientific approach and the idea of expert knowledge as guiding in matters of bodily health in particular, we call the physician's professional activity a "practice" and consider its exercise to involve a degree of "art" involving judgement and discretion (Gadamer 1996: 18–19). Yet, even prior to its transformation by modern science, medicine was always an "unusual art." Unlike any other, the aim of the art of healing is not to produce or make something but rather to maintain or restore a kind of natural equilibrium. Its essence, Gadamer says, is to "re-produce" and "re-establish" a natural state (1996: 32). This means that unlike all other arts and modern science, the basic virtue of the art of healing is its capacity to carefully listen and recognize how and when to support and assist nature and how and when to get out of its path. The art of healing takes place fully within processes of nature that the experts, despite their knowledge, do not control. Nature, not human artisans or technology, does the healing work. The art of healing is an effort of seeking to restore natural processes which have been disrupted (1996: 34).

The Strange Art of Healing

To characterize the moment of health to which the art of healing responds, Gadamer offers a series of approximations using images taken directly from literature and philosophy—demonstrating what, in a sense, has been forgotten in and of the history of the art of healing in their eclipse by scientific methods. The three images Gadamer presents in "Apologia for the Art of Healing" also link his thinking on these topics to his wider philosophical views. They connect his thinking about the art of healing with the central motif of dialogical engagement through which a truth is disclosed and articulated in language. Each is focused on a different aspect of the dialogical circumstance.

In the first of these images, Gadamer explains Rilke's idea of the delicate movements of the acrobat toward and away from the point at which balance is achieved (1996: 36). This is seen as illuminating the moment of health as the equilibrium that emerges suddenly in the exercise of the physician's art. It is not achieved by making or producing something new, or by creating a new space or time in which to balance, but substantially by getting out of the way of the forces and influences that could otherwise knock the acrobat off the tightrope. What the physician knows is somehow like what the acrobat in balancing does without thinking: the forces in play cannot be and are not removed or overwritten in accomplishing the desired result. The knowledge that is valuable is knowing when to let things take their course. The contrast with the usual way we think of art and technology as engaged in step-by-step production of its object is palpable in Gadamer's account of the aptness of Rilke's description:

> [T]he concentrated effort involved in producing and maintaining equilibrium suddenly proves itself, at the very moment when balance is attained, to be the opposite of what it seemed to be. For if the balancing act were to go wrong, it would not be because physical force or power was lacking or too little was exerted, but rather because there was actually too much force in play. But when the act works, suddenly everything seems to happen spontaneously, lightly, and effortlessly. (Gadamer 1996: 36–7)

This almost reverse effort makes the art of healing a "strange art" that foregrounds the idea of health as a moment at which exertion must be let go of rather than as a product or effect created from the application of the physician's craft or skill. Yet "health" has been besieged for centuries now by the development of modern health science, by which it has been radically re-described. What matters for it is the assertion of the powers and means of control accessible to the physician through the knowledge of cause and effect. What matters for it is the reformulation of health into the kind of object that may make itself available to scientific method, quantification, experiment, and calculation. Once the experience of healing has been reduced to these, what is left of the moment of health that is not "treatable" or "operable" in terms of the scientific method is not significant and cannot matter any longer to the physician.

How distorting the health science approach is to the experience of health as a moment is further illuminated with reference to one of the most important and familiar images in Gadamer's work, that of the *Gestaltkreis* or the hermeneutical circle (1996: 38). Gadamer's unidentified ancient text presents an image of the practice of tree-sawing as an illustration of the character of the art of healing. "As one partner draws the blade the other follows in concert, so that the whole sawing process constitutes what Viktor von Weiszacker calls a *Gestaltkreis*, an internally unified configuration in which the respective movements of the two tree-cutters fuse to become a subtle rhythmic flux of movement" (Gadamer 1996: 38). The equilibrium aimed at by the art of healing is and emerges through an *integrated multilateral dialectic*. There is no need to imagine the tree-cutters sawing away eternally to maintain the metaphor, but the use Gadamer wants to make of the image is unmistakably both as a model of the equilibrium of health and of the art of healing. It is an image of health in being like the play in which the players are lost or submerged in response and reaction to one another's moves, in which the back and forth we saw with Rilke's image of the acrobat is central to the complex reality of the experience and movement of teetering, so to speak, in and out of health. It is also an image of the physician's treatment: the art of healing is like the whole movement of the tree-cutters in that the patient's situation and health condition in a sense envelops and submerges physician and patient *in a solicitous whole* in which the receptive openness, care, and delicacy of both "tree-cutters" are essential to supporting, sustaining, and maintaining the movement at or near the moment of balance—the "unified…single rhythmic flux of movement" Gadamer previously characterized as something like the calm eye of a storm. I take this to suggest that we should see health as a dynamic and dialectical state of being which *engages* the medical practitioner. The physician isn't merely standing at the side disinterestedly holding the acrobat's safety net or handing them weights to make them heavier or lighter on one side so as to create a new balance of a new type on a new level. The physician isn't forcing, prescribing, or directing the tree-cutting, as the ancient text observes/warns: should the cutters "employ violent force, then they will utterly fail" (1996: 38).

As Gadamer would have it, the art of healing reflects something real about health, that this strange art can succeed only as a dialogical activity that engages physician and patient in the right way because health is itself a dynamic status: "Hence, the particular solicitude of the doctor who must continue to respect the equilibrium which persists in spite of all disturbance and must stay attuned to the natural process of that equilibrium, just like the tree-cutter in our example" (1996: 38). And the activity of the art of healing occurs among and between humans—unlike the tightrope example—so it is within language and thus has the meaningful aspect that moves toward mutual comprehension and the emergence of the truth of a subject matter—it is a *Gestaltkreis*, a moment in the emergence of a truth through a kind of dialectical movement that is best exemplified in actual dialogue. The integration that is health now shows itself to necessarily include the individual alongside and with others—both in the treatment aimed at health and in being healthy.

Gadamer's interpretation of the tree-cutting example and Rilke's acrobat on the tightrope show us something about health and about healthcare. But they also show in practice how the work of humanistic rendering allows a subject matter to be articulated and understood that starts as something reader and writer know and do not know at the same time. In Plato, this takes the form of Socrates as one for whom the method of successive approximation, often through myth, allegory, and metaphor, captures a substantial aspect of our approach to truth in language. In Plato, as in Gadamer, this activity of allowing the truth to emerge through a kind of back and forth dialectical or dialogical work can be presented through many images, some of them more apt for some purposes and in relation to some experiences than others. The point is that Gadamer wishes the reader to see both in what he says and how he says it the marked contrast with modern science in relation to the truth about health and about healthcare. Health is an *integration* that marks a kind of equilibrium at various levels at which we might say health exists, in which different aspects of our being and experience "hold together" in normally unproblematic ways. These include aspects of the person and their relations with other persons, and their relations with social and political institutions. The key notion is that health and healing refer to larger wholes to which they belong.

This integrative dimension becomes more explicit in the final pages of "Apologia for the Art of Healing" in which Gadamer introduces Plato directly. The passage of *Phaedrus* "illuminates the predicament of the physician who possesses this 'science'," i.e., the Health Science of today, which still bears historical connection to the ancient art of healing, but which has forced it into the mold of modern science (1996: 39). The analogy Plato has Socrates draw between the art of rhetoric and the art of medicine makes the point that neither can be effective at accomplishing its goals if it is unable to understand its subject matter as belonging to a whole from which organically its own essence derives. In the art of healing, this means diagnosis and treatment cannot be reduced to simply a task of bringing particular symptoms in a particular case under a general rule, as they quickly become for health science. In the context of ancient medicine:

> ...all possible climatic and environmental factors were seen to make up the concrete ontological constitution of what it is that the physician helps to restore, namely health....The nature of the whole includes and involves the entire life situation of the patient, and even of the physician...[*T*]*he constitution of the body passes over into the constitution of the human being as a whole*...In this sense Plato's suggestion that the true physician, like the true rhetorician, must take the whole of nature into view remains valid. (Gadamer 1996: 42 emphasis added)

From *Mathesis* to *Anamnesis*

Gadamer's *Phaedrus* reading suggests that *anamnesis* might be a valuable concept in thinking about how we bring the nature and meaning of health to awareness—which under normal conditions remains in concealment and hidden. It also suggests an idea of *diagnosis* that would be dialogical and integrative as opposed to the quantifying, externalized, detached, and abstract logistical kind of interrogation we are forced to endure within the regime of health science. To this view, a kind of dialogical *anamnesis* would be a way of bringing to language a previously inarticulate sense of dis-ease or illness or disharmony. Even keeping with Gadamer's focus on the unconcealment of *health*, the hermeneutical moment Gadamer introduces links his critique with *illness* through the image of diagnosis as a process like *anamnesis* in which the physician plays the role of a solicitous, attentive midwife.

Gadamer's rendering of Plato's "true physician" of *Phaedrus* makes this image clearer, as it is this physician who performs in diagnosis an activity linked to *Gestaltkreis*, which emphasizes receptivity, dialogue, sustenance, and solicitude in assisting the re-emergence and restoration of equilibrium. The result of diagnosis gathers or recollects not something literally "forgotten" but something that is inchoately "known" in the bodily or spiritual sense. What can be and is brought to language in the process is the person's recognition of the contrast between their unthought experience of health and their current status of feeling in the problematic state presenting as illness, anxiety, or dis-ease. Diagnosis in this sense is a fundamentally linguistic dialogical activity of bringing to words from within another person the inchoate truth "known and not known" or unreflected upon and unpacking it through the process of examination. The physician's art in this sense is an attentive and solicitous activity of interrogative Socratic midwifery that attempts to discover something about the patient's condition by articulating it and bringing it to conceptuality.

I wish to press Gadamer here in that along with the image of diagnosis modeled on a kind of Socratic examination comes the prospect of an interrogation/examination of history and collective experience through narrative, artistic, and cultural forms that so often are the repository of the experience of trauma, oppression, violation, and suffering. The idea of the *Gestaltkreis* as a model for the sustenance of health as an equilibrium and also in the particular image of the diagnosis of the "true physician" raises these prospects. Along with the gathering and collecting that allows the discovery and articulation of what is "known/unknown" into something new brought to language is the experienced personal, social, and historical dimensions of suffering beyond the immediate bodily sources of acute and chronic physical and mental trauma.

The ability of diagnosis to bring the condition of the "patient" to recognition respects only the limits set by the questioning art of the physician. The old sophistical paradox that "A student is able to learn only what they already know to look for" is used by Socrates in *Meno* to show how *anamnesis* makes it possible to conceptualize how a large proportion and possibly all of our nontrivial learning in life is more like working out the implications of things we kinda know already than it is really a matter of placing into the mind something utterly foreign to it as Meno or as empiricism would have it. My point here is that the true physician would not set arbitrary boundaries to this learning encounter. In it the individuals engaged in diagnosis would be expected to follow the logic of how they were exposed to a deadly disease because the city was not counting janitorial staff as essential that week and as a result did not provide them with any personal protective equipment, until the Union threatened to strike, but then it was too late for them, or how their chronic degenerative physical condition is related to living on the streets while working two jobs for starvation wages that offer no healthcare, etc. Our broader social need for and implication in one another's lives—which we take for granted and which may be concretely what persons undergoing diagnosis for immediate and acute symptoms are most suffering the loss of, and through which are most directly suffering their diminution of health—also may come to articulation and recognition in this process through their *telling their stories* if it is not arbitrarily prevented. In other words, Gadamer's discussion of health here may provide the basis for a kind of *social recollection* that could be fundamental to a form of institutional critique that flows more naturally from his thinking about health than Gadamer would probably have allowed.

The least we can say is that if Gadamer is correct about health and his notion of health can provide the basis for a critique of current theory and practice, then pursuing the aim of health begins with a kind of conversation that involves putting questions to ourselves and to others with whom we are in a kind of dialogue about the most important and difficult aspects of experience. If the unexamined life is not worth living, it also isn't *healthy*, since it takes a kind of inward-looking interrogation assisted by *maieusis* to sustain and support the kind of equilibrium, balance, and integrity we hope for. I would add that the self-critical moment necessarily implies a broader outward-looking critique of the social and political-economic circumstances in which we live, as they are organically and logically inseparable from the health of individuals. The unexamined life-world is not worth living in. But we may further argue that Gadamer should accept this idea if it can be seen that this kind of collective *anamnesis* is really just what we call the humanities.

This diagnosis of the body politic is a kind of "remembering" the history of everything human including oppression, disenfranchisement, and trauma, an activity of recovering by examining and interrogating our humanity. It is the recovery of what is known/unknown in the bodies and experience of healthy and suffering persons. It is essential to human health and requires the testimony of the arts and humanities. This is just what Gadamer said the true physician knows, that the more carefully one focusses on the health of one, the more we are led beyond to find they are a *subject* that belongs to a totality that is greater than the sum of its many bodies; it leads inevitably to political-economic collectivities and forms of life. Modern science can only say "yes" at this level. Healthcare as such must learn how to say "no" to unhealthful forms of life. It must stop apologizing for and marginalizing individual scientists and medical practitioners who try to do so. It must significantly increase the amount of humanistic study the practitioners of health sciences have real access to at every level of education. Health science must become health*care* and declare independence from the global system of economic incentives that puts profits in the driving seat rather than care.

This leads us back to thinking about the pandemic and the health science response. The vaccine is not a cure for the underlying diseases the virus has exposed. For the urgency to abolish the deadly virus is the urgency to abolish the conditions that have made this virus *so deadly*. The underlying disease of our disintegrated state, our detachment, and mutual disinterest made the tiny virus into a global killer pandemic. And we know this—much of the world's people cannot avoid the reminder every day that the richest people in the world bargain away their lives and futures, about which they care very little. And there are many, perhaps most of us rich who are less than completely deluded about the fact of widespread poverty, hunger, disease, and hopelessness in the world. *Normalcy*. So, these truths, if not evident to all, are in our minds and bones already. They are truths about which we exert ourselves insufficiently. This is the truly critical diagnosis that might be gleaned from the current state of our health sciences in general as the result of the pandemic.

Science, Health Science, and the Humanities

The idea of an integrated dialogical experience of health and healthcare that I have developed here, with an eye toward Gadamer's conception of health as a kind of equilibrium, also has deeper roots in the development and transformation of phenomenology that occurred through the philosophical tradition of his immediate predecessors in phenomenology, Husserl and Heidegger. In a sense, this notion of integrity is most directly related to Gadamer's idea of the humanities as a cultural tradition, which takes Husserl's idea of tradition a step further and closer to practice than Husserl would. The conception of humanistic tradition reflects the depths of the linguistic dimensions phenomenology sees in history and practice. From such a position, the powerful yet problematic situation faced by objective-scientific discourse arises from its home within and without the activity of speaking, which is always situated within history and language. It struggles to remove itself but cannot do so.

Gadamer suggests that natural scientific discourse tends to obscure these practical bases: "[T]he dismantling and reconstructing of everything that is which is carried on by modern science represents simply a particular domain of expansion and mastery…of what exists," in pursuit of which natural science "has and always will come up against a claim of comprehension in the face of which it must fail—and indeed which it should forego" (Gadamer 1986: 12). That is, modern natural science emerges as a discourse unique in being primarily oriented toward an existing, ongoing practical history. This is seen in the tendency of natural science to generate—and police—the illusion of its own self-subsistence as knowledge: "[T]here is implied in every theory of science itself the idea of self-justification, which compels it to go beyond itself…. Hence,…phenomenology undertook to elucidate the constitutive concepts of the natural experience of the world [*Lebenswelt*] that antecedes scientific methodology" (1986: 162–3). As a stance toward practice, modern science is at least disinterested and detached and always potentially subversive with respect to language and its own lifeworld, within which (nonetheless) lie its power, its justification, and also its limit or downfall.

Natural science arises as an abstract totalization of the world of practical engagement that, for Gadamer, it is able at best to re-arrange and constantly re-describe. The world modern science encounters is always already arranged through language, but it displaces language by mathematics and so appears to do more than that. Science is, thus, "unthinking" and "wordless" and forgets the primordial refusal of speech from which it draws its powers. It thus speaks, asserts, and justifies in a sense outside language, upon which its power is premised (1986: 3). But this does not mean modern science must only be seen as having negative impacts on our humanity because we are able to reimagine scientific discourse in a way that would counteract the displacement of language:

> Just as our total experience of the world presents a process of coming to be at home that never comes to an end—to speak with Heidegger—even in a world that appears ever more strange because it has been all too changed by ourselves; so, too, the exigence for a philosophic account of things is an unending process. In it is realized not only the conversation which each of us conducts with ourselves in thinking but also the conversation in which we are all caught up together and never cease to be caught up. (Gadamer 1986: 20)

This is the humanistic tradition to which we have been referring throughout—and it is our principal means not only of understanding ourselves, but also it is essential if we are to understand our understanding of our bodily, mental, and spiritual health, which includes science. In speaking of our "dismantling and reconstructing" of the world, we return to that conversation which recognizes and does not displace for practical exigences our being within language and within nature.

Gadamer suggests we abandon the idea that scientific or any discourse escapes language. Natural science is a peculiar conversation in need of situating itself within a more integrated space, more realistically and comprehensively in relation to society and language:

> [T]he traditions within which we stand—and every tradition that we creatively or appropriatingly pass on—offer less an objective field for the scientific mastery of a subject matter or for the extension of our domination by knowledge of the unknown than a mediation of ourselves with our real

possibilities engulfing us—with what can be and what is capable of happening to and becoming of us. (Gadamer 1986: 166–7)

Conclusions

For Gadamer, "health" is a state of being whole, a kind of balance or integrity like an equilibrium, and this is what makes it enigmatic, in its way: Health is the unexamined and unreflective status of living being, and in this sense, it is unproblematic and requires no reflection or interrogation. Yet, our experience of the world and of the humanistic tradition shows that this balance or calm is also constantly falling away from us in time. Our natural status is not simply to maintain equilibrium indefinitely but to die. Gadamer knows this, but it is important to observe that his viewpoint here has been that of life's enduring and thriving, and not its precarity and vulnerability—the constant tendency of all living things to disintegrate. If this is also a natural part of our condition, solicitude or "letting be" is not only a potential moment of healing, calmness, and restoration but also a real and equally natural moment in which life is engaged in a dynamic struggle to sustain an equilibrium it will eventually lose utterly. Bodies and minds that aren't nourished and exercised tend to fall out of equilibrium. It is not surprising that Gadamer would concern himself so little with this side of the equation in developing the theme of how health science reflects a distorted notion of what it can accomplish. Nevertheless, paying attention to it can help make his point and take it further as I have suggested above. For our awareness of the vulnerability and precariousness of our lives is in some ways the essential insight expressed and retold in the world's traditions of the arts and humanities. To the extent that this may be right, health, far from a purely biological issue, is more consistently "treated" over the course of one's lifetime through the vitality of one's experience in connection with living traditions of culture, mythology, storytelling, conversation, literature, art, expression, etc. Nourishment comes in many forms essential to health. These include provisioning of food and shelter but also the many ways humans share, express, and acquire education, recognition, affirmation, nurturance, solicitude, acceptance, inclusion, and all the ways we express ourselves, desire and feel ourselves to be heard and understood.

I contend that this means Gadamer's conception of health as a kind of equilibrium, or what I have been calling integrity, orients us toward a state that must not be mistaken for inertia. In life as social creatures, the equilibrium (health) of each individual reflects the vitality of their total social environment, implicit in Gadamer's broader idea of the humanities as a tradition we advance historically through encounter, engagement, criticism, and questioning. I conclude from this that authentic health practices such as Gadamer suggests would resist the distorting tendencies of modern health science but will only ever partially restore integrity (health) unless they also address a patient's larger social context in transformative dialogical engagement. In this sense, many who are "healed" of or prevented from getting COVID-19 are not thereby and to that extent "intact" insofar as they may be more deeply entrenched in relations with others that are "sick" even though personally and bodily, they may be "healthy" or at least, for now, do not have the virus.

Finally, despite being currently an almost universally expressed desire, a restorative return to pre-COVID normalcy would not be conducive to health. There is a sense in which this paradox can now be reformulated as a Catch-22: the more we find ourselves threatened by the immediate danger of personal exposure to the disease, the more we are forced to embrace a *normalcy* that exposes us to more deadly dangers. Framing it this way may make it easier to see how escaping from the virus as an immediate and tractable personal threat can be entrenching the more profound and global but less tractable irrationality we the privileged may have come to accept or deny.[2]

Gadamer's equilibrium idea of health can be thought of as expressing the central importance of normal functioning, but while this reinforces Gadamer's conception of health as restorative balance, it also shows its limits. The normal is what has allowed a small controllable pest to become a deadly global killer. The desire for (simple) restoration or return is not so unlike the yearning of the refugee to return home despite the realities

[2] In other words, at this point, the Catch-22 is "resolved" by either denying there is a dilemma at all (doublethink) or ignoring the larger problem by declaring it to be "intractable" (quietism, cynicism, etc.). A related choice between cynicism and doublethink is *rationalization*, well-known in the psychological literature on cognitive dissonance, wherein I preserve my sense of being a rational, honest person by explaining away the significance or reality of one side of the dilemma.

that made them flee, or the false but palpable nostalgia for an abusive family life one might feel all the more intensely the further and freer one becomes from its source, which becomes a fetish, an *ersatz totality*. In cases like these of real emotional contradiction, health is served by confrontation with realities less abstract than those of science, which address us with the clarity and concreteness of human voices. All this does not suggest that more humanistic research and study should be added on to the existing framework of health sciences education. Rather, it recommends that humanistic study and research should continually nourish an ongoing, unending, thorough-going, all-embracing reconsideration of who we are and who we hope to become through the work of healing, considering that "art" in the fullest sense as requiring the diagnosis, treatment, and care of our social institutions as much as of our persons, in the full sense of integrity, while welcoming the prodigal modern science back from its present state of alienation.

Practically, the sketch of a critique outlined here suggests not the abandonment of medicine and public health as reductive health sciences but their expansion as forms of knowledge and practice under the reorientation of theory and practice toward an *integrated* and—dare I say—*holistic* perspective. Health science must be seen as a department of health *service*, or health*care*, whose aim, as Gadamer suggests, can no longer be conceived of as the production of fit working bodies and well-adjusted minds as if commodities but, instead, as the personal and social freedom and full social and historical flourishing of those served, to all of whom as truth they belong.

References

Bloy, Marjie. 2015. *The Irish Famine: 1845–9*. https://victorianweb.org/history/famine.html.

Daly, Mary E. 1997. Historians and the Famine: A Beleaguered Species? *Irish Historical Studies* 30 (120, Nov.): 591–601.

Gadamer, Hans-Georg. 1986. *Reason in the Age of Science*. Cambridge, MA: MIT.

———. 1996. *The Enigma of Health*. California: Stanford University Press.

Woodham-Smith, Cecil. 1962. *The Great Hunger: Ireland 1845–1849*. London: Harper and Row.

3

Ubuntu and COVID-19: A Philosophical Reflection

M. S. C. Okolo

Introduction: The Need for a Philosophical Intervention

The emergence of the coronavirus disease has entered into and re(dis) arranged every aspect of human life. The pandemic has not only raised concerns about the extent to which hitherto-taken-for-granted human activities (touching the eyes, nose and mouth, hugging, handshake and visiting, among others) are no longer viable, and in some cases have become the enemies of humans, but have also fueled discussions and forced immediate changes in human actions and behaviour. Businesses, schools, conferences and church activities among others are conducted online. The new language is "Stay home and stay safe".

These overt issues are, however, not the only crises humanity is grappling with due to the outbreak of COVID-19. There are crises in values, new fears, anxiety, depression, disarranged mental attitude and the need

M. S. C. Okolo (✉)
Department of Communication and General Studies, Federal University of Agriculture, Abeokuta, Nigeria

F. Egbokhare, A. Afolayan (eds.), *Global Health, Humanity and the COVID-19 Pandemic*, https://doi.org/10.1007/978-3-031-17429-2_3

to develop the appropriate critical response that can be applied in helping humanity come to terms with the pandemic and its post-era. It is for this reason that this chapter takes a critical look at the concept of Ubuntu. My interest in Ubuntu is premised on, at least, three claims: First, there is the need to position the defining concern of our time as the recognition that all nations of the world should contribute, should have a say in issues of global concern. The second is that embedded in Ubuntu is a world-view that can help humanity not to wander too far from their human-*humane*-essence. The third is that Ubuntu will provide the needed anchor if all human activities will not fall *prey* to a *techno-centric* world—a world defined, shaped, understood, dissected, maintained, protected, valued, sustained and driven *solely* by the dictates of technology.

The point is not to challenge the medical value of the various preventive measures (social distancing and personal hygiene, among others) stipulated for containing the spread of COVID-19 but to enquire into the effectiveness of those measures for all cultures, the way these measures are affecting the way we think and relate to others and, especially, the way they will continue to influence the way we think and our actions when the pandemic is over. As such, highlighting the essential values embodied in Ubuntu is not just to register a philosophical enquiry but to underscore, at least, three vital points. First is to delineate Ubuntu as a fundamental concept that typifies philosophy's own concern with the fundamentals of existence as captured in philosophy's quest to imbue humans with a sense of value to live a meaningful and purposeful life. Second is to show how Ubuntu can open up a new and better understanding of reality by revealing how humans can approach a new problem. Finally, it is to highlight the crucial role Ubuntu can play to a renewed appreciation of philosophy itself as a constant, critical exploration into whatever issues that are confronting humanity. Besides, it is difficult to discuss a novel pandemic that is redefining human activities without recourse to philosophy and the foundational role it plays in the understanding of other disciplines and *all* issues pertaining to humanity. By examining Ubuntu in connection with COVID-19 and its fallouts, the chapter aims to show what Ubuntu can offer to the arrangement of human interactions that can be useful in the management of the ongoing COVID-19 crises and its post-era.

Ubuntu

Ubuntu is derived from two Bantu words "Ubu", which suggests the notion of being in general, and "ntu", the particular entity or the concrete expression of being. Ubu and ntu, as such, provide a fusion for the adequate conceptualisation of the *totality* of what it means to be truly human (humane, caring, looking out for each other, protecting, nurturing, promoting and sustaining one another). Ubuntu, then, represents the interconnectedness and interdependency of humanity. In other words, one's real humanity is rooted in his communion with others. Without such union, a person can only live the life of an outcast or, at best, exist at the peripheral of existence. To conceive any other sense and way of apprehending humanity, that is, a human that is atomistic and can stand alone outside the humanity of others implies being *inhuman* both in the sense of not having regards for the humanity of others and not being human (Mkhize 2008: 40). Represented aphoristically, Ubuntu means "I am because we are, and since we are, therefore, I am" (Mbiti 1970: 141).

Ubuntu, for Desmond Tutu (2011: 21–24), "is the essence of being human". According to him, the Xhosa expression *Umuntu ngumuntu ngabantu*, which represents Ubuntu, could be best translated as "A person is a person through other person". Our existence has no relevance until it is legitimised "through our recognition of others" and validated through "the collective presence of all". For this reason, "the solitary human being is a contradiction in terms". Ubuntu "speaks of how my humanity is caught up and bound up inextricably with yours". It is the opposite of Descartes' "I think, therefore I am" because it affirms "I am because I belong". To be human is to "need other human beings" for this is the quality that ultimately distinguishes people from animals—"the quality of being human and so also humane", so says Tutu. Fundamentally, Ubuntu "endorses the principle or value of *humanness* and takes the ontological essence of beings as the prime mover within the universe or 'community of beings'" (Etieyibo 2017: 634). Reduced to its essence, a person attains her wholeness through other people (Matolino 2011), not as a rigid subject, but as a dynamic self-constitution dependent on the otherness (Eze 2010).

It should be noted, however, that there are many different (and at times opposed) definitions of what Ubuntu is (Praeg 2017: 494–495). This chapter treats Ubuntu as a philosophical concept that premises the value of humans to live a meaningful and purposeful life through recognising, practising and sustaining the universal bond of cooperation that unites all humanity. At a deep level, the ontological essence of beings which Ubuntu endorses is both what defines humans or humanity and connects them together (Etieyibo 2017: 634). Ubuntu is, therefore, opposed to the Western conception of personhood, against the notion of an atomistic self-sufficient individual, and completely shuns any attempt to propagate an existence that is not rooted in the life of others. It is this communal tie, this ceaseless *flowing into* the life of others, that give *authenticity* to an individual's existence and equips her with the necessary wherewithal to weather life's unending challenges: be it Biafra-Nigeria civil war, Rwandan genocide, Zimbabwe after Mugabe, apartheid and post-apartheid South Africa or a pandemic like COVID-19. Indeed, Ubuntu has served as a guiding ideal in many challenging moments: it was adopted as the political ideology that can carry the weight of differences and conflicts that characterised the transition to majority rule in Zimbabwe and South Africa. Ubuntu, then, offers a platform for humanity to come together, to participate and to respond to a common global challenge as posed by COVID-19. By examining it in connection with COVID-19 and its fallouts, the chapter aims to show what significant contribution Ubuntu can offer to the arrangement of human interactions that can be useful in the management of ongoing COVID-19 crises and a post-pandemic era.

COVID-19: A Brief Summary

The coronavirus disease 2019, also known as COVID-19, came to the world's attention with its emergence in Wuhan, China, in late December 2019. By the end of January 2020, it has spread to most countries of the world, necessitating the WHO to declare it a pandemic on 11 March 2020. According to medical experts, it is highly transmissible. Its primary mode of transmission is mostly via respiratory droplets from an infected person over a short distance such as when the person sneezes, coughs or vomits. If the hands come in contact with these droplets, it can be transmitted through contact with the eyes, nose or mouth. There are also asymptomatic patients who are able to transmit the virus. This imposes more challenge in the fight against the disease. Although there have been major breakthroughs in terms of the development of vaccines, the problem is still far from being over. There are still not enough vaccines to protect everyone. There are still many critical questions: how effective are the vaccines against a reoccurrence of COVID-19? Does getting vaccinated guarantee immunity from the disease for life? Evidence-based answers to these questions can only be available with time, and how long that will take is difficult to conjecture. What is known is that as of 16 March 2021, more than twelve countries, mostly in Europe, had suspended the use of AstraZeneca COVID-19 vaccine over fears of health issues suffered by some of the recipients. Even though the World Health Organization assures that the vaccine is safe, it has done little to alleviate the fears.

Based on above and given the highly contagious nature of the virus, rigorous measures are required to mitigate its spread. Among the strategies include hand hygiene; social distancing; isolation; strong bans on gatherings; closure of schools, churches and businesses; mandatory stay-at-home orders; and lockdowns. These have resulted in fears, anxiety and loneliness for most people. There is also strong emphasis on not visiting the elderly as they are classified as belonging to the vulnerable population. One good reason for this is that the "early death cases of COVID-19 outbreak occurred mainly in the elderly, likely due to a poor immune system that allows for faster viral infection progression" (Tazib 2020: 5).

These measures employed by governments to combat the spread of the virus, especially the lockdowns, have dealt massive blows on the economy of most nations. The resultant effect is that the attention of government across the world is turned to reviving flailing economies caused by COVID-19. This concern, however, leaves out the fears, anxiety and loneliness—and issues of mental health, generally—that the pandemic has forced on a lot of people. It is, therefore, vital that a balanced approach that both caters for the material needs of humans and at the same time takes care of their non-material needs, such as caring for each other, sharing and duty among others, is embraced. With Ubuntu, the dilemma between saving lives and reviving the economy and jobs ceases to exist. Ubuntu resolves both issues on a common dialectic by placing them in an interdependent relationship with each other since both concerns have the best interest of humans at the core. It is imperative, then, that Ubuntu's message is championed and promoted to provide balance for humans who need more than material results. By demonstrating our interdependency, Ubuntu both underscores COVID-19's essential lesson—how interconnected we are—and promotes values that can help combat societal distress occasioned by the pandemic and how we can get through the crises together.

Analyses

What is the purpose of bringing Ubuntu and COVID-19 together in a philosophical reflection? COVID-19 is a new virus that has come to redefine the way humans should interact due to its highly transmissible nature. Ubuntu, as already shown, embodies the interconnectedness and interdependency among humans. To begin with, there is need to constantly examine our life: what are the problems facing humanity, how did they come about, what responses should address them and how can the results be sustained? Socrates cautioned more than two millenniums ago on the futility of the unexamined life. The need for a philosophical reflection on Ubuntu and COVID-19 is to sustain the tradition of critical enquiry into issues affecting humans and their world as well as to usher new ways of thinking, of setting priorities and approaching life.

Let us begin by first enquiring into the "approved" measures for combating COVID-19 and how best to negotiate a flourishing post-pandemic life. A specific example will do in this regard. One of the measures spelt out for the prevention of COVID-19 is the "stay-at-home" order with an additional mandate that elderly people should not be visited during the pandemic as they are more susceptible to the virus. This may well be medically correct. Let us, however, briefly reflect on an elderly person—who in some cases is no longer able to do anything for herself—left alone to cater for herself. What will become of such a person? In states, like those in North America and Europe, with proper documentation and well-developed social welfare system, the government will know of the existence of such a person, and given the fact that the ban on visitation is issued by the government, there will be adequate provision made for the protection and sustenance of such an elderly person. The reverse will be the case in underdeveloped states, like those in Africa, without documentation and poor or in most cases non-existent social welfare. In such societies, the elderly and people living with severe disabilities depend on their families for survival. Their lives, in a sense, more than anything else, are a testimony to the truth of the core value of *entering-into* another person's life, caring and sharing, which Ubuntu represents. What will be the fate of an elderly person in Nigeria, for instance, in the face of messages that promote stereotypes about the virus which allow discrimination and, in some cases, prevent us from the truth about ourselves—an uncaring attitude is easily hidden under the cover of "no visit"?

From the foregoing, while such a preventive measure can adequately cater for an elderly European, the opposite is the case for an elderly African. In preaching the same safety precautions and in accepting and implementing the same preventive measures, African countries overlook the fact that there cannot be a uniform solution to a problem. Indeed, instead of accepting the Western solution in the handling of the elderly, COVID-19 offers a unique opportunity for Africa to position Ubuntu as a more viable alternative in the caring of elderly people. The subjection of the European elderly to social welfare and other technologies of care is not an adequate substitute for the human and familial connection as embodied in Ubuntu. For instance, the Western attitude of consigning the elderly to old people's home fundamentally undermines the essence of belonging to a family: a unit bonded in love and devotion and "bears the primary responsibility for fulfilling the psychic and emotional needs of its members" (Nolan and Lenski 2004: 278). This, however, does not imply that African countries should not have disaster preparation in place. This will act as a guide in knowing what preventive models to accept and which to rework. How this issue is handled can show how the dynamics of globalisation and localisation actually play out.

Based on the above, it is important that the response to the pandemic does not conform only to the European understanding, interpretation and recommendation about safety precautions because as Mogobe Ramose (1999: 33) reminds us, "[t]he European enterprise ... was a philosophical urge to impose and universalize sameness ...". This will no doubt forestall the slipping into what Ernest Wamba dia Wamba (1992: 67) refers to as "the social epistemology of domination". This is a pernicious framework which, for him, Africans urgently need appropriate philosophical paradigms which are capable of refuting and dislodging it. This is not an unreasonable observation if we remember that "[w]e are in a new world of cyberspace" shaped by "the breakup of the USSR, the end of the Cold War, and the cybernetic technological revolution" in which:

> Russia and China had reformed and opened up their economies. It is a new world of convergence of the Western libertarian ideas of democracy and free enterprise. It is a skewed and non-neutral, but metamorphosed imperial philosophy of ... Eurocentric conception of "reality, knowledge, and truth" that is now masquerading as human rights, good governance, democracy, and best practices in conflict resolution among individuals and between nations. (Dauda 2017: 478)

Indeed, the pandemic has positioned this "new world of cyberspace" to infiltrate every aspect of human activity and take over the control. The online platform is the new face of *doing* business and the favourite candidate for future human interactions. COVID-19 is pushing humanity to the edge where human life can be rationally controlled and ordered, down to the very last detail. Accepting the Western solution to COVID-19, and, especially, the subjection of almost all human activities to the dictates of the cyber world, helps to further entrench the "social epistemology of domination". By positioning Zoom meetings, webinars and Google classrooms, among others, as the best solution, African values of caring and sharing, which Ubuntu represents, are gradually eroded and replaced with the Western concept of clinical interaction. This is a limited approach. To reduce human experience to what science and technology can achieve is to discountenance the essence of Ubuntu and, by extension, philosophy in human experience. This will amount to maximum blunder as both Ubuntu and philosophy help humans to make sense of their experience and how to achieve the good life. Helen Lauer

(2017: 541) reminds that "[f]rom a problem-solving perspective, having many alternative approaches outclasses having only one". The Oxford Professor of Medical Ethics, Dominic Wilkinson, argues that "[t]here isn't a single right answer, it depends how you weigh up your choices. You need to distinguish between a number of things" (University of Oxford 2020). He further cautions that "science cannot tell us what values we should put weight on. These are ethical decisions—not scientific ones …". As such, while we embrace webinars and promote teleworking from home, we must also place these within the ambit of the home where these take place. Reports show that domestic violence and rape incidents escalated during the lockdown (Vandekerckhove 2020; Umukoro 2020). Umukoro, in fact, reports that the lockdowns imposed by the federal and states governments in Nigeria and in some other African countries forced vulnerable persons to stay more closely to their tormentors. The statistics produced by the Lagos State government-run Domestic and Gender Violence Response Team demonstrated that domestic violence increased by 60 per cent, sexual violence by 30 per cent and physical child abuse by 10 per cent. This is also the situation in other African countries, according to him. Barbara Sangare, a Cote D'Ivoire gender activist, states that gender violence has increased in her country, while Caroline Peters, a Gender and Community Advocate in South Africa, said that violence against women has gone up to 70 per cent in South Africa. What, then, would be the productivity and psychological disposition of a worker who operates from a violent-suffused home? Moreover, encouraging people to work from home using computer and other technological devices will significantly cut off social ties or reduce them to clinical interactions and transactions, which, on the long run, will affect humans' emotional wellbeing.

In addition, *dwelling* in the world of cyberspace will inevitably force people to recoil from human touch, creating many recluses, and there is no guarantee that this suspicion of each other will not characterise the post-pandemic era. How best can the changing societal values be managed such that humanity does not lose the essence of being human? Addressing this question is pivotal in stemming the tide of the gradual erosion of human values. If this issue is not given the adequate attention it deserves, the future may not be about humans but about post human.

This is why embracing the spirit of Ubuntu is urgently needed to help restore the vital importance of losing oneself in the service of others, of caring, of sharing, of seeing oneself in the other person. Ubuntu exposes the lie in the dominant position of techno-scientific knowledge in contemporary society, which implies a belief that this particular form of knowledge has the last say in establishing all matters of fact and in solving problems of all kinds (Bohme 2012: 45). By embracing the spirit of Ubuntu, the pandemic provides a unique opportunity for *true* interconnectedness and interdependency among nations, for humanity to come together as one: to explore what each culture has to offer, to think through the options and to make choices that best represent the interest of humanity. The philosophy of Ubuntu, then, helps to highlight some important lessons of COVID-19.

The first is the need to enhance peoples' critical thinking and other relevant aspects of rigorous enquiry. Criticism is crucial because it "enables one to reassess one's ideas, beliefs, values, norms, etc., through clarification, argument and persuasion" (Okolo 2015: 112). This does not imply the rejection of the issue under examination "but rational, impartial, and articulate appraisal" that demands a serious evaluation of the ideas in question to know whether they should be "reformed, modified or conserved, and in applying one's entire intellectual and imaginative intelligence to the search for an answer" (Staniland 1979: 4). Indeed, citizens "who think for themselves, rather than uncritically ingesting what their leaders and others with power tell them, are the absolutely necessary ingredient of a society that is to remain free" (Kahane 1995:xv). Such disposition will help people embrace responsible behaviour and be able to strike a balance between overreacting and underreacting due to the challenges posed by COVID-19. This will go a long way in helping to address, and possibly halt, pandemic-induced mental problems that may last beyond the pandemic. To achieve this, there is need for educational sensitisation of the general public on critical thinking. Beyond the pandemic, there is need to sustain this by including critical thinking in school curriculum for all levels of education.

The second lesson is linked to the first. This is the need to prepare ahead for any other global crises and future pandemic. History teaches that from time to time, humanity must face some crises. The response to these crises, how well they are managed and the extent of the damage incurred usually depend largely on the preparations in place before the crises. This can be achieved by training the general public on effective measures to protect them and others during any pandemic and other global challenges in advance. The public must be made to understand why it is necessary to sustain the training received in normal times. For instance, the measures put in place to contain COVID-19 in Nigeria would have been more easily achieved if the training and preventive measures used to contain Ebola in 2014 were sustained. Abraham Rudnick (2020: 1) reminds us that "[s]ocieties are measured in part in relation to how they rise to the occasion of collective crises and learn from them". Indeed, we "are morally obligated to plan for disaster because it affects human life and wellbeing" (Zack 2009: 55). That is, planning is "an integral part of caring for oneself and for others to and for whom we have prior obligations" (Zack 2009: 58). This is what Ubuntu represents.

Ubuntu helps us to better appreciate the ethical aspects of our response and the need for certain ethical considerations to underscore our actions. Given its concern about ethical considerations to underwrite our actions, Ubuntu points to the need for certain things to be in place: what is the level of preparedness to handle crises? Should a caring government wait for crises in the health sector before funding the hospitals and other health institutions? Should a government that understands that government is there because the people are there wait for an outbreak like COVID-19 before educating people on safety measures to prevent a pandemic? This is not to say that preparation will take care of every crisis especially crises that belong to the category of the "unknown unknowns" which Sam Black (1989: 31) views as "sudden calamitous events that cannot be foreseen by anybody". However, with adequate preparation, it would have been easier to respond to the crisis occasioned by the pandemic and any future crises in what conforms to Naomi Zack's (2009) Save All who can be saved (SALL) model in the preparation phase. This is a comprehensive disaster preparation that requires that preparation and prevention, as well as response, be considered in advance. For Zack, being "ready for a pandemic has an element of engagement consisting of being able and willing to act, and an element of having what it takes for a desired outcome" (60). This does not, however, take care of a pertinent issue: what was responsible for the devastation experienced by Western societies given their infrastructural and technological preparedness? The message here is that infrastructural and technological preparedness is not a be-all and end-all in crises management and, indeed, in most challenges of life. Humans need something deeper to cushion the effects of crises and other challenges of life. They need the knowledge that there are others interested in their wellbeing, people who they can share their experiences with. They need to know that they are cared for, sheltered in the common fold that connects all humanity. They need to feel truly human: humane, caring, looking out for each other, protecting, nurturing, encouraging, promoting and sustaining one another. This is what Ubuntu represents. Ubuntu, then, is deeper than providing infrastructural and technological gadgets or, even, rendering material assistance. It acknowledges all these but extends to giving and sharing time, intelligence, experience and all our humane attributes with others.

The third lesson is anchored on the second. COVID-19 teaches that a government that fails to prepare for crisis risks social unrest and uprising during a crisis. The #EndSARS protest, which started in October 2020 in Nigeria, is a good example. The protest that started as a peaceful protest by the youths against countless brutality of law enforcement officers, particularly the Special Anti-Robbery Squad (SARS), on unarmed, innocent civilians in Nigeria was midway hijacked by hoodlums who are mostly unemployed. United Nations deputy Secretary-General, Amina Mohammed, on a solidarity visit to Nigeria to underscore the organisation's support to countries during the COVID-19 pandemic, on Monday 9 November 2020 partly blamed the hardship caused by COVID-19 for the #EndSARS protest. Rudnick (2020) champions the view that unemployment is associated with disrupted mental wellbeing and other personal and societal disruptions such as poverty and crime, among others. Further, he warns that it is easy to have political disruption during a pandemic, particularly in countries where the regime is not democratically robust. To forestall future occurrences like #EndSARS, African governments, especially Nigerian government, must see planning as "a required duty of trustees, stewards, and guardians" (Zack 2009: 58). This entails allowing democracy to work: government that is responsible and responsive to the needs of the people and government that is determined to place itself at the service of the people, in short, a care-oriented government founded on the principles of Ubuntu.

The fourth lesson is the unpredictability of life. Following the outbreak of the pandemic, almost all plans by individuals, groups, churches, schools, businesses, corporations, governments and countries came to a halt. The world looks to science for a solution, for a vaccine that will contain the virus. Even with the production of vaccines for the treatment of COVID-19, there are still many issues (as earlier outlined) waiting for answers. The issues, in fact, demonstrate how impossible it is to box life into the structured, precise and predictable confines of science. COVID-19 is a reminder that lives and the totality of human experiences will never submit to quantifiable data, dissection and causal regimentation. Humanity will always yearn for something more: interactions and connectivity expressed within the fold of looking out for each other, for Ubuntu. It is important to note that there are other non-Ubuntu philosophies, like communitarianism, that speak to looking out for each other. However, communitarianism emphasises the needs of the community over those of the individual in a master-servant kind of relationship. This implies the need to subordinate individual interest to the community. Such an ideology can easily be manipulated against the individual as witnessed under the Nazi regime. While communitarianism called "for constant participation, it aimed to inculcate a spirit of individual attachment to the whole and a readiness not only to obey but also to sacrifice everything for the general interest as defined by the Nazis" (Macridis 1980: 197). Indeed, under this arrangement, the individual's right to think his own thoughts is taken away as the individual becomes a "new individual imbued with communitarian and nationalist beliefs as dictated by the leader and the party" (Macridis 1980: 197). The implication is that the intrinsic freedom of the individual is denied. From this perspective, the looking out for each other embodied in the communitarian ideology is emasculated to the point that it almost resembles Phillips Shively's (1997: 6) "construction of incentives". This is a situation where power is exercised in such a way as to "make the alternative so unattractive that only one reasonable option remains". In contradistinction, Ubuntu invites the individual to participate in the lives of others from a deep knowledge of being a partaker in a common humanity. It represents the essence of humanness that is imbued with ethical consciousness rooted in the ability of the individual to participate in the wellbeing of others. Tutu (2011) maintains that in indigenous African society, Ubuntu was coveted more than anything else because it is seen as the quality that ultimately makes a person both human and humane. Ubuntu's ability to focus humanity on their human-humane essence sets it apart from other philosophies and makes it an ideal candidate to provide direction on how best to ameliorate the adverse effect of COVID-19, especially, on the social relationship of Africans and, by extension, the world. Indeed, COVID-19 brings to the fore the need for a sense of balance as the world becomes more and more scientifically and technologically oriented. Gernot Bohme (2012) suggests that the dominant position of scientific knowledge within contemporary society is leading to a decay of other forms of knowledge and that there are types of problems and types of human needs that scientific and technological knowledge is particularly ill-suited to address. By embracing Ubuntu as the guide for the future, its philosophy of sharing, inclusiveness, interconnectedness, sustainability, caring and wellbeing will balance the clinical approach of science and technology.

The fifth lesson brought to the fore by COVID-19 is that only those who have the key to theory can determine how society is organised and what counts as civilisation. The truth of this becomes evident when we consider that "[w]hat science is can only be settled by looking, among other things, at its many and striking effects on human life" (Bohme 2012: 23). He warns that "[s]cience must be seen as an epoch-defining phenomenon—a cultural form that has shaped a certain period of human history and will in future likely shape the very course of natural evolution". The world is gradually shrinking into a monoculture where technological edge, that is, the institution of cyber world, is being positioned as the most, and gradually the only, acceptable means of human interaction. This wave will increasingly become central to how nations relate to each other. This situation calls for a deeper reflection on Bola Dauda's (2017: 477) discussion on "The philosophical realities of African nation-states in a new world". One way to approach this for him is "for African nation-states to rethink the old paradigms [that impose the European epistemological paradigm upon Africa] and be creative in adapting the evolving cyberspace, global village, and knowledge economies". For African nation-states, it is a wake-up call to rethink their involvement in a world that is fast been converted into a cyberspace. For this reason, there is need to be serious about our destiny: how best to manage our resources in the face of sustained widening economic inequality between the Global North and the Global South, especially given the way this is arranging the relationship between the developed and the developing nations, how to enter equal partnership with other nations bearing in mind that without mutual respect the concept of equality is a farce and how best to craft an authentic African identity considering that "[e]very society, in order to sustain and generate itself, will and must periodically return to the question of what founded it, what gave it a sense of purpose, what is the condition of its own possibility" (Praeg 2017: 497). Using Ubuntu as guide, there is need to set goals that can be evaluated in determining the wellbeing of humanity. Ubuntu allows that there are no final answers and solutions but core values that speak to whatever issues life may throw at us.

The sixth lesson is to underscore the benefits of COVID-19. Difficult as it is to associate the pandemic with gains, yet two advantages clearly stand out. One, it exposes the oneness, unity, bond, fusion and interdependence of all humanity. There are no superior and inferior people, no centres and peripherals. This will go a long way in helping to normalise race relations. These are things which Ubuntu, with its forward-thinking approach to human relationship, has always represented. Its stand on looking out for each other could help prevent superiority and inferiority complexes, which create conditions for some people to victimise or become victims to others. Ubuntu's care-centred philosophy, which prizes the comprehensive wellbeing of people over race and material consideration, has positioned it as the best adequate response to COVID-19 challenges. The philosophy of Ubuntu encourages every individual to see in the other individual a reflection of its self. Two, the lockdown brought about by COVID-19 highlights the urgent need for local solutions. For instance, for once African leaders who favour medical tourism instead of equipping the health sector of their countries were forced to accept medical treatment in their countries. Such situations help to expose the attitude of most African governments towards infrastructural and human capacity development in their country. To address this, there is need for introspective review by the government on how best to re-order the country so as to be able to face life's unexpected challenges. In this, Ubuntu's timeless and unchanging principles can be relied on for guide.

The final lesson, which is also the defining concern of our time, is the recognition that all nations of the world should contribute, should have a say in issues of global concern. COVID-19 has forced humanity to see how closely connected everyone is. For this reason, it is crucial that everyone is involved in finding a solution. This demands a multilateral approach that shuns a mono-cultural ownership of the solution to the pandemic on the one hand and on the other hand favours our collective effort in finding solutions that are both culture specific and culture *generic*. Embracing Ubuntu as Africa's contribution will help to provide the required guide for handling the issue of how best the elderly ones should be taken care of in Africa, where the approved measures are ill-equipped to handle. For instance, even while maintaining social distance, Ubuntu helps us to live within social inclusion by continuously making meaningful difference in other peoples' life through finding out what their needs are and addressing those concerns. Indeed, the pandemic helps to highlight the *pivotal* role of Ubuntu as a guiding principle that should *always* direct the core concerns of humanity.

Conclusion

The pandemic has thrown up many profound and difficult issues. The preventive measures—social distancing, no hugs, no handshakes and no visits, among others—occasioned by COVID-19 are forcing the rethinking of old normal parameters for measuring the things that are truly important. The stringent nature of the safety precaution messages involving COVID-19 is such that can easily destroy human relations. It is for this reason that even while we grapple with a changing world, re-setting our outlook on life and priorities, we should not lose sight of some timeless and unchanging fundamentals such as devotion, care, duty, obligation and integrity, among others, that sustain our humanity. These are what Ubuntu stands for. Ubuntu is about the immersion in and the total entering of an individual into the life of others, such that the "I" pronoun has its meaning only in the company of "they". There is no sole "I" that can embark on any comprehensive experience without the "they" offering one kind of support or the other. To exist, to make sense of the world, is to do so in the company of others, in communion with them. As such, taking lessons from Ubuntu will go a long way to cushion the effect of isolation, fear, anxiety, panic, depression and spike in mental disorder occasioned by COVID-19. What is needed is, perhaps, not more Zoom meetings but more human, humane presence—more spirit of Ubuntu.

In all, the pandemic comes as an opportunity for nations to re-build their confidence, re-think their values and priorities and re-learn the values of mutual respect for each other. The eternal lesson of COVID-19 is that no voice should supersede the other. There are no a priori centres and peripherals, but one humanity, united against a common enemy for the survival and sustainability of the human race.

References

Black, Sam. 1989. *Introduction to Public Relations*. London: Modino Press.

Bohme, Gernot. 2012. *Invasive Technification: Critical Essays in the Philosophy of Technology*. Trans. Cameron Shingleton. London, New Delhi, New York, Sydney: Bloomsbury.

Dauda, Bola. 2017. African Humanism and Ethics: The Cases of Ubuntu and Omolúwàbí. In *In The Palgrave Handbook of African Philosophy*, ed. Adeshina Afolayan and Toyin Falola, 475–491. New York: Palgrave Macmillan.

Etieyibo, Edwin. 2017. Ubuntu and the Environment. In *The Palgrave Handbook of African Philosophy*, ed. Adeshina Afolayan and Toyin Falola, 633–657. New York: Palgrave Macmillan.

Eze, Michael Onyebuchi. 2010. *Intellectual History in Contemporary South Africa*. New York: Palgrave Macmillan.

Kahane, Howard. 1995. *Logic and Contemporary Rhetoric: The Use of Reason in Everyday Life*. 7th ed. Belmont: Wadsworth Publishing Company.

Lauer, Helen. 2017. Philosophy of Science and Africa. In *The Palgrave Handbook of African Philosophy*, ed. Adeshina Afolayan and Toyin Falola, 539–553. New York: Palgrave Macmillan.

Macridis, Roy C. 1980. *Contemporary Political Ideologies: Movements and Regimes*. Cambridge, MA: Winthrop Publishers.

Matolino, Bernard. 2011. Abantu and Their Ethic in the Face of AIDS. In *African Philosophy and the Future Africa*, ed. Gerald Walmsley, 71–81. Washington, DC: The Council for Research Values and Philosophy.

Mbiti, John. 1970. *African Religions and Philosophies*. New York: Doubleday.

Mkhize, Nhlanhla. 2008. Ubuntu and Harmony: An African Approach to Morality and Ethics. In *Persons in Community: African Ethics in a Global Culture*, ed. Ronald Nicolson, 35–44. Scottsville: University of KwaZulu-Natal Press.

Nolan, Patrick, and Gerhard Lenski. 2004. *Human Societies: An Introduction to Macrosociology*. 9th ed. Boulder, London: Paradigm Publishers.

Okolo, M.S.C. 2015. *Philosophy: Contemporary Concerns in Africa*. Owerri: Book-Konzult.

Praeg, Leonhard. 2017. Ubuntu and the Emancipation of Law. In *The Palgrave Handbook of African Philosophy*, ed. Adeshina Afolayan and Toyin Falola, 493–506. New York: Palgrave Macmillan.

Ramose, Mogobe. 1999. *African Philosophy Through Ubuntu*. Harare: Mond Books.

Rudnick, Abraham. 2020. Social, Psychological, and Philosophical Reflections on Pandemics and Beyond. *Societies* 10 (42): 1–4.

Shively, Phillips W. 1997. Power and Choice: An Introduction to Political Science, 5. New York: The MacGraw-Hill Companies, Inc.

Staniland, H.S. 1979. What is Philosophy? *Second Order: An African Journal of Philosophy* VIII (1&2): 3–10.

Tazib, Syed Rahaman. 2020. A Comprehensive Review on COVID-19 and its Prevention and Possible Treatments. *International Journal of Scientific Research* 9 (4): 1–6.

Tutu, Desmond. 2011. *God is Not a Christian: Speaking Truth in Times of Crisis*. London: Rider Books.

Umukoro, Ejiro. June 1 2020. Amidst COVID-19 Lockdown, Nigeria Sees Increased Sexual and Gender Violence. *Premium Times*.

University of Oxford. 2020. The Philosophy of COVID-19: Is it even Possible to do the 'Right Thing'? https://ox.ac.uk/news/arts-blog/philosophy-covid-19-it-even-possible-do-right-thing. Accessed Nov 2020.

Vandekerckhove, Wim. 2020. COVID, Existentialism and Crisis Philosophy. *Philosophy of Management* 19: 127–132.

Wamba dia Wamba, Ernest. 1992. Beyond Elite Politics of Democracy in Africa. *In Quest* 4 (2): 67.

Zack, Naomi. 2009. The Ethics of Disaster Planning: Preparation vs Response. *Philosophy of Management* 8 (2): 55–66.

4

Limits of Science-Based Approaches in Global Health: Sociocultural and Moral Lessons from Ebola and COVID-19

Samuel J. Ujewe

Introduction

This chapter explores the limits of science-based approaches in addressing global health emergencies and outlines the significance of adopting socio-cultural, socioeconomic, and ethical approaches. It uses the 2013–2016 Ebola epidemic in West Africa and the coronavirus global pandemic (COVID-19) to underscore the limits of science-based approaches in tackling deadly infectious disease outbreaks. Against this background, it highlights the valuable effects of humanities measures that have been (or are being) used to show that sociocultural and ethical approaches are crucial to effectively address global health emergencies. Humanities, as used in this chapter, refers to the fields of knowledge and/or expertise that address conceptual and sociocultural aspects of human existence, experi-ences, or global conditions:

S. J. Ujewe (✉)
Global Emerging Pathogens Treatment Consortium (GET-Africa),
Lagos, Nigeria
e-mail: ujewes@mcmaster.ca

F. Egbokhare, A. Afolayan (eds.), *Global Health, Humanity and the COVID-19 Pandemic*, https://doi.org/10.1007/978-3-031-17429-2_4

> ...those branches of knowledge that concern themselves with human beings and their culture or with analytic and critical methods of inquiry derived from an appreciation of human values and of the unique ability of the human spirit to express itself. As a group of educational disciplines, the humanities are distinguished in content and method from the physical and biological sciences and, somewhat less decisively, from the social sciences. The humanities include the study of all languages and literatures, the arts, history, and philosophy. (Britannica 2021)

This is different from the commonly understood usage of humanities to refer to the human race, collective human co-existence, or acts of benevolence (Oxford 2021). The point is not to minimize the invaluable contributions of science to global health but to demonstrate the need for adopting a harmonized approach toward addressing current and future global health emergencies.

COVID-19 raises questions regarding the sufficiency of science-based approaches in addressing global health emergencies, especially those relating to deadly infectious disease outbreaks. Despite rapid scientific advancements and technological innovations in biomedicine, the virus engulfed the world in phases with the most devastating health costs to-date borne by high-income countries (HICs) (Ritchie et al. 2021), where scientific advancements in biomedicine are most entrenched. Within one year into the COVID-19 pandemic, several vaccines were rapidly developed and distributed around the world in a desperate effort to end the pandemic. Yet, while some countries vaccinated most of their populations within a short period, others are yet to vaccinate a significant proportion of their frontline workers—especially in low- and middle-income countries (LMICs) (Ritchie et al. 2021). Alongside the hospitalization of acute COVID-19 cases, social measures like lockdowns and physical distancing became key strategies for fighting the virus. LMICs that could not bear the economic costs of lockdowns were the same ones having limited access to COVID-19 vaccines (Ritchie et al. 2021). At the same time, some of the worst affected by COVID-19 and its allied impacts in HICs were historically marginalized groups or populations (APM Research Lab n.d.; CDC 2020; Williamson et al. 2020).

While science has provided advanced biomedical tools for fighting COVID-19 and other global health crises, science-based approaches are not sufficient toward effectively securing a healthy world. Scientific measures need to be considered alongside other crucial approaches in order to have better chances at securing global health. Recent experiences of Ebola epidemics in the Democratic Republic of Congo and the West African region and global experiences of COVID-19 have shown that science-based approaches need to be bolstered by sociocultural, socioeconomic, and ethical approaches to be successful. It has also been shown that global health emergencies can be addressed sooner if other approaches are deployed alongside the science based. For instance, science has shown that wearing of face masks is effective in breaking the transmission chain of COVID-19 (Howard et al. 2021). However, social, cultural, and ethical measures, among others, are needed to motivate the population to wear masks, as upholding values such as rights and freedom, and communal responsibility and solidarity come into fierce contention in effecting compliance (BBC 2020; Taylor and Asmundson 2021). The successful approaches toward addressing global health emergencies will be ones that adequately harmonize science-based approaches with sociocultural, socioeconomic, and ethical approaches.

This chapter provides a brief overview of advances in science and biomedicine and explores the limitations of science-based approaches in the light of recent global health emergencies, including Ebola in sub-Saharan Africa and the COVID-19 global pandemic. Analyzing these in the light of sufficiency theory and its application in global health, the chapter situates the need to include humanities-based approaches. This will ensure that in addressing global health emergencies, social, cultural, and moral realities of affected populations are accounted for. The chapter concludes by proposing three humanities-based approaches that could consolidate science-based approaches if the latter are to be effective toward addressing global health emergencies.

Advances in Science and Biomedicine Since the Spanish Flu

The 1918 Spanish Flu killed between 20 and 100 million persons globally by the time it ended (Dickin et al. 2020). While total deaths in the United States was estimated at 675,000 (Billings 1997), the death toll in India was between 12 and 18 million ((BBC News 2020; Chhun 2021). By contrast, as of September 2021, total COVID-19 deaths in the United States stands 638,632, and India had total deaths of 43,895 (WHO 2021b). Diagnostic science and biomedical remedies were deployed as valuables tools in tackling the Spanish Flu pandemic and vaccines played a major role (Billings 1997). In just over a century after the Spanish Flu, the world is still in the grips of another flu pandemic, COVID-19. The current total global deaths due to COVID-19 stand at 4,539,723—as of September 2021 (WHO 2021b). Between these two historical events, intermittent deadly epidemics have occurred around the world, with the West African Ebola being one of the most devastating (BBC 2016). Despite Ebola's deadly nature, it took around four decades from the emergence of the virus for the world to come up with effective vaccines (History of Vaccines 2021).

It is important to note that the COVID-19 global pandemic took place in an era where scientific and biomedical advancements are at historic peak. Many infectious diseases have been successfully eradicated from many parts of the world, and others like smallpox have been eliminated globally (Strassburg 1982). A major milestone was reached in the global polio eradication when Africa was declared polio-free in the early months of the COVID-19 pandemic in 2020 (Guglielmi 2020) . The triumph of science and biomedicine is made more visible with COVID-19, as the world has advanced in genomic sequencing of disease organism and real-time data sharing that enhances prompt global research and development of effective control measures, drugs, and vaccines. Of note is the pace with which scientists mobilized across the globe to develop several COVID-19 vaccines in less than one year, surpassing the traditional decade-long vaccine development timeline (Zimmer et al. 2020; WHO 2021a). A number of these vaccines were used around the world in a race to attain herd immunity among populations, contributing towards ending the COVID-19 pandemic. Some of the leading vaccines have deployed a new genetic technology in their development, including those developed by Pfizer BioNtech and Moderna (Corum and Zimmer 2020a, 2020b).

Among other things, life expectancy in HICs has heightened due to advancements in science and biomedicine (World Bank 2021). This is partly a reflection of the successful suppression or eradication of infectious diseases, but also amidst rising incidences of noncommunicable diseases (Ho and Hendi 2018). By contrast, LMICs, especially in the global south, with less advanced science and biomedicine, continue to record relatively lower life expectancies and higher mortalities and morbidities from infectious diseases, including malaria, tuberculosis and HIV/AIDS, among others (Roser and Ritchie 2016). These may also be attributable to the relatively slow advancements in biomedicine, arguably. Yet, HICs have been worse hit by the COVID-19 pandemic than LMICs in terms of infection and mortality rates, as is most visible when comparing the rates from Europe and North America with those of sub-Saharan Africa (WHO 2021b). The unanswered questions remain: how and why did COVID-19 emerge as a global pandemic mostly affecting HICs despite historical advancements in science and biomedicine, and why are COVID-19 infection and mortality rates significantly lower in LMICs? What is obvious is that advanced biomedicine, by itself, did not avert the COVID-19 global pandemic.

Limits of Science-Based Approaches

Scientific innovations have been crucial in navigating the global COVID-19 response, starting with the rapid genome sequencing of the virus in the early moments of the pandemic and sharing real-time data from the originating country of the virus (Behrmann and Spiegel 2020; Van Noorden 2021). Rapid knowledge development about the virus was advanced through rapid scientific analysis with real-time data as the virus spread across the globe (Guillou 2020). This informed the rapid development of a variety of COVID-19 testing kits and vaccines, leading to the record one-year vaccine development timeline attained by several COVID-19 vaccines (Cui et al. 2020; Zimmer et al. 2020). The rollout of the vaccines is being accompanied by global aggregation of data to enable continuous analysis to determine the efficacy and safety of the vaccines (Mathieu et al. 2021). It is also worth noting that the now globally normalized use of face masks was informed by scientific evidence around the transmissibility of the virus (Howard et al. 2021).

Despite these advancements and deployment of new scientific and biomedical innovations in tackling COVID-19, the virus spread across the globe almost unhindered and continues to mutate. The most scientifically and medically advanced nations were found unprepared to deal with the pandemic at the onset. While global COVID-19 mortalities rates have been generally higher among older populations, severe mortalities were recorded among older people living in care homes in many of the affected countries (Amore et al. 2021). In some countries, like the United Kingdom, COVID-19 has disproportionately affected racialized minority groups who are already largely systemically disadvantaged in terms of access to healthcare (Kirby 2020).

While these scientifically informed measures are crucial, it has also become evident that these alone are insufficient for ending the Covid19 pandemic. Vaccine hesitancy was made manifest, as doubt and fear surrounded the safety of the vaccines being rolled out globally (Sallam 2021). Past experiences of populations with health interventions and significant vaccine shortage in sub-Saharan Africa raised more questions, implanting doubts and facilitating hesitation among populations to take the limited vaccines available (MENEZES et al. 2021). Despite the scientific evidence around the use of face masks, mask resistance and anti-mask movements persisted in North America (Stewart 2020; Shivaram 2021). The lack of broad cooperation by the United States' public to use face mask has been attributed to as a key factor in the spread of the disease and the rise of the Delta variant (Wilner 2021).

Finally, one of the major problems that has followed the successful development of COVID-19 vaccines is "vaccine nationalism"—a situation whereby few-producing or rich countries amassed large supplies of the available vaccines, when other non-producing or low-resourced countries have few or no doses (Lock 2021). For instance, as of March 2021,

78% of the 447 million doses of COVID-19 vaccines deployed globally were administered in only ten countries, and about a quarter of the world's population was forecast to not have access to the vaccines until 2022 (So and Woo 2020; Beyrer et al. 2021). And by September 2021:

> 41.3% of the world population [had] received at least one dose of a COVID-19 vaccine. 5.6 billion doses [had] been administered globally, and 30.38 million [were being] administered each day. [Yet] only 1.9% of people in low-income countries [had] received at least one dose. (Ritchie et al. 2021)

The COVID-19 Vaccines Global Access (COVAX) Facility was developed by the World Health Organization (WHO) in conjunction with the Global Alliance for Vaccines and Immunizations (GAVI) to ensure that COVID-19 vaccines are available and accessible to non-producing and low-resourced countries across the globe who signed up to the initiative (BBC 2021; WHO 2020). The main aim of the COVAX Facility is to ensure equitable access to COVID-19 vaccines globally, so that self-financed and funded countries can have access to the battery of proven vaccines (Berkly 2020).

However, despite the unprecedented pace of the COVID-19 vaccine development and with several vaccines being administered around the world, it is evident that science-based approaches have been insufficient in tackling the pandemic and more humanities-based approaches are needed to ensure an end to the pandemic globally. The growing global health inequities and lack of trust in global health stakeholders exposed and perpetuated by COVID-19 have also demonstrated this conclusion.

Sufficiency Theory and Global Health Emergencies

The limitations of science-based approaches can be understood in terms of sufficiency theory, where the primary focus of justice is to achieve a descent minimum quality of life for the worse off populations, groups, and persons:

> …the sufficiency principle also holds that the duty to improve the condition of the worse off applies only until the point that the worse off rise above some level of absolute deprivation … [as] justice requires that everyone has enough, or a sufficient amount, of what contributes to a good life, not that everyone has an equal share. (Powers and Faden 2006, 55)

The idea of sufficiency and health aims to ensure that in situations where persons or populations are relatively disadvantaged, the varied factors, beyond their biological functioning or disease conditions, contributing to their inability to attain a certain level of health outcome are addressed. Hence, this approach is also concerned with the totality of the social structures and relative income inequalities, which profoundly and pervasively affect the well-being of the disadvantaged populations and which keep them below the acceptable threshold of good health (Powers and Faden 2006).

From the humanities perspective of global health emergencies, a sufficiency approach would require that while the pathogenic elements of a deadly disease are being addressed through drug or vaccine development, the social, cultural, and systemic issues that bear on the overall health of the affected populations are equally addressed. For instance, it has been established that the 2013–2015 Ebola epidemic in West Africa was not only a factor of the virus but also of weak health infrastructure and poor healthcare systems in the affected countries (Moon et al. 2015). In addition, sociocultural factors and moral experiences of affected communities invariably contributed to the spread of the Ebola Virus Disease (EVD) and truncated the response strategies toward ending the epidemic (Aggrey and Shrum 2020; Mitman 2014; Le Marcis et al. 2019).

From a sufficiency theory outlook, scientific innovations alone would not be enough to end the epidemic: "…a sufficiency approach would [aim to] understand the background social, cultural, anthropological and economic conditions influencing the spread of a disease" (Ujewe and Mungwa 2019, 175–76) and crucially seek ways to address them. In the light of the COVID-19 pandemic, a sufficiency approach would require that while global health actors are mobilizing vaccine development and distribution, social and cultural factors that would enhance or deter the acceptance or distribution of these great innovations are addressed. The development of efficacious vaccines is futile if the targeted populations reject them. This has been proven by the escalation of polio in West Africa when populations in Northern Nigeria boycotted the mass polio immunization program and set back polio eradication by years (Ujewe 2020). The pervasive anti-vaccine, anti-lockdown, and anti-mask movements during the COVID-19 (Stewart 2020; Dror et al. 2020) have further shown that innovative scientific measures, including the record time vaccines developed, can have no real impact on the pandemic if the social, cultural, moral, and other allied issues are not addressed. Sufficiency in global health emergencies would entail relative levels of social organization and scientific development that will be enough to address or prevent deadly infectious disease outbreaks, epidemics, and pandemics (Ujewe and Mungwa 2019).

Against this background, a sufficiency approach is crucial toward ensuring the great innovations that have emerged, including rapid sequencing of the virus, real-time development of test kits, and rapid vaccine development, make immediate impact in the fight to end the pandemic. For instance, the global inequities in access to personal protective equipment (PPE) exposed in the earlier waves of the pandemic demonstrated that some parts of the world had more, while others had little to none. And as the use of vaccines became imminent toward ending the pandemic and the global vaccine rollout continues, it is no longer news that while a large proportion of the global population barely has access to a single dose of any of the vaccines available, others are being privileged with third doses (Ritchie et al. 2021; Lieber 2021). The sufficiency approach would require that beyond simply increasing global production of vaccines, for instance, global equity in access would be achieved that accounts for social and cultural outlooks and moral experiences of disadvantaged populations across the globe. Likewise, the unprecedented pace with which COVID-19 vaccines were developed would be required to be similarly replicated in the global distribution and access, especially for non-producing and poorer countries that could not compete in the race to procure the vaccines.

Need for Humanities-Based Approaches

The Covid-19 pandemic was met with sensational resilience by advancements in medicine and health technology, where the isolation and genetic sequencing of the coronavirus were done and shared globally in real time (Behrmann and Spiegel 2020). Epidemiological data were also collected, analyzed, and distributed across the board in real time, allowing for close analysis of the global situation (Guillou 2020). This has remained crucial in detecting the new more virulent variants of COVID-19 that are becoming the dominant strains (Abutaleb and Sun 2021). Also, there have been rapid development of various COVID-19 vaccines, which were done in record time, outpacing any previous vaccines ever developed in the delivery timeline—as noted above.

However, underlying socio-political and socio-ethical resistance have been emboldened by events surrounding stringent COVID-19 measures, which science and technology alone cannot address. For instance, various forms of vaccine hesitancy advanced across the globe, perhaps as rapidly as the COVID-19 vaccines were developed. Vaccine hesitancy is the situation where certain populations do not accept to use scientifically validated vaccines due to experiential, moral, or other ideological reasons: "…[it] occurs on the continuum between high vaccine demand and complete vaccine refusal, i.e. no demand for available and offered vaccines" (MacDonald 2015, 4162):

> Vaccine hesitancy is not a superficial issue with a universal solution. … Rather, it is a multifaceted, deeply complex construct that may be rooted in the moral composition that guides our daily decision making … Several distinct values are associated with vaccine hesitancy—particularly purity, liberty, and anti-authority. … Combined with the historical amnesia of the consequences of vaccine preventable diseases, vaccine hesitancy becomes easier to understand as a belief system grounded in certain moral values. (McAteer et al. 2020, 703–4)

While there may be significant differences in the rates of vaccine acceptance or hesitancy, as noted in a systematic global review of COVID-19 vaccine hesitancy (Sallam 2021), its broad presence means that regardless of the advancements in science to fast-track vaccine development, the successful deployment of vaccines as a critical solution to the COVID-19 and others pandemics lies outside of the confines of science alone. Likewise, the sustained global inequity in COVID-19 vaccine access cannot be addressed by purely scientific approaches, as inequity is defined and determined by several social, political, and cultural determinants, and addressing them would require an ethically embedded framework. Humanities approaches become crucial toward addressing the underlying issues of liberty, purity, anti-authority, and other moral values that influence the non-acceptance of scientifically validated vaccines.

Sample Humanities Approaches to Complement Science

Effectively addressing issues like vaccine hesitancy as buttressed by sociocultural realities and moral experiences of populations would require approaches that are embedded with similar frames of references. Two key relevant approaches include community engagement, which accounts for the sociocultural and socioeconomic realities, and addressing the moral experiences of populations. These approaches have been previously demonstrated as having great potentials to ensure acceptance of health intervention measures among hesitant populations.

Community Engagement

Community engagement has emerged as one of the most promising strategies toward gaining trust in responding to public health emergencies. Its deployment has proved to be a valuable resource in addressing epidemics, as shown by the associated gains in the conduct of research in affected communities during the Ebola epidemic in West Africa (Afolabi et al. 2021). Community engagement is an emerging process ethics approach that requires community members to be consulted in an open and collaborative manner throughout the course of research or health intervention processes, from planning through implementation to eventual feedback on the outcomes, and in a culturally sensitive manner (Folayan et al. 2016; Kombe et al. 2019). People's reactions or opposition to early emergency response plans and efforts imposed by governments and other response agencies demand a responsibility to build a network of relationships with various communities and enter into various forms of negotiations with the affected populations (Le Marcis et al. 2019).

These forms of dialogue ensure that the concerns and perspectives of affected communities are accounted for in developing and implementing emergency response strategies. For instance, following a series of oppositions to Ebola response in Guinea, the World Health Organization (WHO) facilitated a community mediation process that led to reconciliation and enabled community mobilization and empowerment, constituting a joint effort to end the epidemic (Le Marcis et al. 2019). In Liberia, community liaisons, as nominated by community members, were chosen to lead the Ebola task forces, in order to legitimize Ebola response strategies; in Sierra Leone, where local chiefs were losing legitimacy, community youths were variously involved in the consultations, paving ways for acceptance of emergency response initiatives (Le Marcis et al. 2019). Openness, reflexivity, and accountability have been highlighted as crucial elements to successful community engagement for emergency response during the West African Ebola epidemic (Ryan et al. 2019). These are valuable attributes that can enhance the acceptability of scientific evidence and advancements in medicine during health emergencies and maximize their impact in the restoration of health and normalcy.

Additionally, the need for open-ended consultations and cultural appreciation of affected communities was pointed out by local researchers and consortia, as a crucial aspect of engagement. In the early stages of clinical trials on the use of convalescent plasma to treat Ebola, the Global Emerging Pathogens Treatment Consortium (GET-Africa), for instance, pointed to the need for community engagement and patient advocacy in a culturally appropriate manner (F. Kombe et al. 2016). It placed weight on a special protection of the Ebola survivors' network, in order to avoid potential exploitation of community engagement by researchers. To ensure robust involvement of communities and avoid undue inducement and exploitation in Ebola research, community engagement was positioned as a strategy to increase community education on Ebola and reduce the risk of therapeutic misconceptions; address myths and misconceptions about Ebola and vaccines that engender distrust; and facilitate negotiations for post-trial access to potential Ebola therapies and vaccines, given the historical exclusion of trial communities from accessing the Hepatitis B vaccine (Molyneux and Geissler Molyneux 2008; Folayan et al. 2016; Franco et al. 2012). This is not to say that community engagement is the perfect approach for addressing health emergencies but that its attributes would provide a viable platform to ensure the success of scientific measure, like testing and innovative vaccines.

Addressing Moral Experiences of Communities

Underpinning community engagement are the moral experiences of communities in relation to interventions and research during health emergencies. This leads to the need to address moral residue in, and through, health research and interventions (Ujewe 2020). Moral residue in the context of global health research and intervention refers to:

> ...the moral experience following events or situations where health interventions or research carried out amongst communities, population groups or regions leave traces of harm or exploitation that engender feelings of guilt, remorse, or regret, anger, frustration, anxiety or self-blame among those affected or global health actors. The urgency to meet one healthcare need could result in another equivalent or even worse problem, for which the affected population also needs urgent intervention, but which remains unaddressed. (Ujewe 2020, 4)

Public oppositions and non-compliance to Ebola response initiatives during the West African epidemic, for instance, were linked to historical experiences of the affected populations with exploitative research and other engagements and/or knowledge of communities in other parts of sub-Saharan Africa that had had these experiences. For instance, ethnographic studies show that local resistance in Guinea, Liberia, Sierra Leone, and Ghana were informed by a number of factors related to history and international political economy (Le Marcis et al. 2019; Aggrey and

Shrum 2020; Tangwa et al. 2018), ranging from legacies of the transatlantic slave trade and colonialism to economic structures built around international extractive industries and aid dependencies (Benton and Dionne 2015). These historical experiences were re-inscribed in the nature of emergency responses under the WHO's Public Health Emergency of International Concern (PHEIC) declaration (WHO 2014). For instance:

> In each of the three countries, humanitarian interventions or clinical trials were largely run through national institutions with direct ties to former colonial powers—France intervened in Guinea, the UK in Sierra Leone, and US organisations were the first in Liberia. (Le Marcis et al. 2019)

Explanations to the emergency response oppositions and other challenges encountered in the three countries are deemed to be associated to these political configurations, rather than on culture alone, as was often implied (Chandler et al. 2015).

The opposition to Ebola vaccine trials in Ghana was based on a mixture of knowledge and experience of previous exploitative medical research and the role of politics in advancing such agendas, in addition to the history of colonialism and the slave trade (Aggrey and Shrum 2020; Tangwa et al. 2018). In a more recent cultural memory was the dubious meningitis vaccine trial in Nigeria in 1996 by Pfizer, which instigated the halting of a mass polio eradication campaign in 2003 (Ujewe 2020). This background, combined with insufficient public information provided to the public about the scheduled Ebola vaccine trials, led to a wariness in the Ghanaian population that the trials were being undertaken in secret in their communities. The wariness was strengthened by the public uncertainties surrounding the specific nature of the clinical trials with fears linked to suspicions that the trial vaccines could bring Ebola to Ghana (Kummervold et al. 2017).

Underlying these reactions was the political context in which the vaccine trials were attempted, which was linked to the design and implementation of the vaccine trials (Aggrey and Shrum 2020). Politicians charged with the responsibility of reviewing the trial protocols and providing oversights were suspected to have had vested personal interests in the research and were accused of non-declaration of conflict of interest by the public (Tangwa et al. 2018). These accusations led to a total collapse of the Ghana arm for Ebola vaccine trials, which may have provided greater gains toward the future eradication of the virus, if the clinical trials had been successful.

In the light of the outlook of moral residue in global health and considering their applications for science in COVID-19 response, it is imperative to address relevant underlying socio-ethical issues to ensure the effectiveness of scientific innovations. This kind of harmonized approach will provide avenues for greater success in the global search for an effective solution to future pandemic.

Conclusion: Toward a Harmonized Science and Humanities Approach

It may be inconceivable to overcome global health emergencies like Ebola and COVID-19 without the substantive contributions of science in isolating and sequencing viruses, tracing the epidemiological pathways, and developing cures and vaccines. Yet, these scientific achievements remain mute unless they are accepted and/or utilized by human communities across the globe. For instance, it is not sufficient to simply develop a COVID-19 vaccine that is 98% efficacious; the actual effectiveness of the vaccine is ultimately determined by the conviction of populations around the world to accept to be immunized with it. Vaccine hesitancy and anti-vaxxers' beliefs are conceptualized against moral outlooks like human rights and trust that cannot be resolved by science, but which must be addressed for vaccines to even gain marginal success. Specific ethical tools are needed to address these kinds of underlying vaccine issues and achieve success of scientific innovation in tackling global health emergencies.

As a way forward, harmonized science and humanities approaches are needed. These will include context-relevant application of science, building trust and respect, and addressing inequities, among others. Science and its medical advancements are without use if they fail to address specific health conditions around the globe. For instance, during the first wave of COVID-19, lockdowns were recommended globally in the light of the scientific evidence that they would slow and help to eradicate the virus. However, while these measures were largely sustainable in high-income countries (HICs) in Europe, North America, and Austral-Asia, they were barely effective in LMICs like sub-Saharan African countries (Eyawo et al. 2021). A scientifically based lockdown that is informed by the social, economic, and cultural realities of the LMICs would achieve greater benefit for global health.

Likewise, there is a history of medical atrocities, especially in the trials of new drugs, that stalls trust in science and its health benefits for marginalized populations across the globe. These are aspects that cannot simply be wished away by rapid advancements in science and medicine. And new advances in medicine cannot have impact where these historical burdens persist. Humanities approaches like community engagement and addressing moral residue can be used to resolve these burdens and pave a path for the impact of scientific innovations on the health of populations globally.

Finally, various forms and levels of inequities persist across the globe, which scientific advancements in medicine help to perpetuate. The case of the global COVID-19 vaccine distribution is a testament to this effect. For instance, while most HICs have vaccinated most of their eligible populations, LMICs have yet to achieve significant milestones in vaccinating their high-risk populations (Mirza and Rauhala 2021; Ritchie et al. 2021). The key underlying factor is the global inequity in access to the COVID-19 vaccines. COVID-19 may not end until proportionate vaccination rates are achieved in all parts of the globe. Science alone cannot address this problem. Scientific innovations and humanities approaches underpinned by ethical agility and political will can provide a clear pathway out of this and other global health crisis. In short, a harmony of science and humanities measure is a prerequisite for ending global health emergencies.

References

Abutaleb, Yasmeen, and Lena H. Sun. 2021. How CDC Data Problems Put the U.S. Behind on the Delta Variant. *Washington Post*, 19 August 2021. https://www.washingtonpost.com/health/2021/08/18/cdc-data-delay-delta-variant/.

Afolabi, Muhammed O., Morenike Oluwatoyin Folayan, Nchangwi Syntia Munung, Aminu Yakubu, Gibril Ndow, Ayodele Jegede, Jennyfer Ambe, and Francis Kombe. 2021. Lessons from the Ebola Epidemics and Their Applications for COVID-19 Pandemic Response in Sub-Saharan Africa. *Developing World Bioethics* 21 (1): 25–30.

Aggrey, John K., and Wesley Shrum. 2020. Politics and Trust in Ebola Vaccine Trials: The Case of Ghana. *Politics and the Life Sciences* 39 (1): 38–55.

Amore, Stefano, Emanuela Puppo, Josué Melara, Elisa Terracciano, Susanna Gentili, and Giuseppe Liotta. 2021. Impact of COVID-19 on Older Adults and Role of Long-Term Care Facilities during Early Stages of Epidemic in Italy. *Scientific Reports* 11 (1): 12530. https://doi.org/10.1038/s41598-021-91992-9.

APM Research Lab. n.d. Color of Coronavirus: COVID-19 Deaths Analyzed by Race and Ethnicity. APM Research Lab. Accessed 3 September 2021. https://www.apmresearchlab.org/covid/deaths-by-race.

BBC. 2016. Ebola: Mapping the Outbreak. *BBC News*, 14 January 2016, sec. Africa. https://www.bbc.com/news/world-africa-28755033.

———. 2020. Hundreds Gather in Madrid for Anti-Mask Protest. *BBC News*, 16 August 2020. https://www.bbc.com/news/av/world-europe-53802226.

———. 2021. Covax: How Will Covid Vaccines Be Shared around the World? *BBC News*, 3 May 2021, sec. World. https://www.bbc.com/news/world-55795297.

BBC News. 2020. Coronavirus: What India Can Learn from the Deadly 1918 Flu. 18 March 2020, sec. India. https://www.bbc.com/news/world-asia-india-51904019.

Behrmann, Ole, and Martin Spiegel. 2020. COVID-19: From Rapid Genome Sequencing to Fast Decisions. *The Lancet Infectious Diseases* 20 (11): 1218. https://doi.org/10.1016/S1473-3099(20)30580-6.

Benton, Adia, and Kim Yi Dionne. 2015. International Political Economy and the 2014 West African Ebola Outbreak. *African Studies Review* 58 (1): 223–236.

Berkly, Seth. 2020. COVAX Explained. *GAVI: The Vaccine Alliance*. September 2020. https://www.gavi.org/vaccineswork/covax-explained.

Beyrer, Chris, Pascale Allotey, Joseph J. Amon, Stefan D. Baral, Mary T. Bassett, Harriet Deacon, Lorraine T. Dean, Lilianne Fan, Rita Giacaman, and Carolyn Gomes. 2021. Human Rights and Fair Access to COVID-19 Vaccines: The International AIDS Society–Lancet Commission on Health and Human Rights. *The Lancet*.

Billings, Molly. 1997. The 1918 Influenza Pandemic: Responses. Human Virology at Stanford. 1997. https://virus.stanford.edu/uda/fluscimed.html.

Britannica, The Editors of Encyclopaedia. 2021. Humanities. *Encyclopedia Britannica*. 2021. https://www.britannica.com/topic/humanities.

CDC. 2020. Health Equity Considerations and Racial and Ethnic Minority Groups. Centers for Disease Control and Prevention. 11 February 2020. https://www.cdc.gov/coronavirus/2019-ncov/community/health-equity/race-ethnicity.html.

Chandler, Clare, James Fairhead, Ann Kelly, Melissa Leach, Frederick Martineau, Esther Mokuwa, Melissa Parker, Paul Richards, and Annie Wilkinson. 2015. Ebola: Limitations of Correcting Misinformation. *The Lancet* 385 (9975): 1275–1277.

Chhun, Maura. 2021. 1918 Flu Pandemic Killed 12 Million Indians, and British Overlords' Indifference Strengthened the Anti-Colonial Movement. *The Conversation*. http://theconversation.com/1918-flu-pandemic-killed-12-million-indians-and-british-overlords-indifference-strengthened-the-anti-colonial-movement-133605.

Corum, Jonathan, and Carl Zimmer. 2020a. How Moderna's Vaccine Works. *The New York Times*, 5 December 2020, sec. Health. https://www.nytimes.com/interactive/2020a/health/moderna-covid-19-vaccine.html.

———. 2020b. How the Pfizer-BioNTech Vaccine Works. *The New York Times*, 5 December 2020, sec. Health. https://www.nytimes.com/interactive/2020b/health/pfizer-biontech-covid-19-vaccine.html.

Cui, Zhanfeng, Hong Chang, Hui Wang, Boon Lim, Chia-Chen Hsu, Yejiong Yu, Huidong Jia, et al. 2020. Development of a Rapid Test Kit for SARS-CoV-2: An Example of Product Design. *Bio-Design and Manufacturing*, May, 1–4. https://doi.org/10.1007/s42242-020-00075-7.

Dickin, J., Patricia G. Bailey, and Erin James-Abra. 2020. 1918 Spanish Flu in Canada. *The Canadian Encyclopedia*. https://www.thecanadianencyclopedia.ca/en/article/1918-spanish-flu-in-canada?gclid=EAIaIQobChMI6LOosMqc7wIVGjeGCh2mkAdIEAAYASAAEgLoH_D_BwE.

Dror, Amiel A., Netanel Eisenbach, Shahar Taiber, Nicole G. Morozov, Matti Mizrachi, Asaf Zigron, Samer Srouji, and Eyal Sela. 2020. Vaccine Hesitancy: The next Challenge in the Fight against COVID-19. *European Journal of Epidemiology* 35 (8): 775–779.

Eyawo, Oghenowede, A.M. Viens, and Uchechukwu Chidiebere Ugoji. 2021. Lockdowns and Low- and Middle-Income Countries: Building a Feasible, Effective, and Ethical COVID-19 Response Strategy. *Globalization and Health* 17 (1): 13. https://doi.org/10.1186/s12992-021-00662-y.

Folayan, Morenike Oluwatoyin, Aminu Yakubu, Bridget Haire, and Kristin Peterson. 2016. Ebola Vaccine Development Plan: Ethics, Concerns and Proposed Measures. *BMC Medical Ethics* 17 (1): 1–8.

Franco, Elisabetta, Barbara Bagnato, Maria Giulia Marino, Cristina Meleleo, Laura Serino, and Laura Zaratti. 2012. Hepatitis B: Epidemiology and Prevention in Developing Countries. *World Journal of Hepatology* 4 (3): 74.

Guglielmi, Giorgia. 2020. Africa Declared Free from Wild Polio—But Vaccine-Derived Strains Remain. *Nature*, August. https://doi.org/10.1038/d41586-020-02501-3.

History of Vaccines. 2021. Ebola Virus Disease and Ebola Vaccines. *History of Vaccines*. https://www.historyofvaccines.org/content/articles/ebola-virus-disease-and-ebola-vaccines.

Ho, Jessica Y., and Arun S. Hendi. 2018. Recent Trends in Life Expectancy across High Income Countries: Retrospective Observational Study. *BMJ* 362 (August): k2562. https://doi.org/10.1136/bmj.k2562.

Howard, Jeremy, Austin Huang, Zhiyuan Li, Zeynep Tufekci, Vladimir Zdimal, Helene-Mari van der Westhuizen, Arne von Delft, et al. 2021. An Evidence Review of Face Masks against COVID-19. *Proceedings of the National Academy of Sciences* 118 (4): e2014564118. https://doi.org/10.1073/pnas.2014564118.

Kirby, Tony. 2020. Evidence Mounts on the Disproportionate Effect of COVID-19 on Ethnic Minorities. *The Lancet Respiratory Medicine* 8 (6): 547–548. https://doi.org/10.1016/S2213-2600(20)30228-9.

Kombe, Francis, Morenike O. Folayan, Jennyfer Ambe, Adaora Igonoh, and Akin Abayomi. 2016. Taking the Bull by the Horns: Ethical Considerations in the Design and Implementation of an Ebola Virus Therapy Trial. *Social Science & Medicine* 148: 163–170.

Kombe, Francis K., Jennyfer Ambe, and Gibril Ndow. 2019. Scientific Response to Deadly Novel Epidemics: The Role of Health Research Ethics. In *Socio-Cultural Dimensions of Emerging Infectious Diseases in Africa*, 215–228. Springer.

Kummervold, Per Egil, William S. Schulz, Elizabeth Smout, Luis Fernandez-Luque, and Heidi J. Larson. 2017. Controversial Ebola Vaccine Trials in Ghana: A Thematic Analysis of Critiques and Rebuttals in Digital News. *BMC Public Health* 17 (1): 1–24.

Guillou, Ian Le. 2020. Covid-19: How Unprecedented Data Sharing Has Led to Faster-than-Ever Outbreak Research. *The EU Research and Innovation Magazine*. 23 March 2020. https://ec.europa.eu/research-and-innovation/en/horizon-magazine/covid-19-how-unprecedented-data-sharing-has-led-faster-ever-outbreak-research.

Le Marcis, Frédéric, Luisa Enria, Sharon Abramowitz, Almudena-Mari Saez, and Sylvain Landry B. Faye. 2019. Three Acts of Resistance during the 2014–16 West Africa Ebola Epidemic: A Focus on Community Engagement. *Journal of Humanitarian Affairs* 1 (2): 23–31.

Lieber, Dov. 2021. In Israel, Being Fully Vaccinated Now Means Three Shots. *The Wall Street Journal*. 31 August 2021. https://www.wsj.com/articles/in-israel-being-fully-vaccinated-now-means-three-shots-11630426257.

Lock, Helen. 2021. Vaccine Nationalism: Everything You Need to Know. *Global Citizen*. 11 February 2021. https://www.globalcitizen.org/en/content/what-is-vaccine-nationalism/.

MacDonald, Noni E. 2015. Vaccine Hesitancy: Definition, Scope and Determinants. *WHO Recommendations Regarding Vaccine Hesitancy* 33 (34): 4161–4164. https://doi.org/10.1016/j.vaccine.2015.04.036.

Mathieu, Edouard, Hannah Ritchie, Esteban Ortiz-Ospina, Max Roser, Joe Hasell, Cameron Appel, Charlie Giattino, and Lucas Rodés-Guirao. 2021. A Global Database of COVID-19 Vaccinations. *Nature Human Behaviour* 5 (7): 947–953. https://doi.org/10.1038/s41562-021-01122-8.

McAteer, John, Inci Yildirim, and Ann Chahroudi. 2020. The VACCINES Act: Deciphering Vaccine Hesitancy in the Time of COVID-19. *Clinical Infectious Diseases* 71 (15): 703–705.

Menezes, Neia Prata, Muloongo Simuzingili, Zelalem Yilma Debebe, Fedja Pivodic, and Ernest Massiah. 2021. What Is Driving COVID-19 Vaccine Hesitancy in Sub-Saharan Africa? *World Bank Blogs*. 11 August 2021. https://blogs.worldbank.org/africacan/what-driving-covid-19-vaccine-hesitancy-sub-saharan-africa.

Mirza, Atthar, and Emily Rauhala. 2021. Here's Just How Unequal the Global Coronavirus Vaccine Rollout Has Been. *Washington Post*. 22 April 2021. https://www.washingtonpost.com/world/interactive/2021/coronavirus-vaccine-inequality-global/.

Mitman, Gregg. 2014. Ebola in a Stew of Fear. *New England Journal of Medicine* 371 (19): 1763–1765.

Molyneux, Sassy, and P. Wenzel Geissler. 2008. Ethics and the Ethnography of Medical Research in Africa. *Social Science & Medicine* 67 (5): 685–695.

Moon, Suerie, Devi Sridhar, Muhammad A. Pate, Ashish K. Jha, Chelsea Clinton, Sophie Delaunay, Valnora Edwin, Mosoka Fallah, David P. Fidler, and Laurie Garrett. 2015. Will Ebola Change the Game? Ten Essential Reforms before the next Pandemic. The Report of the Harvard-LSHTM Independent Panel on the Global Response to Ebola. *The Lancet* 386 (10009): 2204–2221.

Oxford. 2021. Humanity. Oxford *Advanced Learner's Dictionary*. https://www.oxfordlearnersdictionaries.com/us/definition/english/humanity?q=humanities.

Powers, Madison, and Ruth R. Faden. 2006. *Social Justice: The Moral Foundations of Public Health and Health Policy*. New York: Oxford University Press.

Ritchie, Hannah, Edouard Mathieu, Lucas Rodés-Guirao, Cameron Appel, Charlie Giattino, Esteban Ortiz-Ospina, Joe Hasell, Bobbie Macdonald, Diana Beltekian, and Max Roser. 2021. Coronavirus Pandemic (COVID-19). *Our World in Data*, September. https://ourworldindata.org/covid-deaths.

Roser, Max, and Hannah Ritchie. 2016. Burden of Disease. *Our World in Data*, January. https://ourworldindata.org/burden-of-disease.

Ryan, Molly J., Tamara Giles-Vernick, and Janice E. Graham. 2019. Technologies of Trust in Epidemic Response: Openness, Reflexivity and Accountability during the 2014–2016 Ebola Outbreak in West Africa. *BMJ Global Health* 4 (1): e001272.

Sallam, Malik. 2021. COVID-19 Vaccine Hesitancy Worldwide: A Concise Systematic Review of Vaccine Acceptance Rates. *Vaccines* 9 (2): 160.

Shivaram, Deepa. 2021. The Topic of Masks in Schools is Polarizing Some Parents to the Point of Violence. *NPR*, 20 August 2021, sec. Back to School: Live Updates. https://www.npr.org/sections/back-to-school-live-updates/2021/08/20/1028841279/mask-mandates-school-protests-teachers.

So, Anthony D., and Joshua Woo. 2020. Reserving Coronavirus Disease 2019 Vaccines for Global Access: Cross Sectional Analysis. *BMJ* 371 (December): m4750. https://doi.org/10.1136/bmj.m4750.

Stewart, Emily. 2020. Anti-Maskers Explain Themselves. *Vox*. 7 August 2020. https://www.vox.com/the-goods/2020/8/7/21357400/anti-mask-protest-rallies-donald-trump-covid-19.

Strassburg, Marc A. 1982. The Global Eradication of Smallpox. *American Journal of Infection Control* 10 (2): 53–59. https://doi.org/10.1016/0196-6553(82)90003-7.

Tangwa, Godfrey B., Katharine Browne, and Doris Schroeder. 2018. Ebola Vaccine Trials. In *Ethics Dumping*, 49–60. Cham: Springer.

Taylor, Steven, and Gordon J.G. Asmundson. 2021. Negative Attitudes about Facemasks during the COVID-19 Pandemic: The Dual Importance of Perceived Ineffectiveness and Psychological Reactance. *PLOS ONE* 16 (2): e0246317. https://doi.org/10.1371/journal.pone.0246317.

Ujewe, Samuel J. 2020. Moral Residue and Health Justice for the Global South: Addressing Past Issues through Current Interventions and Research. *Developing World Bioethics* 20 (2): 96–104.

Ujewe, Samuel J., and Alice Mungwa. 2019. Insufficiency of Pathogen Focused Approaches Towards Managing Deadly Epidemics in Africa: Harmonising the Roles of Governments, Health Systems and Populations. In *Socio-Cultural Dimensions of Emerging Infectious Diseases in Africa*, 173–188. Cham: Springer. https://doi.org/10.1007/978-3-030-17474-3_13.

Van Noorden, Richard. 2021. Scientists Call for Fully Open Sharing of Coronavirus Genome Data. *Nature* 590 (7845): 195–196. https://doi.org/10.1038/d41586-021-00305-7.

WHO. 2014. Statement on the 1st Meeting of the IHR Emergency Committee on the 2014 Ebola Outbreak in West Africa. http://www.who.int/mediacentre/news/statements/2014/ebola-20140808/en/.

———. 2020. COVAX: Working for Global Equitable Access to COVID-19 Vaccines. https://www.who.int/initiatives/act-accelerator/covax.

———. 2021a. Timeline: WHO's COVID-19 Response. https://www.who.int/emergencies/diseases/novel-coronavirus-2019/interactive-timeline.

———. 2021b. WHO Coronavirus Disease (COVID-19) Dashboard With Vaccination Data. https://covid19.who.int.

Williamson, Elizabeth J., Alex J. Walker, Krishnan Bhaskaran, Seb Bacon, Chris Bates, Caroline E. Morton, Helen J. Curtis, et al. 2020. Factors Associated with COVID-19-Related Death Using OpenSAFELY. *Nature* 584 (7821): 430–436. https://doi.org/10.1038/s41586-020-2521-4.

Wilner, Michael. 2021. CDC Director Blames COVID Setbacks in Spread of Delta Variant on Unvaccinated People. *McClatchy Washington Bureau*. 30 July 2021. https://www.mcclatchydc.com/news/coronavirus/article253156748.html.

World Bank. 2021. Life Expectancy at Birth, Total for High Income Countries. *FRED, Federal Reserve Bank of St. Louis*. 7 September 2021. https://fred.stlouisfed.org/series/SPDYNLE00INHIC.

Zimmer, Carl, Jonathan Corum, and Sui-Lee Wee. 2020. Coronavirus Vaccine Tracker. *The New York Times*, 10 June 2020, sec. Science. https://www.nytimes.com/interactive/2020/science/coronavirus-vaccine-tracker.html.

5

The Vaccination Mandate Debate Revisited

Peter Aloysius Ikhane

Introductory Remarks

For clarity, the vaccination debate centres on whether, and in what condition, individuals may justifiably exempt themselves (or refuse) to be vaccinated, given that vaccination is a means to prevent, especially, the spread of communicable diseases. With the outbreak of COVID-19 and the rollout of vaccines that was expected to follow (or has followed), the debate has again received some heightened attention. Before taking up a discussion of the debate, beginning with the epistemics of the debate, let me first present a scenario that grounds my eventual analysis of the rationale for which vaccination may be refused.

In April of 2020, a month-plus into the country's lockdown as part of government's measures to curtail the spread of the coronavirus (COVID-19) that was hitting hard in other parts of the world and was speedily finding its way to countries on the African continent, Nigerians

P. A. Ikhane (✉)
Department of Philosophy, University of Ibadan, Ibadan, Nigeria

F. Egbokhare, A. Afolayan (eds.), *Global Health, Humanity and the COVID-19 Pandemic*, https://doi.org/10.1007/978-3-031-17429-2_5

woke up to the troubling news of a proposed bill, "Control of Infectious Disease, 2020", being sponsored by the Speaker of Nigeria's House of Representative. The troubling aspect of the news was that part of the proposed bill contained statements intended to give the Nigerian state the powers to impose determined fines and jail term on any citizen who refuses vaccination that it believed would help in curbing the spread of infectious diseases in the country, including COVID-19, perhaps when the vaccine(s) become available. For a little more emphasis, the bill, which was proposed as a replacement of the "Quarantine Act", sought to impose a penalty of between N200,000 and N5,000,000 as well as a jail term for violators, as against the N500:00 fine that the Quarantine Act imposed. While the Speaker of the House claimed that the proposed bill was intended to develop what is in existence (i.e., the Quarantine Act) towards strengthening the management of Nigeria's public health system, many human rights advocates, as well as some members of the Federal House of Representative itself, questioned the sincerity of the proposed bill, wondering why it was quickly taken through the first and second readings, with no plans for public hearing. Indeed, "[m]any human rights advocates, as well as a member of the Federal House of Representative, … called the bill 'draconian' and if passed, could further stifle human rights freedom in Nigeria" (Olurounbi 2020).

Part of the responses that greeted the state's attempt to pass the bill was the question of whether the state had the prerogative to enact law(s) that would impose vaccination on citizens and punish them if they refused to comply.[1] Nigerians wondered whether the state could so regulate the choices of individuals in such matters as the freedom to choose to be vaccinated or not on the claims that it was its duty to ensure the safety of all in society: "don't people have the right and freedom to determine how their health care should be handled?" they asked. The Nigerian experience of the state's intent to legislate (and impose penalties where

[1] I would like to state here that there are ethical concerns raised by the use of punitive/incarceration measures to address public health issues, such as mandating vaccination. Indeed, several authors have examined some of these ethical concerns related to the use of punitive/incarceration measures to deal with public health problems. The focus of the chapter however is not to turn attention to these; rather, it examines an instance that may legitimately question the state's "right" to act in certain ways, albeit, in the context of the vaccination mandate debate.

necessary) on the vaccination of her citizens, and the citizen's outcry against that intent and its proposed execution, echoes the vaccination debate. It does so by resonating with the claims of the state that it bears the burden of ensuring that individuals are able to achieve their good and, so, can mandate vaccination and the counter-claims of citizens that they each have the right to determine how their health care would be managed.[2]

In the light of the foregoing, the epistemics of the vaccination debate refers to the rationale that is assumed to ground the claims of the state and the counter-claims of citizens. Whereas the rationale of the state's claim relates to the obligation that accrues to it from the "social contract" it entered with the citizen, and which legitimises its government, that of the citizen turns on the rights to freedom of choice. Evident, then, in the Nigerian experience, is the supposition by the state that on the grounds of its obligations to ensure an enabling condition for individuals to achieve their good, it could mandate vaccination. In the same vein, the citizen may be read to have assumed that they have right to determine their choices, rather than being compelled to accept certain choices. This is what has supposedly informed the sort of response that they put up against the state's attempt to so legislate on vaccination. Aside this, the Nigerian experience also reveals grounds on which the rationale of the state intent may be put to question. That is, the basis on which the citizens responded to the state's intent to legislate on compulsory vaccination provides ample reasons for examining the epistemics of the claims of the vaccination debate.

In the literature, however, proponents of these claims have provided more nuanced dimensions to the arguments for and against mandating

[2] The literature on the vaccination debate sometimes classifies vaccines into those that are "medically necessary" and those that are "practically necessary". Vaccines that are "medically necessary" are those that are the only known viable defenses against diseases taking hold in a community, while those that are "practically necessary" are those to which there are alternatives, but which alternatives are, in practice, not used by a significant number of people. I am more interested in vaccines that are "medically necessary".

vaccination than I have presented here. In broad terms, supporters[3] of the view that the state can mandate vaccination in certain instances such as with COVID-19 argue that since empirical observations have shown that as more and more individuals are allowed to refuse the vaccination by choosing what they suppose is in their individual interests, there is the likelihood that the collective public health will weaken as herd or community immunity diminishes. Thus, they argue further, the rational thing to do is, at least, to get a higher percentage of the population vaccinated. To this end, the state may be described as acting according to what Garrett Hardin refers to as the "tragedy of the commons", by employing various legal measures to mandate individuals to be vaccinated.

Counter-arguments in support of citizens' freedom of choice to accept vaccination or otherwise insist that the individual's right to self-determination provides sufficient grounds for citizens to refrain from vaccination.[4] The proponents ground their argument for individual self-determination on the science of vaccination,[5] which has shown that vaccination does not work in similar ways for everyone. There are, indeed, pertinent questions regarding the efficiency and efficacy of vaccines and their use in minimising and eliminating the spread of infectious diseases.[6] Supporters of this view also raise issues relating to bodily deformation,

---

[3] Proponents of this view provide argument in defense of different extent to which such mandate that be enforced. Roland Pierik (2018), for instance, provides an unqualified defense, while Jessica Flanigan (2014) and Alberto Giubilini (2020) provide qualified or limited defense for mandating vaccination.

[4] For extensive discussions of this, see Leask et al. (2010); Moran et al. (2006); Omer et al. (2009); Wolfe and Sharp (2002).

[5] I take the science of vaccination to concern the systematic research and knowledge that goes into the production of vaccines as well as its use in eliminating infectious diseases. This science grew from inoculation, which was the initial method of immunization that involved the use of smallpox material transferred from the arm of an infected sick person to that of a healthy person to induce a milder form of the illness. Much of the initial challenges with vaccination were associated with inoculation which investigations showed inadvertently contributed to the spread of smallpox and other bloodborne diseases. My comments here are drawn from a reading of the science of the history vaccination as a means to prevent the spread of communicable diseases. See, for instance, Colgrove (2005: 168).

[6] It is pertinent to however note that since the beginning of the use of vaccination, rather than inoculation, in the nineteenth century, the science has grown, reducing the occurrence of the risks of other contagions that were associated with it at its inception. This has been found to be particularly the case since "the use of vaccine made from glycerinated calf's lymph began to replace arm-to-arm transfer of disease material in the 1860s …"

such as swollen and abscessed arm, arising from vaccination (Colgrove 2005: 168; Malone and Hinman 2007).

In the Nigerian experience, however, there is a twist that necessitates and drives my concerns with the debate. This may be aptly described as the challenge of political distrust in relation to gaps in health information-sharing on the part of the state. An instance of this may be seen in the events that led to the altercation between the US/EU and Chinese governments regarding the failure of the Chinese government to send timely warning to the global community, perhaps through the WHO, regarding the infectious rate of the COVID-19 (Colgrove 2005).[7] It is indeed the handling of vital information at the early beginnings of the COVID-19, particularly in China, that has generated many uncertainties. For example, a research carried out by the PEW Research Centre reveals that two-thirds of Americans (64%) say that China has done a bad job dealing with the coronavirus outbreak. Around three-quarters (78%) place a fair amount of the blame for the global spread of the coronavirus on the Chinese government's initial handling of the COVID-19 outbreak in Wuhan (Silver et al. 2020). Furthermore, Beijing's reluctance to agree to an independent inquiry, after many months of negotiations for the WHO to have access to the city, also created room for political distrust. The point here is that the manner in which governments across the world have handled information and information-sharing regarding COVID-19 has left many, both in the more and less developed worlds, questioning the sincerity of governments to ensure their good.

In brief, political distrust describes the condition of the lack or absence of citizens' confidence in government regarding its sincerity to ensure their good; it may be empirically determined by taking the ratio of citizens' evaluation of government performance in relation to their expectations of how government ought to perform (Hetherington 1998; Hetherington and Husser 2012). In relation to this and the context of the

[7] An interesting reporting that looks back at how the Chinese government tried to silence social media report of the outbreak of a deadly SARs-like virus done by BBC's Kerry Allen and Zhaoyin Feng may be read here: https://www.bbc.com/news/world-asia-china-55355401. They report of how the country's government censors worked harder than ever to suppress negative online information and how the citizens managed to break through the Great Firewall.

paper, political distrust relates to citizens' misgivings that government has its best interest in mandating vaccination.

From the foregoing, the fundamental concern that I examine in the chapter is whether the state, given its duty to ensure and bring about the conditions to enable individuals achieve their good in the society, *still* holds the right to mandate vaccination in the context of the challenge of political distrust? It is obvious, here, that I have assumed the following: (1) that the state holds a certain right to mandate vaccination and (2) that such right may be put to question on, say, the basis of the condition I allude to in the second part of the paper. I take (1) to be my argument for the government's default position regarding the vaccination debate and (2) to be a limitation to what I present in (1), and, hence, the reason for my examining the debate.[8]

In the default condition, I suppose that there is sufficient empirical record about the efficacy of vaccination, such as records about increase in herd immunity and evidence of the eradication of disease, as recently demonstrated with the case of polio in Nigeria and Africa.[9] The default position also assumes the absence of any significant situations that may result in political distrust, such as gaps in information-sharing. With respect to (2), I draw on the notion of political distrust as regards information-sharing *in the time of a health pandemic*. I intend, in this regard, to examine the terms of the vaccination debate not by essentially questioning the science of vaccination but showing that information asymmetry, between the state and the citizen that results from the state's preferences, provides persuasive grounds that challenge the state's legitimate use of law to enforce vaccination.[10] In addressing my focus in the first section of the chapter, I will elaborate on the epistemics of the vaccination debate. This is to enable me to identify what I take to be the default position. On the assumption that I succeed with showing that in

---

[8] My response to (1) can be read as a reiteration of the 1905 US Supreme Court decision that established the constitutionality of state compulsory vaccination laws when such laws are considered necessary for the public health and safety. See Walloch (2015): 187–214. Suffolk Woodbridge (2008): 1820–1841. https://doi.org/10.7722/j.ctt18kr6pf.15.

[9] Nigeria was recently declared polio-free; as the last country in Africa to be so declared, the entire continent was declared free of wide polio. This is a feat that is attributable to vaccination.

[10] I do not so much as question the science of vaccination because it is obvious that it has developed much as compared to its early beginnings before the use of glycerinated calf's lymph.

the default condition, the state has the obligation to ensure the safety and wellbeing of all in society, and, hence, that it holds the prerogative to mandate vaccination, I however argue that the exercise of such prerogative may be limited by the condition necessitated by political distrust.

The Vaccination Mandate Debate

In the vaccination debate, two strongly opposed camps may be identified, with a third camp taking a rather moderate position. For clarity, let us refer to those who support the view that government has the right to enforce vaccination as "vaccination advocates (VAs)", those who aver that individuals enjoy the right to self-determination in such matters and may decide to opt against vaccination as "individual rights advocates" (IRAs) and the group of theorists who take a moderate position as "moderationists of vaccination" (MOVs). Following from this, the contending claims of the debate may be stated thus: while VAs assert that vaccination represents the more sustainable answer to curbing the impact or spread of infectious diseases, and so push for making vaccination mandatory, IRAs argue that vaccination need not be made mandatory as this goes too far to intrude on individual's right to self-determination.

In support for their position, VAs see vaccines and vaccinations as public good. A testament to this is the declaration by the Centres for Disease Control and Prevention (CDC) in the United States that vaccines are one of the ten great public health achievements of the twentieth century (Malone and Hinman 2007: 338). On the contrary, the IRAs suppose that in peculiar situations, experience shows that the use of vaccination can have various side effects that may affect the wellbeing of individuals, leading them to conclude that this may result in the invasion of the capacity of individuals to the pursuit of their life's goals.[11] The MOVs, for their part, canvas for some form of exemption that allows individuals to stay away from vaccination. They however propose that such exemptions,

[11] For an extended reading on the debate, see Cole and Swendiman (2014) and Malone and Hinman (2007): 262–284.

which are to be a form of government's regulation, may be made difficult to get through government's legislation.

Furthermore, the conflict between the claims of the IRAs and VAs, which has been well documented in the literature, may be illustrated with, say, the work of Garrett Hardin. In "The Tragedy of the Commons," Hardin makes analogous allusion to the decrease in the community's interest in maximising food production in a common cattle pasture because each individual member of the community is allowed, without restrictions or measures of control, to continue to pursue their own individual interests for more benefits by adding additional numbers of cattle to an already saturated common cattle pasture. Hardin notes that when such is permitted to go on, the consequence of an inevitable ruin of the common pasture for cattle grazing is similar to the herd or community immunity that vaccination is meant to procure, unless some measures are put in place to ensure individuals get vaccination as against permitting the pursuit of individual interests. Indeed, VAs claim that "a community free of an infectious disease because of a high vaccination rate can be viewed as a common" (Malone and Hinman 2007: 339).

From the foregoing, the terms of the vaccination debate, in relation to the issue at stake, may be normatively stated thus: which ought to have prior status between the pursuit of the conditions for individuals to attain their good in society through vaccination that ensures herd immunity, on the one hand, and the assertion of individual autonomy given the uncertainties associated with the science of vaccination, on the other? The terms of the debate, so understood, generate some dilemma in choice-making regarding mandating vaccination or whether the choice to make such mandate violates the rights of individuals. Malone and Hinman aptly capture this seeming impasse:

> As disease rates drop, the risks associated with the vaccine come even more to the fore, providing further incentive to avoid immunization. Thus, when an individual … chooses to go unimmunized, it only minimally increases the risk of illness for that individual, while conferring on that person the benefit of avoiding the risk of vaccine-induced side effects. At the same time, however, this action weakens the herd effect protection for the entire community. As more and more individuals choose to do what is in the

> 'best' individual interest, the common eventually fails as herd immunity disappears and disease outbreak occurs. To avoid this 'tragedy of the commons', legal requirements have been imposed by communities (in recent times, by states) to mandate particular vaccinations. (Malone and Hinman 2007: 339)

The dilemma alluded in the statement above may be illustrated in this way: suppose that someone, x, leaves in a community, C, and x alone remains unvaccinated for a certain infectious disease. The argument of IRAs is that if x has decided to stay away from being vaccinated on the grounds of personal choice or exercise of individual' right to self-determination, it would amount to an infringement on x's personal preferences to force or legally bound x to get vaccination on the argument of the pursuit of either the common or collective good of all in C by providing the enabling conditions for individuals to attain their good, since the herd immunity of C, which is part of the collective good in this instance, is high and it is only x who is left unvaccinated. Even if it is supposed further that if an infectious disease finds its way into C, and because x is unvaccinated, x is prone to be infected, a situation that may affect the herd immunity of C, IRAs could still respond that x's choice against vaccination does not put to jeopardy C's herd immunity. Part of statement quoted from Malone and Hinman that "when an individual … chooses to go unimmunized, it only minimally increases the risk of illness for that individual, while conferring on that person the benefit of avoiding the risk of vaccine-induced side effects" further shows that when the herd immunity is high, individuals may justifiably pursue their interests in choosing to stay away from vaccination on the grounds that it has been shown that the risk of vaccination is significantly high. And if such persons can be exempted, what is the warrant to mandate individuals, particularly when the herd immunity is high and when there is the risk of side effect?[12]

---

[12] I express many thanks to the reviewer and the editors who drew my attention to the implication of my argument here. It was noted that my claim here is cogent because I am arguing with regard to just one individual. What happens if there are more than an individual, say a million, who refuse to refuse to be vaccinated? Does the size of the unvaccinated change the terms of the debate? My response to this is that if the size of the numbers refusing to be vaccinated threatens the herd immunity, it will very well affect the debate as drawn from the statement of Malone and Hinman.

But the question that remains unanswered concerns how the high levels of the herd immunity are to be attained if individuals are not made to see the benefits of vaccination and sometimes compelled to be vaccinated, when the need arises. If, on a different approach, we assume that there are other members of C that are not able to get vaccination for one health condition or another, in reply to the earlier assertions of IRAs, VAs may argue that x's choice to remain unvaccinated puts the health of these others in danger and, so, affects the herd immunity of C. And because the latter condition of there being individuals that are not able to get vaccination and so be immune to particular infectious diseases is the more apt description of most human communities, VAs argue that there is the need for legal regulation to enforce vaccination, if the need arises.

Whereas my submission with respect to the debate as examined so far aligns with the claims of VAs, my argument is nuanced by what I refer to as the default condition. In this vein, my submission is that barring any condition created by government that may have consequences for achieving its obligation to ensure the common or collective good of all in society, the government or state retains the right to enforce vaccination, if the need arises. This is because I take the state's right that derives from its obligation to procure the collective good of all in society to be grounded on the "social contract" that exists between the state and the citizen. My assertion here is that if the state has not created the grounds for individuals to raise questions about the sincerity of its pursuit of the collective good of all, there are no justifiable bases on which individuals can place premium on the exercise of their individual rights to stay away from vaccination, if there are no medical grounds for doing so. In the light of this, and as long as the "minimal terms" of the contract are in place, the state retains the right to pursue the attainment of the collective good of all in society.[13] As an extension of the ground for my submission, I take the sort of "social contract" between the state and the citizen to be aptly denoted

[13] I assume here an ideal rendition of the "social contract", without paying much attention to the situation of realpolitiking, which calls into focus how the social contract has always been circumvented by racial and sexist underpinning. Works such as *The Racial Contract* by Charles W. Mills and *The Sexual Contract* by Carole Pateman are key in this regard. My reason for this is to be able to identify what may be taken as the minimal requirement of the state in being part of that contract, which is essential for my analysis in the chapter.

by the notion of commutative justice. As a matter of commutative justice, which is "understood as the principle to give each person that to which he or she is entitled" (Koslowski 2001), I take the state's right as grounded on reciprocal plus-sum relation with citizens that entitles it, as a "just due", to mandate vaccination as a duty on the part of citizens towards ensuring the safety of society. In this sense of the state's right, I refer to this as the "entitlement sense" of right, as it places emphasis on the state's moral faculty to exact its "just dues" from citizens. In this sense of entitlement, "just dues" imply that right is a proper object of justice; and as such, if someone has the right to exact certain just dues, someone else has the "duty" to render such just dues (Bittle 1950: 274–275).

Revisiting the Vaccination Mandate Debate

My revisiting the vaccination mandate debate turns on the epistemics of the debate with particular attention on the condition I provided as grounds for why the right to mandate vaccination held by the state, in relation to fulfilling its duty/obligation of ensuring the wellbeing of all in society, may be questioned. For clarity, I argued in the preceding section of this chapter that in the debate between VAs and IRAs, the state enjoyed the prerogative to enforce the vaccination of individuals, barring the presence of any condition resulting from the state's activities that necessitates political distrust. As such, my analysis, in what I referred to as the default situation, is that the state possesses such right and can compel, by legislation, its citizens to present themselves for vaccination.[14] But when state action genuinely warrants or generates grounds to politically distrust the state's intent to bring about the collective good of its citizens, the state's retainership of such right can be put to question.

Let me explicate what I mean by "genuinely warrant". There are recorded instances where the state's actions have not aligned with its stated goal to actualise the good of all in society. In instances as these, a

[14] My claim here is made even with the awareness that vaccination may result in adverse side effects for some individuals. The medicine of vaccination realises and provides for the exemption of persons in certain conditions. Moreover, in making this supposition, I take it that it is enough to have a higher percentage of the populace vaccinated to achieve herd immunity.

case for the state's action genuinely warranting individuals or citizens to doubt or distrust the intents of the state can be made. A case that can be made here refers to the political distrust resulting from the state's failure—as seen with the attempt to pass the "Control of Infectious Disease, 2020" bill without provision for public hearing—in information-sharing, particularly in relation to matters of health care. The failure of the Nigerian state, in this regard, supervenes on the nature of the workings of the state and government in postcolonial Nigeria. To be sure, the workings of the state are inflected by its postcolonial and modern realities, which include biting poverty, an unrelenting neo-colonialism, high levels of illiteracy, a nascent democracy and a clipping occurrence of fraud.[15] These realities also include the tensions of modernity and development, mismanagement and corruption, political apathy, violence and ethnic and religious rivalries (Falola 2021). These realities coupled with how they inflect on the state's action circumscribe the understanding of rights or commutative justice between the state and the people. And in the light of these, serious questions have been raised regarding the moral limits of the state's power in various contexts. This can be seen in the case, stated above, of the attempt of the legislative arm of the state to pass a bill criminalising refusal of vaccination without consideration for the extent of consultations it has to engage in before such is done. Particularly worrisome is that this was a time where there were no vaccines that had been found for COVID-19, and people were refusing to take the vaccines, hence, the need for such hurried passage of the bill. Of immediate concern to my analysis, however, is the state's mismanagement of information regarding COVID-19. Rather than concerning itself with addressing and dousing the fears and worry emanating from the many conflicting and discouraging information going around, particularly on the Internet regarding the emergence and spread of the virus, the state bothered itself with hurriedly passing a bill that criminalises refusal of a vaccine/vaccines that was/were yet to see the light of day.

[15] Authors such as Peter P. Ekeh (1975): 91–112; Achille Mbembe (2001); Adeshina Afolayan (2012). Ekeh, for instance, argues that the experiences of colonialism in Africa have led to the emergence of a unique historical configuration in colonial Africa: the existence of two publics instead of one public, as in the West. He further asserts that many of Africa's political problems are due to relationships between the two publics.

To push my case here, let me state that information is a public good.[16] As a public good, information is a social commodity and cannot be taken simply as a private property; this indicates how it is to be handled. That information is a social commodity is seen in the way people seek it as means to achieve some overall or ultimate good for their lives. In the light of this, it could be asserted that in the way our social condition inflects our private world, information is at the centre of this. As a public good, information can lift the collective life of a community. And as information is a public good, it can be viewed a right; and, in my consideration of information-sharing, this is where I suppose it derives its being a right for individuals as citizens of a state. In relating citizens' right to the right or correct information, reference cannot but be made to the duties or obligation of the state to provide the same, in the context of our consideration of the information. That is, as we make reference to the rights of individuals, in this regard, we equally make allusion to the duty of the state to ensure the same. It is, indeed, the balance of rights (whether of the state or of individuals), on the one hand, and duties (again, of the state or individuals), on the other, that results in justice in the commutative sense.

Every right in one person involves a corresponding duty in others to respect this right and not to violate it. And as rights are meant to achieve certain ends in society, the purpose of rights is the establishment and maintenance of social order among humans. In this vein, rights and duties are understood to always go together as a consequence of the law's attempt to institute justice in society. That is, citizens have the right to be provided with the "right" information. The "right" information is to be viewed not as just the correct information—which is a key defining feature of the right information—but also the timely information. To put it simply, the right information is the correct information that is timely. Citizens have a right to this, more so "in the time of a health pandemic".

For me, "in the time of a health pandemic" signifies the time when the most significant value is life, that is, the value of being alive. In such time, other values such as economic gains, political advancement and even

[16] Information, which may be taken as a cognate concept of knowledge, meets the requirements of what public goods are. See Razzolini (2003): 782–784.

educational growth become, in economic terms, the opportunity costs or forgone alternatives to the value of keeping alive. But in the time of the current health pandemic of COVID-19, the state (not only in Nigeria but in the global space) seems to have failed in this realisation, a failure that necessitated political distrust. Indeed, a characterisation of how the state has handled information and information-sharing with its citizens in the times of the current health pandemic can be likened to protectionist attitudes in trade; states in the comity of nations in the global space have been protectionists about information and information-sharing, such that information that is a supposed public good became a political tool to gain certain state advantages. It is in the light of this that I argue that the state's right to legislate on mandating vaccination, like it intended to do in Nigeria, can be put to question and shown not to meet the demands of commutative justice. Indeed, my argument in the preceding section that the state's right derives from commutative justice, which itself is a reflection of the "social contract" between the state and the citizens, comes to play in support of individuals affirming the pursuit of their interests when there is a genuine warrant that the state has failed to do so.

In concluding this section of the chapter, let me address myself to some possible rejoinders to the argument I have made in the section. To begin, from my argument that political distrust arising from gaps in information-sharing provides some ground on which the state's prerogative to enforce vaccination, if the need arises, may be questioned, it would seem that I have inadvertently canvassed for the exercise of the rights to self-determination by individuals who may choose to refrain from vaccination when such situations arise. This is, perhaps, on the suggestion that as the major contending camps in the debate are VAs and IRAs, it would seem implied that when the argument in favour of VAs is flawed, then the position of IRAs prevails. And since I have provided grounds for why the claims of VAs may not be sustained, then I have equally provided evidence that make the claims of IRAs plausible. While this is a possible reading of my argument, I suppose that the inference—from my argument to the assumption that the position of IRAs prevails—is not a necessary one. That is, I do not take my argument to necessitate the position that when the claims of VAs are shown to be defective, then the opposite claim of IRAs becomes credible.

For one, the issue at core of this debate is not "white or black", that when one position in the debate is rejected, the other side is unintentionally accepted; there are other possible outcomes that may be arrived at when one side of the major contending position is shown to be inconsistent. Also, I take herd or community immunity to be some public good that ought to be striven for; and if the exercise of individual rights in choosing to refrain from vaccination would put this to jeopardy, then the exercise of such rights should be regulated. Indeed, in relation to my analysis, a possible outcome is that in showing that there are possible limitations to the state's entitlement to enforce vaccination in instances like when the state's actions lead to the emergence of political distrust, I have also indicated that the state not only has the obligation to ensure the enabling conditions for individuals to attain their good of all in society—an obligation from which its prerogative to enforce vaccination derives—it also has the added obligation "to show" that it is pursuing the good of all in society. What the state may therefore do when such scenario of political distrust poses challenges for the exercise of its right is to seek ways to redress the events that may have resulted in the emergence of such political distrust.

But the question may however be raised regarding how to determine when the state is no longer in the pursuit of the collective good. Put differently, it may be asked how to determine if government's intentions are sincere: that is, when the government is not just deceiving, but withholding relevant information. This is because (political) sincerity "is perfectly compatible with people keeping secrets, withholding information, or more broadly, being entitle to privacy" (Loriaux 2017: 1). Though, addressing this would stretch the essay beyond its focus, in brief, it may be significant to state that experts in the field employ such methods as thematic content analysis (TCA). This method develops from the knowledge of how easy speech may be manipulated and, hence, the need to device a truth detector. It "consists of a fairly large—and expandable—number of coding systems for analysing nonobvious aspects of verbal behaviour. TCA coding systems do not rely on analysing manifest content; they look at underlying characteristics that are less easy to manipulate, as least until politician becomes familiar with the system" (Suedfeld et al. 2007: 60). Along with this, it suffices to say here that the possibility of political distrust, which is different from how it may be determined, provides enough grounds for the analysis that has been done in the essay. Moreover, political distrust extends beyond just the withholding of information; there is, at least, the added question of the intent behind withholding information. As regards the concern of the essay, my reference to gaps in information-sharing alludes to, among others, government's withholding of vital information that should bring about the collective good of all.

Concluding Remarks

My analysis has followed a path from first defending the state's obligation to ensure the collective good of all in society as a right that permits it to, if the need arises, mandate vaccination so as to curb the spread of infectious diseases, to showing that such right may however be limited on certain grounds. The ground indicated in the chapter, however, concerns the state's action about health relating to the use of vaccination, which has resulted in some doubts about the state's sincerity in the pursuit of the collective good. In the former instance, the question was whether the government had the right bequeathed to it by its duty to ensure the good of society to legislate in such matters that bother on individuals being vaccinated; and in the latter instance, the question was whether the state, as a result of its duty to ensure and bring about the collective good of all in society, still holds the right to mandate its citizen to be vaccinated even in the context of the challenge of political distrust. My analysis was driven by the assumption that government has the duty (hence, right) to ensure the collective good. This is for the sake of the good of all. This is even more so in the time of a health pandemic, when government is expected to ensure the safety and wellbeing of all its citizens. In this case, it is tenable to argue that government's duty holds prior to individual rights to self-determination. But when there is inkling that the state is no longer after the pursuit of the common or collective good, such right of the state may be questioned.

What I did in the first section of the essay then was to uphold the position that in the vaccination debate between supporters of the state's use of some legal means to enforce vaccination and advocates of the exercise of individual rights in choosing to refrain from vaccination, the former's claims take priority over that of the latter on the grounds that the "social contract" that exists between the state and citizens, which in turn gives the state the obligation to ensure the collective good of all in society, privileges the state with the right to enforce vaccination when the need arises if this becomes a means to achieve the collective good in this instance. Again, I referred to the right of the state in this regard as deriving from commutative justice that allows the state to mandate vaccination as a reciprocal response on the part of individuals in guaranteeing that it is able to ensure the collective good of all in society. In brief, my argument included (1) the state's duty to ensure and bring about the collective good of all in society; (2) from (1) the state's right to mandate its citizens to be vaccinated; and (3) from (2) the citizen's corresponding duty, over their right to self-determination, not to reject vaccination. In the second section of this chapter, I drew on the notion of commutative justice (earlier employed to defend the state's right) that emphasises reciprocal and equitable exchange among entities to show that the condition generated by political distrust in relation to health information-sharing is a limiting one for the state's exercise of its prerogative to mandate vaccination, which itself derives from its obligation to ensure the collective good of society. The claim here is that when the state fails in its duty to citizens, it relinquishes whatever prerogative it has in such contexts.

References

Afolayan, Adeshina. 2012. Postcolonialism and the Two Publics in Nigeria: Rethinking the Idea of the Sceptical Public. *Ogirisi: A New Journal of African Studies* 9: 44–68. https://doi.org/10.4314/og.v9i1.2.

Bittle, C.N. 1950. *Man and Morals: Ethics*. Milwaukee: The Bruce Publishing Company.

Cole, J.P., and K. Swendiman. 2014. Mandatory Vaccinations: Precedent and Current Laws. *Congressional Research Service Report*. Congressional Research

Service: 1–14. Accessed 2 April 2021. https://fas.org/sgp/crs/misc/RS21414.pdf.

Colgrove, J. 2005. Science in a Democracy: The Contested Status of Vaccination in the Progressive Era and the 1920s. *Isis* 96 (2): 167–191.

Ekeh, Peter. 1975. Colonialism and the Two Publics in Africa: A Theoretical Statement. *Comparative Studies in Society and History* 17 (1): 91–112.

Falola, Toyin. 2021. *Understanding Modern Nigeria: Ethnicity, Democracy, and Development*. Cambridge: Cambridge University Press.

Flanigan, J. 2014. A defense of compulsory vaccination. *HEC Forum* 26: 5–25.

Giubilini, A. 2020. An argument for compulsory vaccination: the taxation analogy. *Journal of Applied Philosophy* 37 (3): 446–466.

Hetherington, M.J. 1998. The Political Relevance of Political Trust. *The American Political Science Review* 92 (4): 791–808.

Hetherington, M.J., and J.A. Husser. 2012. How Trust Matters: The Changing Political Relevance of Political Trust. *American Journal of Political Science* 56 (2): 312–325.

Koslowski, P. 2001. Commutative Justice. In *Principles of Ethical Economy*, 184–210. Dordrecht: Springer. Accessed 14 May 2021. https://doi.org/10.1007/978-94-010-0956-0_9.

Leask, J., S. Chapman, and S.C.C. Robbins. 2010. 'All Manner of Ills': The Features of Serious Diseases Attributed to Vaccination. *Vaccine* 28: 3066–3070.

Loriaux, S. 2017. Introduction. In *Sincerity in Politics and International Relations*, ed. S. Baiasu and S. Loriaux. London: Routledge.

Malone, K.M., and A.R. Hinman. 2007. Vaccination Mandates: The Public Health Imperatives and Individual Rights. In *Law in Public Health Practice*, ed. Richard A. Goodman, Mark A. Rothstein, Richard E. Hoffman, Wilfredo Lopez, Gene W. Matthews, and Karen L. Foster, 338–360. New York: Oxford University Press.

Mbembe, Achille. 2001. *On the Postcolony*. Berkeley: University of California Press.

Moran, N.E., et al. 2006. Are Compulsory Immunisation and Incentives to Immunise Effective Ways to Achieve Herd Immunity in Europe? In *Ethics and Infectious Disease*, ed. M. Selgelid, M. Battin, and C. Smith, 115–131. Malden, MA: Blackwell.

Olurounbi, R. 2020. Coronavirus: Nigeria's Proposed COVID-19 Law Tears the Country Apart. Accessed 2 March 2021. https://www.theafricareport.com/27969/coronavirus-nigerias proposed-covid-19-law-tears-the-country-apart/.

Omer, S.B., et al. 2009. Vaccine Refusal, Mandatory Immunisation, and the Risks of Vaccine Preventable Diseases. *New England Journal of Medicine* 360 (19): 1981–1988.
Pierik, R. 2018. Mandatory vaccination: An unqualified defense. *Journal of Applied Philosophy* 35 (2): 381–398.
Razzolini, L. 2003. Public Goods. In *The Encyclopedia of Public Choice*, 782–784. https://doi.org/10.1007/978-0-306-47828-4_166. Accessed 3 March 2021. https://www.researchgate.net/publication/226579607_Public_Goods.
Silver, L., K. Delvin, and C. Huang. 2020. Americans Fault China for Its Role in the Spread of COVID-19. *Global Attitudes & Trends*: 1–12. Accessed 13 April 2021. https://www.pewresearch.org/global/2020/07/30/americans-fault-china-for-its-role-in-the-spread-of-covid-19/
Suedfeld, P., P.E. Tetlock, and R. Jhangiani. 2007. Assessing the Sincerity of Politicians: The Case of President George W. Bush. *Psicologia Politica*, no. 35.
Walloch, K. 2015. Jacobson v. Massachusetts. *In the Antivaccine Heresy: Jacobson v. Massachusetts and the Troubled History of Compulsory Vaccination in the United States*. Rochester, NY: 187–214.
Wolfe, R.M., and L.K. Sharp. 2002. Anti-vaccinationists Past and Present. *BMJ* 325 (7361): 430–432.
Woodbridge, S. 2008. Toward a Twenty-First-Century Jacobson v. Massachusetts. *Harvard Law Review* 121 (7): 1820–1841. https://doi.org/10.7722/j.ctt18kr6pf.15.

Part II

Critical Framing of the Pandemic in Africa

6

An African Perspective on the Ethics and Politics of Foreign Medical Aid in a Pandemic

Adeolu Oluwaseyi Oyekan
and Ademola Kazeem Fayemi

Introduction

Early in January 2020, the world became aware of the spread of COVID SARS 2, a strain of coronavirus, in the Chinese city of Wuhan. About two months later, not only had it became obvious that the virus was contagious, but the spread had also gone across the world enough for the World Health Organization (WHO) to declare it a pandemic (WHO 2020). While the figures of infection and mortality resulting from COVID-19 virus have continued to rise across the world, amid second, third waves and beyond, several topical issues have already arisen and are emerging that warrant scholarly considerations.

A. O. Oyekan (✉)
Identities and Social Cohesion in Africa (ISCIA), Nelson Mandela University, Port Elizabeth, South Africa

A. K. Fayemi
Institute of African and Diaspora Studies, University of Lagos, Lagos, Nigeria
e-mail: kfayemi@unilag.edu.ng

F. Egbokhare, A. Afolayan (eds.), *Global Health, Humanity and the COVID-19 Pandemic*, https://doi.org/10.1007/978-3-031-17429-2_6

One of the fundamental issues that has arisen is how China conducted itself in terms of handling the outbreak. There are so many reasons to believe that the Chinese government made efforts to suppress information about the outbreak of the virus, including the arrest of a doctor who first made its contagious nature public. The doctor himself eventually became infected and died of the virus (Hegarty 2020). The opacity of the Chinese government, it is believed in many quarters, made it difficult for the rest of the world to at least prepare effectively for the mitigation of the virus as it eventually became a pandemic.

It is within this context that one must situate the subsequent actions of the Chinese government and the reactions it has elicited across the world. While China has deployed enormous human resources around the globe in terms of healthcare workers, as well as medical materials such as masks, ventilators, and personal protective equipment (PPE), in what can be partly described as pandemic philanthropy, the gesture has been received with mixed feelings. In Nigeria, where there is a notable shortage of test kits and other resources, there has been a vehement opposition to the efforts of government to leverage on Chinese expertise and generosity in combating the epidemic (Ayitogo 2020; Shaban 2020). For instance, reputable professional bodies such as the Nigeria Medical Association (NMA), National Association of Resident Doctors (NARD), and the Nigerian Union of Journalists (NUJ) were at the vanguard of a campaign that led to the drastic scaling down of the level of intervention contemplated in government circles (see NARD Press Release 2020; NMA Press Release 2020).

This development, no doubt, generated issues that are of political and ethical interests. Questions have been raised, for instance, on whether China ought to be trusted to provide medical assistance when the extent of its cover-up of the virus remains unknown. There are also questions on whether China is using pandemic philanthropy to buy leverage as a superpower to vitiate efforts holding it accountable for the negligence and concealment that have resulted today in the deaths of thousands of COVID-19 victims across the world. One question that is of more interest to this chapter is: Was Nigeria right to accept foreign medical aid from China?

In a bid to register its displeasure with China on the one hand and assert its sovereignty on the other, ought Nigerian government reject or accept medical philanthropy from China? A moral conundrum ensues here—choosing between accepting foreign medical aid from China to bridge to some degree the shortage in the resources needed to contain and manage the virus, when such will likely save lives in Nigeria, and opting for a rejection of pandemic philanthropy from China despite being needed for the timely and efficient management of the public health crises posed by COVID-19 in Nigeria. In other words, should the overriding desire for accountability take precedence over accessing the kind of assistance needed in the immediate, even when the same is likely to whittle down the capacity to demand accountability from China and deter future re-occurrence? To what extent does China's pandemic philanthropy extenuate its culpability as a nation whose avoidable choices have led to the spread of the pandemic and its consequences? Under what moral considerations can assistance be accessed without compromising the needed latitude to demand accountability from an erring superpower? These questions are fundamental to a better understanding of the ethics and politics of foreign medical aid in a pandemic.

This chapter provides a fundamental evaluation of the ethics and politics of foreign medical aid in COVID-19 management in Nigeria using insights from the principles of African ethic of communion. The choice of this framework is informed by the dearth of literature evaluating pandemic philanthropy in general from an African ethical perspective and in particular an absence of literature on the African ethical values relevant to evaluating the act and politics of foreign medical aid from China to Nigeria in the wake of COVID-19. This chapter fills this gap as it considers important understanding, from an African perspective, the values both at play and absent in choosing foreign medics as a complementary strategy in tackling the challenges of COVID-19 in Nigeria.

The chapter is organized into five sections. The first section briefly traces the historical evolution of the outbreak of the virus in China, and the spread across the world, to such a point that it became a pandemic. The second section is an overview of Nigeria's healthcare system in relation to its level of preparedness for managing a health crisis of the present magnitude. The third section examines the nature of Chinese medical philanthropy. Section four is an exploration of an African moral theory and an application of its principles of relationality, equity, and harmony to the act of COVID-19 foreign medical aid from China to Nigeria. The core position defended in this section is that while the values of transparency, trust, relationality, consultation, dialogues, and harmony are lacking in the decision-making process that brought the Chinese foreign medics' aid to Nigeria, the act in itself is morally justified. This chapter contends that a viable ethics of pandemic philanthropy can be considered morally acceptable, in such a way that prioritizes the safety of lives and preserves the collective and individual integrity of a recipient third-world nation, from a culpable superpower. In light of an African ethic of communion, the chapter concludes in the fifth section with what developing nations like Nigeria ought to do to be better prepared for not only future pandemics but also the obligations that lie on other nations, China inclusive, that are part of the global health ecology, for collective survival.

The Virus: From Outbreak to Pandemic

COVID-19 is a highly transmittable and pathogenic viral infection caused by severe acute respiratory syndrome. The virus responsible for the disease is Coronavirus 2 (SARS-CoV-2) (Shereen et al. 2020). It derived its name based on phylogenomic analysis of the genomic data of 2019-nCoV, which showed that the 2019-nCoV is a zoonotic, enveloped single-stranded virus that is most closely related to severe respiratory syndrome (SARS)-like CoV sequences isolated in bats during 2015 to 2017 (Guo et al. 2020). This strongly suggests that the bats' CoV and the human 2019-nCoV share a recent common origin. Both epidemics emerged in China, in a region with high dietary consumption of wildlife, and occurred during cold dry winter seasons.

The new coronavirus was first isolated from traders at the South China seafood market, commonly referred to as "wet markets" in Wuhan, China (Lau et al. 2020). This market also sells wild animals or mammals, suspected to be the likely intermediate hosts of 2019-nCoV, after their origination from bat hosts. It seems much probable from several accounts that the intermediate hosts (wild mammals) were sold to the seafood market in Wuhan, from where the virus began to spread. In December 2019, patients with viral pneumonia due to microbial agent were reported in Wuhan (Lu et al. 2020), with a number of them having a history of exposure to the seafood market in Wuhan, suspected to be the infection source. As other patients who had not been to the market itself but to its vicinity reported their illnesses, preliminary pointers to human-to-human transmission of the virus emerged and were eventually affirmed by evidence of clusters of infected family members and medical workers (Chan et al. 2020). Within one month, the virus had spread throughout China during the Chinese New Year—a period when there is a high level of human mobility, social gathering, and festivity (Adhikari et al. 2020).

The Context of Philanthropy in China

Philanthropy is defined by Payton (1988: 7) as "voluntary action for the public good." Or, as Van Til argues, philanthropy is the act of "voluntary giving and receiving of time and money aimed (however imperfectly) toward the needs of charity and the interests of all in a better quality of life" (Til 1990: 1). This definition lays emphasis on the autonomy of choice by both the benefactor and the beneficiary, and the ultimate objective of improving the lives of the latter, even if there are reasons to consider the act as imperfect. Perhaps one of the most popular definitions of philanthropy is Lester Salamon's (Salamon and Anheier 1992) conception, which holds it as the private giving of time or valuables (money, security, property) for public purposes.

Historically, philanthropy has been a part of traditional Chinese society, as it is much compatible with Confucianism, Taoism, and Buddhism (Baocheng and Mengsha 2017). Upon the institutionalization of socialism in the 1950s, however, the control and distribution of resources became centralized, with the State having the primary responsibility of providing amenities to all citizens regardless of class. According to the *Chinese Encyclopedia*, philanthropy is performed "through sympathy, pity, or religious belief, sending money or material goods to those in need, or provide other practical aid to social programs ... with a heavy religious and superstitious hue, its aim is to do good things for good press. ... [F]or a small number of people it is only a kind of temporary passive relief. ... [T]he social consequences are still disputed" (quoted from Baocheng and Mengsha 2017: 34). In the 1990s, however, as China began to open up more, its disposition toward philanthropy evolved more toward accommodation (Baocheng and Mengsha 2017). Today, not only is China more open toward philanthropy within; it has embraced external philanthropy as a state policy.

After containing the spread of the virus through a lockdown of Wuhan and a mass contact tracing operation driven by high level of surveillance, China began to send medical assistance in the form of kits and personnel to affected countries where the virus continued to spread in a way that overwhelmed the healthcare systems. Some of the beneficiaries of China's pandemic philanthropy include Italy, Serbia, Iran, Venezuela, Iraq, and the Philippines, among others. According to Wang Yi, the State Councilor and Minister of Chinese Foreign Affairs (2020), the two motivating reasons for the assistance of pandemic-stressed countries are first to show gratitude for the assistance received when the infection became an epidemic in China and second to demonstrate its commitment to "international humanitarianism and to implement the vision of a community with a shared future for mankind."

Chinese philanthropy has been two-pronged, coming from both the government and the private sector. Jack Ma, Alibaba's founder, has not only contributed about $14 million through his foundation to develop a COVID-19 vaccine, but he has also donated millions of masks and test kits to Japan, all 54 African countries, Europe, Latin America, Russia, and other parts of Asia. In all, Chinese donors and foundations have contributed close to a billion dollars, about a fifth of the estimated $4.3 billion of worldwide donations raised as of April 2, 2020, to deal with COVID-19 and its many repercussions (The Conversation 2020).

China and the Politics of Pandemic Philanthropy

The above-stated objective of Republic of China's pandemic philanthropy notwithstanding the State's reasons for pandemic philanthropy have been met with skepticism, rejection, and outright condemnations in some quarters. China's supply of protective masks to some countries suffering severe shortage especially for frontline health workers is qualified as "mask diplomacy" by several critics (Alton 2020; Seaman 2020; MERICS 2020). China has been accused of using its assistance to pursue the twin goal of seeking political goodwill on the one hand and attaining global leadership role on the other. The goodwill being sought is meant to deflect responsibilities and accountability arising from references to China as the source of the virus, while as a second objective, it seeks to consolidate its own position as the dominant superpower. These alleged objectives are regarded as unethical and opportunistic on the part of China, which at the outbreak of the virus in Wuhan had enjoyed an outpour of assistance from Western countries, even going as far as requesting that such philanthropic gestures be downplayed out of respect for its own dignity and sensitivity. China's publicized philanthropy across different parts of the world appears thus to have failed the test of reciprocity of moderation and altruism as undergirding principles (Seaman 2020).

There are two popular narratives about China's alleged complicity. The first is that China deliberately engineered the virus and spread it across the world to create a devastation and disruption that would change the current global order in its favor. This allegation, while farfetched and unsubstantiated, has gained traction as one of the most propagated conspiracy theories about the pandemic. Senior American officials, including former President Donald Trump, have made comments that give credence to this belief (Singh et al. 2020). The second allegation is that China is culpable for the outbreak of the pandemic, not because it engineered the virus but because it suppressed vital information that could have helped the rest of the world take more proactive measures in good time. This allegation is predicated on information that emerged later that China had arrested a doctor who first raised alarm about the contagious nature of the virus and had suppressed information even as its transmission escalated. The whistleblower subsequently died of the virus (Hegarty 2020).

In relation to Africa, the foray of China into the continent since the 1950s, which has accelerated over the last two decades, has continued to generate diverse reactions in scholarly and policymaking circles. As the continent sought aid as well as alternative funding partnership for developmental projects, criticism of the Bretton Woods institutions over some of their austere lending policies had made possible a pivot toward China. Still, Sino-African relations have not ceased to be an issue for serious debates. After some respite, the interest dwindled but was revived when the West in the 1990s decided to ostracize China yet again on issues bothering on human rights abuses (Hirono and Suzuki 2014: 444). While some works have analyzed the Sino-African relationship from the perspective of dependency and exploitation, others have tried to argue for a more nuanced view that accommodates African agency (Berhe and Hongwu 2013; Mohan and Lampert 2013; Ayabei 2017).

At the outset, Chinese relations with Africa have been motivated by the need to mitigate the isolations of the 1950s and 1960s, by associating with emerging African states seeking to break from imperialism. This relation is undergirded by the stated principles of non-interference and respect for state sovereignty, often presented as a contrast to the overbearing disposition of Western countries that continue to treat Africa as a colony even after independence. Chinese investment in Africa is reported to have grown to about 15 trillion dollars between 2005 and 2019 (Smith 2020).

In Nigeria, Chinese investments continue to spread sectorally, from manufacturing to Fintech, hospitality, construction, and, more recently, transportation. These investments are estimated to be worth about 20 billion dollars and still rising (Odutola 2019), amid accusations in some quarters that local industries are being crowded out with local labor outsourced to Chinese. It is within this context that the announcement by the government of Nigeria that Chinese medical assistance will be arriving the country to cope with the pandemic ignited a huge opposition. The Federal Government together with the China Railway Construction Corp (CRCC), which had initially said the Chinese medics were coming to help, subsequently backtracked, saying they would only be coming to attend to the needs of some Chinese expatriates working in Nigeria (Nan 2020).

The Nigerian Medical Association (NMA), the National Association of Resident Doctors (NARD), and the Nigerian Union of Journalists (NUJ) were the three opposition groups with the most strident objections. The NMA, in a release expressing its disappointment on the government's decision to seek Chinese assistance, claimed among others that:

1. The Federal Government is ... inviting the Chinese who from available accounts are not out of the woods themselves. The spike in cases and the death toll from COVID -19 in Italy coincided with the arrival of the Chinese in the guise of offering assistance.
2. The Government did not take into consideration the extant laws regulating the practice of medicine in Nigeria as enshrined in the Medical and Dental Council Act. This is one such circumstance where the Medical and Dental Council of Nigerian should be consulted to grant necessary approvals to foreigners to interact with Nigerian patients.
3. The Association is aware of a large pool of general medical and specialist practitioners who are either unemployed or underemployed that can be engaged instead of bringing foreigners who, aside from national security concerns, may not be conversant with the cultures, terrains and peculiar challenges Nigeria will definitely present.
4. The Association believes that the invitation is ill-timed and of no overbearing significance considering that whatever experiences the Chinese have can be shared by digital technology through conferencing.
5. It is a great disservice to the morale of the long-suffering frontline health workforce if the Government goes ahead to invite these Chinese doctors. The invitation demeans their sacrifices so far in this pandemic.
6. The government is expected to rescind the decision, employ more Nigerian doctors, and also provide kits and protective equipment. The Association would consider the withdrawal of the services of its members from attending to COVID 19 patients should the government go ahead with the invitation of the Chinese medics. (NMA 2020)

The position of the NMA was strengthened by that of NARD which stated:

> We find it rather curious that our government would contemplate to throw open her international borders to Chinese nationals having watched how similar action in Italy proved socio-economically suicidal. ... The crafty Chinese scientists should be the last group of friends to trust at this time, given how unreliably and covertly they have managed the information around the pandemic beginning from the data around its origin, characteristics, and other virulence features to help the nations yet to experience the surge to be better prepared. ... We should not lose sight of the fact that conspiracy theories have it that COVID-19 is a possible tool for both sociopolitical and economic manipulation and domination. (NARD 2020)

The NUJ issued a release which went further to predicate its objections on the possible linkage between the coronavirus and 5G technology, hence the danger in trusting Chinese philanthropy (Iftikhar 2020).

From the above, it is evident that oppositions to Chinese philanthropy were triggered by remote and immediate factors bothering on pre-COVID suspicions of expansionism and exploitation and perceived culpability in the spread of the virus, whether on account of poor decisions or deliberate acts of sabotage. Thus, while a Chinese delegation and medical materials eventually arrived the country on April 8, 2020, it was obvious they would not be allowed to offer their expertise or assistance in the country's pandemic response. By the time they arrived, their mission had been modified to be the treatment of Chinese workers in Nigeria, especially those who work with CCECC (A Chinese construction firm with huge footprints across Nigeria). Evidently, the coming of the Chinese medics in spite of the hostile reaction to the gesture was a face-saving effort on the part of the Nigerian and Chinese governments to ensure that Nigerian medics do not carry out their threats while saving China the embarrassment of having its offer of assistance turned down. Meanwhile, the pandemic continues to spread as Nigeria appears to be reaching the peak because of community transition.

Healthcare in Nigeria and the Dearth of Infrastructures

The healthcare system in Nigeria has undergone a tremendous evolution in the last five decades, in terms of policies and initiatives, "but without the desirable quality of health care delivery to advance the health of Nigerians" (Asakitikpi 2019: 1). Healthcare in Nigeria is among the poorest, coming at the low level of 142 out of 195 countries in terms of access and quality (Fullman et al. 2018). With an average life expectancy of 52 years in Nigeria, compared to other African countries such as Ghana (61 years) and South Africa (57 years), more than 90% of the Nigerian population live without health insurance (Medic West Africa 2019). It is no surprise, therefore, that the prevalence of infectious diseases is high in Nigeria. "Nigeria ranks poorly on the incidence of tuberculosis (128 out of 138 countries) and the prevalence of HIV (123 out of 138 countries). On under-five child mortality, there are 89 deaths per 1,000 live births, a level far above the target of 64 deaths per 1,000 live births set in the UN Sustainable Development Goals (SDGs)" (Medic West Africa 2019: 2). Besides tuberculosis and HIV, Nigeria has in the past suffered several severe infectious diseases including cholera, Ebola, and Lassa fever and continues to lack public healthcare facilities to monitor and control the disease outbreak with no exception to the current SARS COVID-19 pandemic. The public healthcare system in Nigeria is poorly managed with inadequate resources and equipment for quality primary and specialty care needed for most serious health issues such as cancer, maternal care, bone marrow, eye surgeries, maternal and infant mortality, and other infectious diseases.

The continuous decline in the healthcare sector despite the rich economy and resources is greatly disturbing. The state of healthcare is due to several factors and challenges. There is a severe lack of human resource as the doctor-patient ratio is 1:3,500 (Igoni 2020), which is significantly low when compared with the World Health Organization's recommended doctor-patient ratio of 1:600. Many Nigerian medical professionals, in search of greener pastures, choose not to work in Nigeria's public health centers due to poor remuneration and welfare; rather, they prefer to seek employment in the Global North with standard medical facilities, stable income, good working environments, and attractive living conditions. The consequence of this is a shortage of skilled health professionals in the country's health sector. Also, the lack of adequate and enabling infrastructures such as stable electricity supply and state-of-the-art hospitals and infectious disease isolation centers makes the country healthcare system more vulnerable in the wake of unplanned epidemics and pandemics. More fundamental is the poor clinical governance of meagre funding and shortage of medical resources, drugs, and supplies provided by the government in managing the primary, secondary, and tertiary healthcare in Nigeria. Ultimately, such clinical maladministration opens patients to risks, especially when hospitals are incapable of providing patients with basic medication and optimal care. Poor clinical governance, which makes irregular and non-remuneration of health workers pronounced in Nigeria, shows a healthcare system in crisis. Largely, funding of the Nigerian health sector is a fundamental problem yet to be given deserved attention.

Nigeria's budgetary allocation for health is far below the Abuja Declaration that insists on the allocation of at least 15% of annual national budget toward improving the public health sector in different African states (Olalere and Gatome-Munyua 2020). Little wonder then that there is an alarming rate of medical tourism from Nigeria to other parts of the world for "kidney transplants, open heart or cardiac surgeries, neurosurgeries, cosmetic surgeries, orthopedic surgeries, eye surgeries and other health conditions, and even delivering babies" (Medic West Africa 2019: 10). Political leaders who are supposed to develop the national health sector also seek medical treatment outside the country, spending millions of the state resources on medical tourism leaving the public health centers in severe conditions at the detriment of the poor masses who cannot afford the cost of medical care at private health centers.

From the COVID-19 pandemic, it is evident that over the years, there have been no infrastructures and resources set in place to monitor, track, or counter the spread of infectious disease outbreak. Isolation centers and molecular laboratories are just being created when the pandemic is hitting hard. Unequivocally, the level of preparedness for the appropriate management of a health crisis of the COVID-19 magnitude was poor. Just like many existential issues affecting Nigerians that the government plays so much politics with, there is so much crisis of trust and lack of imagination in the government's preparedness for and management of the COVID-19 pandemic. An important question to raise and address at this point is: Is the decision to opt for medical aid from China a moral right or wrong? The next section addresses this concern.

Toward an African Moral Theory of Pandemic Philanthropy

The ethics of pandemic philanthropy is usually discussed from the dominant Western views (Singer 2010, 2015; Illingworth et al. 2011) with a near-complete absence of perspectives from African ethics. To provide varying perspectives that may foster understanding of philanthropy across diverse contexts, and especially during pandemics such as the COVID-19, this chapter would be using a specific interpretation of an African ethic of communion. Some theoretical grounding in support of the duty to engage in philanthropy includes effective altruism defended by Peter Singer (2015) and positive deontology articulated by Immanuel Kant (2005). Based on a commitment to utilitarian framework, effective altruism focuses on helping to reduce or prevent suffering in areas of the world with worst hit through scientific and calculated philanthropy. Positive deontological thinking holds that "we all, in virtue of our shared humanity, have a moral duty to aid others in great need..." (Malm et al. 2008). The humanity formula that requires respect for others as moral equals, and not any other special relationship, is the ground for duty-based obligations of philanthropy.

To the extent that these perspectives have their strengths and shortcomings, the primary concern of this chapter is not the evaluation of effective altruism and deontologism. It is not to even compare these perspectives in relation to the Afro-communal option. Rather, this chapter is motivated by the urgent need to develop an African moral theory of pandemic philanthropy in order to add to the theoretical ethical diversity of understanding aid while also applying such constructed perspective to the context of medical aid from China, or any other nation for that matter, to Nigeria in the midst of the COVID-19 pandemic. To be able to achieve this task, it is apt to provide a brief exposition of what an African ethic of communion entails.

The phrase "an African ethic of communion" is traceable to Thaddeus Metz's (2017, 2018, 2020) reading and interpretation of characteristic ethics dominant in the African space, most significantly, in the South of the Sahara. Roughly, ethic of communion is a philosophic reflection on and articulation of the dominant characterization of living morally well commonly found among the black Africans where emphasis is on communion. Communion is understood as values deriving from accepting "fellowship," "harmony," and "cohesion" as the ultimate moral paradigm and focus of human relationships. "Metz traces his African ethical theory to the *ubuntu* understanding of the traditional African worldview" (Samuel and Fayemi 2020: 3), which places emphasis on communal relationships as the basis of self and societal organization. Metz identifies two interpretations of a typical relationship of communion that instructs moral thinking and judgment among Africans South of the Sahara—shared identity and solidarity. According to him:

> On the one hand, there is considering oneself part of the whole, being close, sharing a way of life, belonging and experiencing oneself as bound up with others [shared identity]. On the other hand, there is achieving the good of all, being sympathetic, acting for the common good, serving others (in one's community) and being committed to the good of others (in one's society) [solidarity]. (Metz 2020: 9)

> The point in the above is that communal and harmonious relationship is anchored on distinct and overlapping notions of identity that involves sharing a way of life and caring for others' quality of life in ways that show solidarity with one another. To the extent that relationship is important in African moral worldview, in Metz's reconstruction of such worldview, his emphasis is not on "the relationship in itself as a basic value but rather on an individual's natural capacity for it". (Metz 2018: 53)

According to Fayemi, "a communal relationship is an interpersonal connection governed by norms based on harmonious, relational, interdependent, and cooperative values of existence" (Fayemi 2020: 12). To identify with others is to have the psychological belongingness of membership of a group. Concomitant to such disposition is sharing one's lifeworld through cooperative behavior. To exhibit solidarity is to act in ways that evince the common good through "mutual concern for the welfare of others" (Masolo 2010: 240). Solidarity in this sense is thus defined by actions and positive dispositions "oriented towards other people's good, including an empathetic awareness of their condition and a sympathetic emotional reaction to this awareness. The actions are those likely to be objectively beneficial, that is, to meet others' biological and social needs, and not merely to promote their pleasure or desire satisfaction" (Metz 2020: 10).

Necessary conjunction of identity and solidarity, therefore, entails a cooperative enterprise and behavioral actions between or among moral agents. Regarding communion as a cooperative and mutual relationship, Masolo (2010: 115) makes the point that the moral values involved include "being transparent about the terms of interaction, allowing others to make voluntary choices, acting on the basis of trust, adopting common goals, and, at the extreme end, choosing for the reason that 'this is who we are'." In deducing moral principles of actions from the African understanding of relationship, it is reasonable to infer that "any action that undermines harmonious relations is wrong, while actions that respect communion are considered right prima facie" (Fayemi 2020: 13). As communal beings, we have obligations to honor persons in a relationship of communion. It is instructive to quote Metz on what respecting relationship entails:

> Respecting or honouring a person insofar as she can be [a] party to a communal relationship with us in the first instance means communing with her, rather than ignoring her, let alone subordinating and harming her, which are the discordant or anti-social opposites of communion. Hence, insofar as the capacity to commune has a dignity, sometimes honouring it will include actions that seek to promote the capacity, i.e. creating more

> people, as well as its actualization, fostering communion with them. (Metz 2020: 11)

In light of the foregoing expose of an African ethic of communion, especially with its emphasis on other-regarding virtues, it seems reasonable to deduce that there are aspects of it that qualify it as a potential candidate for constructing an African moral theory of pandemic philanthropy and for evaluating the China model of philanthropism during COVID-19 in Nigeria.

Consider the nature of philanthropy, which entails empathy, doing good for the sake of others, and acting in beneficent ways that are not driven by self-interest. This understanding of philanthropy is connected to an African ethic of communion. Core values of an Afro-ethic of communion are foundational to a cogent framing of the ethic of pandemic philanthropy. In a pandemic, everyone is vulnerable, and the virtues of "might," "rights," and "oppression" are less forceful. Moral values of "generosity, kindness, compassion, benevolence, respectfulness, concern for others" (Gyekye 1992: 109); "charity, politeness, benevolence" (Masolo 2010: 251); and "a sense of togetherness, participating on a cooperative basis, engaging in mutual aid and doing so out of sympathy and for one another's sake" (Metz 2020: 12) are incredible credentials for framing an ethic of philanthropy in general and pandemic philanthropy in particular.

The ethic of philanthropy is about providing moral justification for the obligations that relational beings and entities have toward reducing suffering and protecting the most vulnerable during and post-pandemic. Afro-communion ethic is an "other-regarding" orientation that emphasizes relationships of humans in general as a community deserving cooperation and respect for collective survival. As a prescriptive ideal, Afro-communion ethic is not oblivious of the warranted partialism undergirding diplomatic relations in international politics where actions are weighed and taken on the maxim of "what is most beneficial to homeland." To the extent that existential realities in global politics reflect such partialism, Afro-communion ethic is premised on a subtle principle of precedence that holds that universal human nature of communion and the capacity to be part of a relationship of communion tend to have a substantially greater moral impact and obligations than the political realism of interests and opportunism that defines relations in international circles. Thus, Afro-communion ethic entails common identity of vulnerabilities and solidarity toward collective curtailment of a pandemic. Understood in this sense, Afro-communion ethic of pandemic philanthropy is a sympathetic impartially driven aid to a fellow human in need of help owing to their worst-off existential condition when compared relative to the aider's situation. In a situation like a pandemic where the spread of disease is beyond boundaries and places of origin, an ethic of pandemic philanthropy insists that both the aider and the aided are vulnerable, except that the resources at the disposal of the aider are considerably better to those of the aided. Afro-communion philanthropy ethic, therefore, involves a non-symmetrical relational term where the aided *may or may not* have the capacity to reciprocate the philanthropic gestures of the aider at present or in the future.

Central to pandemic philanthropy in Afro-communal framing is the treatment of others (the aided) in ways that respect the dignity of all parties as relational beings. Respecting relationship that would foster harmony in philanthropy entails that calculated opportunism in the form of commercial returns or financial bargaining of profit and losses from the act of philanthropy would be a moral wrong. In the light of African ethic of communion, a philanthropic act, whether triggered by a pandemic or not, would qualify as morally allowed when it is intended and reasonably executed in ways that promote harmonious relations and respect communion between the aider and the aided. Afro-communal ethic of pandemic philanthropy is about mobilizing available resources that would not bring greater harm to the aider in the interest of the aided that is helplessly in need in order to save highly vulnerable lives in a pandemic.

In the context of the China-Nigeria bilateral relationship pre- and during the COVID-19 pandemic, the question is: to what extent can it be argued that the emergency medic philanthropy by China to Nigeria reflects an action done out of the principles of relationality, friendliness, equity, and harmony definitive of the Afro-ethic of communion? To what extent can Afro-ethic of communion explicated above be instructive in the assessment of whether or not an asymmetry of power does imperil or substitute the well-being and sovereignty of Nigeria in the face of a pandemic aid? Carefully assessed, not every act of supposed philanthropy would unequivocally qualify as morally right within the prism of Afro-communion ethic of philanthropy insofar as the core values elemental to the theory are undermined. In the recent China-Nigeria context, the values of transparency, trust, relationality, consultation, dialogues, and harmony were lacking in the decision-making process that eventuated the pandemic philanthropy of medics and medical supplies to curtail the spread of COVID-19 in Nigeria. Notice that Afro-communion ethic places emphasis not only on the intention of philanthropy but also on the process of carrying out the act. In this regard, it is one thing for the act in itself to be morally justified, prima facie, that it is done out of the impulse of promoting harmonious relations between the two sovereign states; yet it is another for the process involved in the culmination of the foreign aid decision to be corrupted or vitiated in ways capable of creating disharmony among stakeholders.

The act of supporting Nigeria with medics of different specializations can be considered morally acceptable where the intention is primarily that of securing the lives of Nigerians exposed to danger on account of the inadequacies of the country's medical capacity and preserving the collective and individual integrity of a recipient third-world nation from COVID-19. To the extent that unpacking the underlying intention of such state policy by China is herculean, history of Sino-Africa relations seems to backstop the assumption of an imperialistic expansionism in Africa. Even if such an assumption, among others, is farfetched, the process leading to the decision rendered the action morally questionable. What appeared to have worsened the crisis of confidence and trust is the fact that the Chinese offer was announced and defended by the Minister of Health alongside the Secretary to the Federal Government, who chaired the Presidential Taskforce on COVID-19. These government officials, unlike the Director of the Nigerian Centre for Diseases Control (NCDC), are seen more as politicians rather than as medical experts. The impression created with the disregard for the scientific and medical community in Nigeria, therefore, is that the idea of medical philanthropy was exclusively political and devoid of expert input as to what was needed the most and in what area. This was further interpreted as not only disparaging the professional competence of Nigerian medics but also an attempt to sacrifice Nigeria's integrity by creating a window for China whose supposed altruism which is under intense global scrutiny as an image laundering and instrumental gesture.

As earlier noted, government has since modified its position to claim that the Chinese medics were only coming to attend to the need of Chinese expatriates in Nigeria. Post the arrival of Chinese expatriates, their whereabouts and the true nature of their mission were a subject of growing discussion on social media and in the public space. China's efforts at combating the virus within its territory has been criticized as discriminatory against blacks in general and Nigerians in particular, with reports of dehumanizing and humiliating measures including forced evictions and denial of essential services even in public places (Aljazeera 2020). The Nigerian government's opacity and inconsistency have created a situation that increases public distrust and presented the political class as captives of Chinese expansionist agenda.

In a desperate bid to force the government into a retreat and correct what it perceives as an undesirable outcome of power asymmetry, the medical community in Nigeria resorted to unfounded allegations against China, suggesting not only that it was responsible for the virus but that its medical personnel had been using pandemic assistance to spread the virus. It claimed, without evidence, that Chinese doctors were responsible for the rise in death tolls in Italy, as an instance (NARD Press Release 2020). The allegations further fueled the conspiracy theories about the origin and purpose of the virus, which had gained considerable acceptance within the populace. Such a dangerous tactic equally negates the idea of African communal ethic, as it involves the use of manipulation and populism by the very experts whose opinions ought to guide the public's response to the pandemic. The Nigerian medical community in negation of this ethic has prioritized its own professional integrity, not only at the expense of whatever expertise and experience the Chinese medics could have provided as complements to Nigeria's effort but also at the expense of truth and scientific facts.

The implication of the current situation is that China's medical philanthropy, which at a time like this ought to have been of immense benefit to Nigeria, became enmeshed in the politics of hegemony and resistance at a time when hospitals are in dire shortage of test kits and experienced hands in pandemic management. On the other hand, the possibly anticipated improvement in the image of China on account of the philanthropic effort has achieved the opposite result of pitting a considerable section of Nigerians, including the medical community, against it. This could have been avoided if the principles of respect, harmony, openness, and regard for others, as features of Afro-communal ethics, had undergirded the gesture between the powerful donor and the developing recipient nation.

Conclusion

This chapter concludes that developing nations like Nigeria ought to be better prepared for future pandemics to avoid being potential preys of dark philanthropy during a pandemic. Also, developed states and the global community have obligations to promote collective survival of lives through pandemic philanthropy and other initiatives that can reduce suffering of the most vulnerable in the global health ecology. Such altruistic efforts, when offered within the ethical framework of relationality, and underpinned by values of generosity, kindness, compassion, benevolence, respectfulness, concern for others, charity, and politeness, are likely to result in mutually benefitting outcomes for the aider and the aided. While domination and exploitation are perceived rightly or wrongly as the primary motivation for altruistic gestures between unequal parties, the moral and utilitarian benefits of such philanthropic efforts are at the risk of being lost, while the challenge which motivated the effort, as in the case of COVID 19, deteriorates.

Though the science of mitigating the current pandemic continues to unfold, it seems apparent that the interconnectedness of the world, as well as the impact the virus has had globally, makes it a challenge that can best be confronted in solidarity, unity, and cohesion. This requires the coming together of all stakeholders, including the powerful nations of the world, with resources and ideas on how to address the health, economic, political, and social challenges arising from the pandemic. Such cohesion and solidarity are best forged with transparency, respect, openness, and generosity, best encapsulated in Afro-communal ethic of pandemic philanthropy.

One potential criticism of the African ethic of communion in grounding philanthropism in general, and pandemic philanthropy in particular, is how to address the clash of values and objectives between the aider and the aided in the context of intercultural and international philanthropy. The possibility of super-imposing the values of the aider (China, for instance) on the aided (Nigeria in this specific context) is high, given that the aider is the source of the philanthropy. An ensuing paradox that an African ethic of communion introduces in the context of pandemic philanthropy is that of investing the values of the aided on the aider. One way to address this is to argue that avoiding the exposure of the more vulnerable to the weighty burdens of the pandemic, to which the countries in the global south are more susceptible, is possible, given that the normative values underpinning philanthropic gestures are not at variance with those of transparency, respect, and generosity, which undergird Afro-communal ethics.

Acknowledgments The contribution of Adeolu Oyekan to this work is based on the research supported by the National Research Foundation of South Africa (Grant Number 99188, SARChI Chair in Identities and Social Cohesion in Africa, Nelson Mandela University). Opinions, findings, conclusions, and recommendations expressed in this work are those of the author's alone, and the NRF accepts no liability whatsoever in this regard.

The contribution of Ademola K. Fayemi to this work is based on part of the outcome of research conducted within the Africa Multiple Cluster of Excellence at the University of Lagos-ACC, funded by the Deutsche Forschungsgemeinschaft (DFG, German Research Foundation) under Germany Excellence Strategy—EXC 2052/1—390713894.

References

Adhikari, S., S. Meng, Y. Wu, et al. 2020. Epidemiology, Causes, Clinical Manifestation and Diagnosis, Prevention and Control of Coronavirus Disease (COVID-19) during the Early Outbreak Period: A Scoping Review. *Infectious Diseases of Poverty* 9: 29. https://doi.org/10.1186/s40249-020-00646-x.

Aljazeera. 2020. 'Unacceptable': Nigeria Condemns Treatment of Citizens in China. April 4. Accessed 28 September 2020. https://www.aljazeera.

com/news/2020/4/14/unacceptable-nigeria-condemns-treatment-of-citizens-in-china.

Alton, Tom. 2020. *China's Global Aid Blitz and "Mask Diplomacy"*. Alberta: China Institute, University of Alberta.

Asakitikpi, A.E. 2019. Healthcare Coverage and Affordability in Nigeria: An Alternative Model to Equitable Healthcare Delivery. In *Universal Health Coverage*, ed. Aida Isabel Tavares. Intech Open.

Ayabei, C. 2017. The Rise of China and Conflicts in Africa: The Case of Sudan. *African Journal of Political Science and International Relations.* 11 (2): 29–35.

Ayitogo, N. 2020. Chinese Doctors: Hold Buhari Responsible for Any Coronavirus Upsurge—PDP. *Premium Times*, April 8. Accessed 6 September 2020. https://www.premiumtimesng.com/news/more-news/386799-chinese-doctors-hold-buhari-responsible-for-any-coronavirus-upsurge-pdp.html.

Baocheng, L., and Z. Mengsha. 2017. *Philanthropy in China Report of Concepts, History, Drivers, Institutions*. Geneva: Globeethics.net.

Berhe, M.G., and L. Hongwu. 2013. *China-Africa Relations Governance, Peace and Security*. Addis Ababa: Institute for Peace and Security Studies, Addis Ababa University.

Chan, J.F.W. et al. 2020. A Familial Cluster of Pneumonia Associated with the 2019 Novel Coronavirus Indicating Person-to-Person Transmission: A Study of a Family Cluster. *Lancet*, Published Online Jan 24. https://doi.org/10.1016/S0140-6736(20)30154-9.

Fayemi, A.K. 2020. Is Skin Bleaching a Moral Wrong? An African Bioethical Perspective. *Theoretical Medicine and Bioethics* 41: 1–22.

Fullman N, Yearwood J, Abay S.M, Abbafati C, Abd-Allah F, Abdela J, Abdelalim A, Abebe Z, Abebo T.A., Aboyans V. 2018. "Measuring Performance on the Healthcare Access and Quality Index for 195 Countries and Territories and Selected Subnational Locations: A Systematic Analysis from the Global Burden of Disease Study 2016." *Lancet.* 391: 2236–2271.

Guo, Y.R., Q.D. Cao, Z.S. Hong, et al. 2020. The Origin, Transmission and Clinical Therapies on Coronavirus Disease 2019 (COVID-19) Outbreak—An Update on the Status. *Military Medical Research* 7: 11. https://doi.org/10.1186/s40779-020-00240-0.

Gyekye, K. 1992. Person and Community in African Thought. In *Person and Community: Ghanaian Philosophical Studies*, ed. K. Gyekye and K. Wiredu, vol. 1, 101–122. Washington, DC: Council for Research in Values and Philosophy.

Hegarty, S. 2020. The Chinese Doctor Who Tried to Warn Others about Coronavirus. *BBC News*, 6 February. Accessed 30 August 2020. https://www.bbc.com/news/world-asia-china-51364382.

Hirono, M., and S. Suzuki. 2014. Why Do We Need 'Myth-Busting' in the Study of Sino–African Relations? *Journal of Contemporary China* 23 (87): 443–461. https://doi.org/10.1080/10670564.2013.843889.

Iftikhar, P. 2020. Corona and 5G Conspiracy Theories. *The Express Tribune*, May 4. Accessed 5 October 2020. https://tribune.com.pk/story/2213294/corona-5g-conspiracy-theories https://tribune.com.pk/story/2213294/corona-5g-conspiracy-theories.

Igoni, D. 2020. Nigeria's Doctor-Patient Ratio Is 1:3, 500. *Punch*, January 23. Accessed 13 June 2020. https://punchng.com/nigerias-doctor-patient-ratio-is-13500-nuc/.

Illingworth, Patricia, Thomas Pogge, and Leif Wenar. 2011. *Giving Well: The Ethics of Philanthropy*. New York: Oxford University Press.

Kant, I. 2005. *Groundwork of the Metaphysics of Morals*. Trans. T.K. Abbott and L. Denis. Peterborough: Broadview Press.

Lau, S.K., H.K. Luk, A.C. Wong, K.S. Li, L. Zhu, Z. He, and P.C. Woo. 2020. Possible Bat Origin of Severe Acute Respiratory Syndrome Coronavirus 2. *Emerging Infectious Diseases 26* (7): 1542.

Lu, R., X. Zhao, J. Li, P. Niu, B. Yang, H. Wu, et al. 2020. Genomic Characterisation and Epidemiology of 2019 Novel Coronavirus: Implications for Virus Origins and Receptor Binding. *The Lancet 395* (10224): 565–574.

Malm, H., T. May, L.P. Francis, S.B. Omer, D.A. Salmon, and R. Hood. 2008. Ethics, Pandemics, and the Duty to Treat. *The American Journal of Bioethics 8* (8): 4–19.

Masolo, D.A. 2010. *Self and Community in a Changing World*. Bloomington: Indiana University Press.

Medic West Africa. 2019. *2019 Healthcare Market Insights: NIGERIA*. Accessed 15 May 2020. https://www.medicwestafrica.com/content/dam/Informa/medic-west africa/english/2019/HealthcareInsights.pdf.

MERICS. 2020. The Consequences of Corona in China: The End of the Crisis Is the Beginning of the Next One. *China Update* No. 6/2020 March 13–25.

Metz, Thaddeus. 2017. Ancillary Care Obligations in Light of an African Bioethic. *Theoretical Medicine and Bioethics* 38: 111–126.

———. 2018. A Bioethic of Communion: Beyond Care and the Four Principles with Regard to Reproduction. In *The Ethics of Reproductive Genetics: Between Utility, Principles, and Virtues*, ed. Marta Soniewicka, 49–66. Cham: Springer.

———. 2020. African Communitarianism and Difference. In *Handbook of African Philosophy of Difference*, ed. Elvis Imafidon, 31–51. Cham: Springer.

Mohan, G., and B. Lampert. 2013. Negotiating China: Reinserting African Agency into China–Africa Relations. *African Affairs* 112 (446): 92–110. https://doi.org/10.1093/afraf/ads065.

Nan, Z. 2020. CRCC Task Force to Look After Its Employees in Nigeria. *China Daily*, August 4. Accessed 2 October 2020. https://www.chinadaily.com.cn/a/202004/08/WS5e8d3342a310aeaeeed50b2e.html.

NARD. 2020. COVID-19: Invitation to Chinese Doctors Suicidal, NARD Warns. April 5. Accessed 30 August 2020. https://www.vanguardngr.com/2020/04/invitation-to-chinese-doctors-suicidal-nard-warns/.

NMA. 2020. COVID-19: NMA Press Release Rejecting FG's Invitation of Chinese Doctors into the Country. April 5. Accessed 30 August 2020. https://nationalnma.org/2020/04/05/covid-19-nma-press-release-rejecting-fgs-invitation-of-chinese-doctors-into-the-country/.

Odutola, A. 2019. How the Chinese Are Taking Over Nigeria's Economy. *Nairametrics*, November 28. Accessed 14 May 2020. https://nairametrics.com/2019/11/28/how-the-chinese-are-taking-over-nigerias-economy/.

Olalere, N., and A. Gatome-Munyua. 2020. Public Financing for Health in Africa: 15% of an Elephant Is Not 15% of a Chicken. *Africa Renewal*, October 2020. Accessed 25 October 2020. https://www.un.org/africarenewal/magazine/october-2020/public-financing-health-africa-when-15-elephant-not-15-chicken.

Payton, R.L. 1988. *Philanthropy: Voluntary Action for the Public Good*. New York: American Council on Education/Macmillan Publishing.

Salamon, L.M., and H.K. Anheier. 1992. In Search of the Non-Profit Sector I: The Question of Definitions. *Voluntas* 3 (2): 125–151.

Samuel, O.S., and A.K. Fayemi. 2020. A Critique of Thaddeus Metz's Modal Relational Account of Moral Status. *Theoria*, Issue 162, 67 (1): 28–44.

Seaman, J. 2020. *COVID-19 and Euro-China Relations: A Country Level Analysis*. European Think-Tank Network on China (ETNC): French Institutes of International Relations (IFRI).

Shaban, A. 2020. Chinese Experts Arrive to Help Nigeria in Coronavirus Fight, Opposition Kicks. *Africanews*, April 9. Accessed 7 September 2020. https://www.africanews.com/2020/04/09/chinese-experts-arrive-to-help-nigeria-in-coronavirus-fight-opposition-kicks/./

Shereen, M.A., et al. 2020. Origin, Transmission, and Characteristics of Human Coronaviruses. *Journal of Advanced Research* 24: 91–98.

Singer, Peter. 2010. *The Life You Can Save*. New York: Random House.

———. 2015. *The Most Good You Can Do: How Effective Altruism is Changing Ideas about Living Ethically*. London: Yale Press.

Singh, M., H. Davidson, and J. Borger. 2020. Trump Claims to Have Evidence Coronavirus Started in Chinese Lab but Offers No Details. *The Guardian*, May 1. Accessed 20 September 2020. https://www.theguardian.com/us-news/2020/apr/30/donald-trump-coronavirus-chinese-lab-claim.

Smith, E. 2020. Zambia's Spiraling Debt Offers Glimpse into the Future of Chinese Loan Financing in Africa. Accessed 3 October 2020. https://www.cnbc.com/2020/01/14/zambias-spiraling-debt-and-the-future-of-chinese-loan-financing-in-africa.html.

The Conversation. 2020. China's Big Donors Are Pitching in to Deal with the New Coronavirus—And Not Just in Their Own Country. April 3. Accessed 18 September 2020. https://theconversation.com/chinas-big-donors-are-pitching-in-to-deal-with-the-new-coronavirus-and-not-just-in-their-own-country-134777.

Til, J.V. 1990. *Critical Issues in American Philanthropy: Strengthening Theory and Practice*. Glenview, IL: AAFRC Trust for Philanthropy.

WHO. 2020. WHO Director-General's opening remarks at the media briefing on COVID-19—11 March. *World Health Organization*, 16.2.

Yi, W. 2020. Following Xi Jinping Thought on Diplomacy to Build a Community with a Shared Future for Mankind Through International Cooperation Against COVID-19. April 19. Accessed 29 September 2020. https://www.fmprc.gov.cn/mfa_eng/zxxx_662805/t1771257.shtml.

7

Disease Discourses, African Knowledge Systems, and COVID-19 in Senegal

Karen S. Barton, Jieun Lee, and Ivan J. Ramírez

Introduction

Too often discussions surrounding best practices in global public health exclude or altogether ignore geographies of Africa south of the Sahara. This is especially true for the discourse surrounding severe acute respiratory syndrome coronavirus 2, known commonly as COVID-19 (SARS-CoV-2). Some African states—including Senegal—have made impressive strides in coronavirus management by harnessing the power of science and

K. S. Barton (✉) • J. Lee
Department of Geography, GIS, and Sustainability, Greeley, CO, USA
e-mail: karen.barton@unco.edu

I. J. Ramírez
Department of Health and Behavioral Sciences, University of Colorado, Denver, CO, USA
e-mail: ivan.ramirez@ucdenver.edu

F. Egbokhare, A. Afolayan (eds.), *Global Health, Humanity and the COVID-19 Pandemic*, https://doi.org/10.1007/978-3-031-17429-2_7

community-based response systems.[1] Yet Africa's COVID success stories have been largely downplayed by a global media that amplifies coronavirus triumphs in developed countries over those of emerging states. Much of this oversight is rooted in prevailing misconceptions of Africa "the diseased continent" in which sub-Sahara is seen as a breeding ground for emerging pathogens (Afolayan 2020). Certainly the continent's tropical climate is responsible for creating some physical geographies that are conducive to infectious diseases. Pathogens such as malaria, dengue, and Ebola are endemic across portions of Africa, and their diffusion can be exacerbated by poor infrastructure, malnutrition, high population densities, and limited access to health care. But these narratives fail to account for the diversity of infectious conditions that exist between and within African states. Such language (Campbell 2020; Fink 2020) ignores spatial nuances in favor of gross generalizations while reifying the disease-disaster tropes about the continent.

Our growing ability to harness spatial quantitative data on coronavirus case counts can shed critical light on recent public health failures (United States) and successes (Senegal) around the world, causing us to reevaluate the administrative winners and losers in this global battle. In particular, the process of accurately relaying disease information has been deftly facilitated by mapping technologies such as geographic information systems (GIS), which allow us to disseminate stories in visually engaging and digestible ways. A vast majority of the globe, for instance, is reliant upon the geospatial data of the Johns Hopkins Coronavirus Resource Center, whose GIS maps of the pandemic received 1 billion hits as early as April (GIS Lounge 2020). These maps provide ongoing evidence that Senegal's low case count relative to other developed states is both exemplary and impressive. To be fair, hallmark research by Monmonmeier (1991) has shown us that despite their immense value, some maps lie and that they must do so. Yet Monmonmeier's work also suggests that rather than dismiss all cartographies, we should evaluate them critically, employing a healthy skepticism given how easy they are to manipulate

[1] Rwanda enlisted anti-epidemic robots, contact tracing, and an early lockdown system in response to the COVID-19 pandemic, which has resulted in some of the lowest case counts and deaths in the world. Ghana also has similarly low COVID-19 death counts. This is due in part to an extensive system of contact tracing, the use of community health workers and volunteers, and innovative new techniques such as "pool testing" where multiple blood samples are analyzed and then followed up as individual tests only if a positive result is found.

(Monmonmeier 1991, 10). His concerns with maps stem in part from colonial era policies which served to carve up the African continent in ways that were both capricious and haphazard.

For West Africa, specifically, portions of what were once the Mali Kingdom were parceled out between the British (The Gambia) and the French (Senegal), literally dividing communities in half. Yet, whereas Senegal's origin story was a product of colonial cartography, today's coronavirus maps can serve to *amplify* Senegal's successes instead of its subjugation (Barton 2020a). Thus, it is possible to be skeptical of maps while also utilizing them to explain important geographical phenomena. Scholars can simultaneously ground-truth mapping data in conjunction with qualitative materials on health, disease, and its diffusion by using a mixed methods approach to disease studies. That said, this chapter draws from both the growing corpus of coronavirus GIS data *and* qualitative research on Senegal's pathogen management to address its unique handling of COVID-19. A deeper dive into the work of Dakar's Center for Infectious Diseases and Pasteur Institutes will illustrate whether Senegal's successes are a collective, multicausal by-product of the country's (1) rapid response plan and existing community health systems; (2) widespread public support for social distancing; (3) enduring treatment of elderly populations; and (4) geographical position along the tropical belt. Theoretically, we also offer a framework that this global crisis has forced us to interrogate (Ihekweazu and Agogo 2020). That is, what if—in the case of pandemic management—some African solutions are just *better* ones? Using maps and qualitative data, this work underscores the ways in which public health experts can (and should) draw from the indigenous expertise of African nations in managing and responding to pandemics like COVID-19.

Field Context: Geography of Health and Resources in Senegal

That Senegal—a small West African nation once carved up by colonial powers—can be held up as a model of coronavirus containment success is particularly impressive and ironic given its geographic location, existing health resource base, and capital limitations. First, it straddles what the Pew Foundation objectively terms the "religious fault zone" of the African Sahel where, despite national conflicts, Senegal's diverse faith-based communities converge and coalesce (Barton 2020b). Senegal is often recognized for its exceptionalism due to the country's relative political stability; it stands in sharp contrast to adjacent states like Mali and Guinea-Conakry where internal conflict is rife (Pew Forum 2010). Certainly, the Mouvement des Forces Démocratiques de Casamance (MFDC)—an ongoing separatist struggle based in the south—has challenged Senegal's peaceful coexistence, but villages and communities have generally learned to adapt and coalesce (Ojeda 2012).

Second, with a population of roughly 16 million people, the country possesses a relatively fragile health-care system, scarcity of hospital beds, and about seven physicians per 100,000 people (World Bank 2020). Although Senegal launched an ambitious hospital reform program in 1998 that included a large injection of government funds, many of these institutions were soon close to bankruptcy (Lemière et al. 2012). Equity of access to hospital care, particularly for the poorest, had also deteriorated, which is problematic given that a large number of individuals live below the poverty line (World Bank 2020). This fragile health landscape has also been exacerbated by long-standing gender norms across Senegal, particularly in the semi-arid north of Saint Louis, where women have been largely excluded from local politics, civil society, and local health committees for many decades (Foley 2001; Paul et al. 2020). Yet Senegalese people make do, and despite these systematic and systemic roadblocks, the government has tackled COVID-19 aggressively and thus far effectively. By February 2021, one year into the pandemic, this densely populated country had reported only 35,000 coronavirus cases and 896 deaths, and yet it still has not been adequately recognized for its best practices (Johns Hopkins University 2021). Figure 7.1 provides a geographical view of COVID-19 case counts and incidence for Senegal's fourteen districts as of January 2021. Note that some rural districts in the east have been relatively unaffected by the coronavirus pandemic, a spatial process that will be addressed at a later point in this chapter.

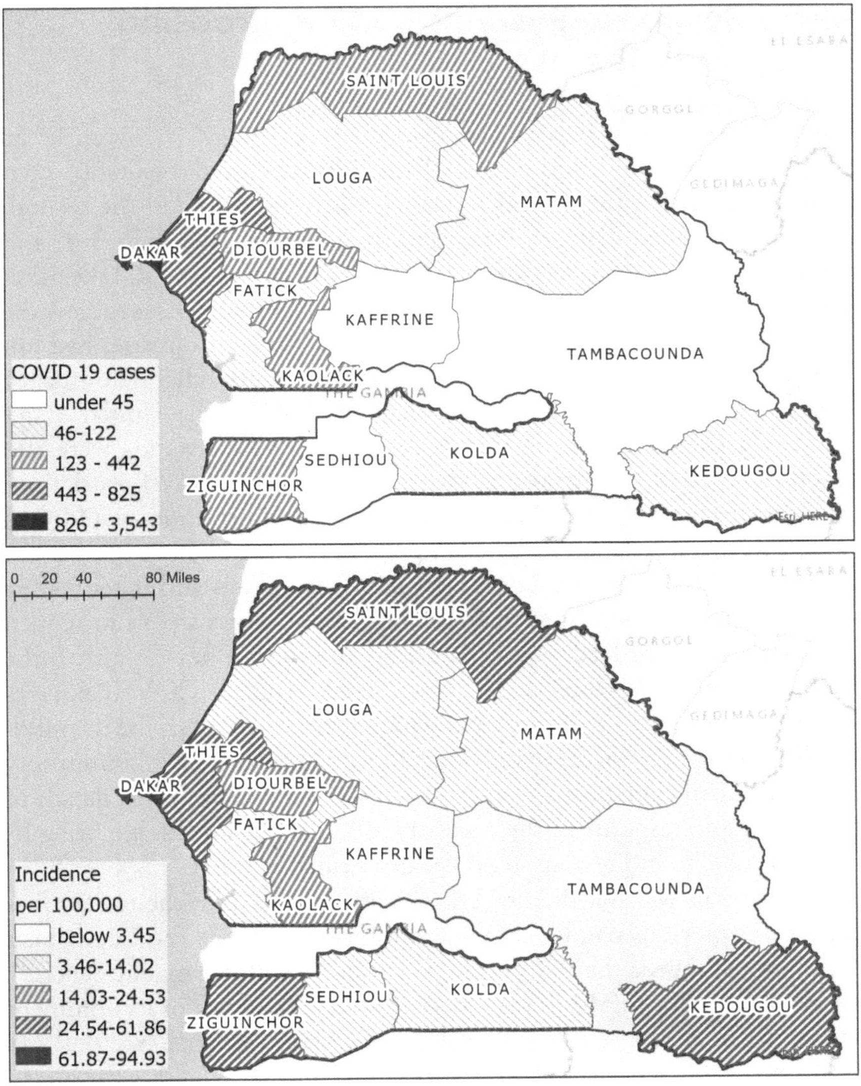

Fig. 7.1 Senegal's COVID-19 cases by regions; COVID incidence per 1000

Rapid Response Systems and Repurposing Community Teams

Senegal's 2020 coronavirus narrative, not surprisingly, is rooted in its colonial era connections to France. While Egypt boasted the first coronavirus case to strike the African continent, Senegal recorded the second, when a Frenchman living in Dakar returned from holiday with fever and was ultimately quarantined for the duration in Fann Hospital. Like other African states, Senegal took rigorous measures from the outset to slow the spread, and by mid-March, some 25 out of 54 African countries had put in place sweeping restrictions to manage the crisis, ones that far outpaced the glacial sequence of restrictions that unfolded in the United States (CGD 2020). South Africa, Kenya, Mauritania, and Rwanda were also among the list of countries that swiftly set in motion travel restrictions and closed local schools. But the American administration would take several weeks to institute widespread policies to safeguard its citizens. On March 24, 2020, just two weeks after many businesses and schools were shuttered, then-President Donald Trump announced his plan to reopen the country by April 12, citing that the "cure cannot be worse than the problem itself" (Al Jazeera 2020). In contrast, Senegal's COVID policies set the bar not just for the speed at which it responded but for its philosophical approach to the pandemic, in which village and community needs trumped capitalism. The following section lays out these details of Senegal's rapid response in the wake of COVID-19 while highlighting its cultural roots in indigenous West African health systems.

Coronavirus was not the first crisis to affect Senegal in the twenty-first century, as previous pandemics would ultimately serve as cautionary tales for other pathogens that lay ahead on the horizon. Undeniably, Senegal's particular handling of the Ebola virus laid the foundations for its imminent management of the 2020 COVID-19 pandemic (UNAIDS 2020; US Embassy 2020). Senegal is no stranger to the challenge of halting the spread of infectious diseases within its borders despite high case fatalities across the other parts of the subcontinent. Dr. Moussa Seydi, Head of Infectious Diseases at the Centre Hospitalier Universitaire de Fann, worked alongside a team of specialists to treat the country's only Ebola patient in 2014. This figure was critical, given that between 2015 and 2016, more than 11,000 people died from Ebola, the majority of whom were Africans, yet Senegal was largely unscathed (WHO 2020). Discovered in 1976 near the Ebola River in what is now the Democratic Republic of the Congo, Ebola is both contagious and deadly, and Senegal's first case was confirmed when a man who had been in contact with an Ebola patient traveled by road from Guinea to Dakar. The Senegalese government responded immediately, aided in part by existing health institutions such as the world-class Pasteur Institute and Laboratory enabling the state to test quickly and reliably for viral hemorrhagic fevers using contact tracing. A separate center was designated for Ebola, which freed up the health system to deliver routine services. Public information campaigns were engaged, and this lessened public anxiety and encouraged health cooperation with control measures. The author had the privilege of touring the Center for Infectious Disease facilities in Dakar, and this visit made clear that despite limited capital, Senegalese disease experts had marshalled all resources to help slow the spread (Seydi, personal communication 2018). In many ways, the Ebola outbreak across Africa would serve as a dress rehearsal for Senegal's encounter with coronavirus in 2020. The state would prove that it could meticulously organize a response through sound science, quick action, strong communication, and innovation, despite the events that were unfolding in adjacent states. That the Health Ministry was able to quickly repurpose Ebola and polio response teams as coronavirus unfolded provided the jump start officials needed to drastically slow the pathogen's spread.

One of the most striking features of Senegal's 2020 pandemic response plan was its ability to conduct rapid testing in order to step up COVID-19 diagnoses despite the nation's limited supply of health resources (Bensaid and Grine 2014). During the first few months of the crisis, three major strategies anchored the state's efforts to bolster COVID testing:

1. Senegal delivered testing results within one day once samples were received by medical laboratories, and these labs operated 24 hours per day using an automated process, which ensured safety of front line health-care workers.
2. The health ministry developed digital platforms through which health workers received results from surveillance teams; many of these exem-

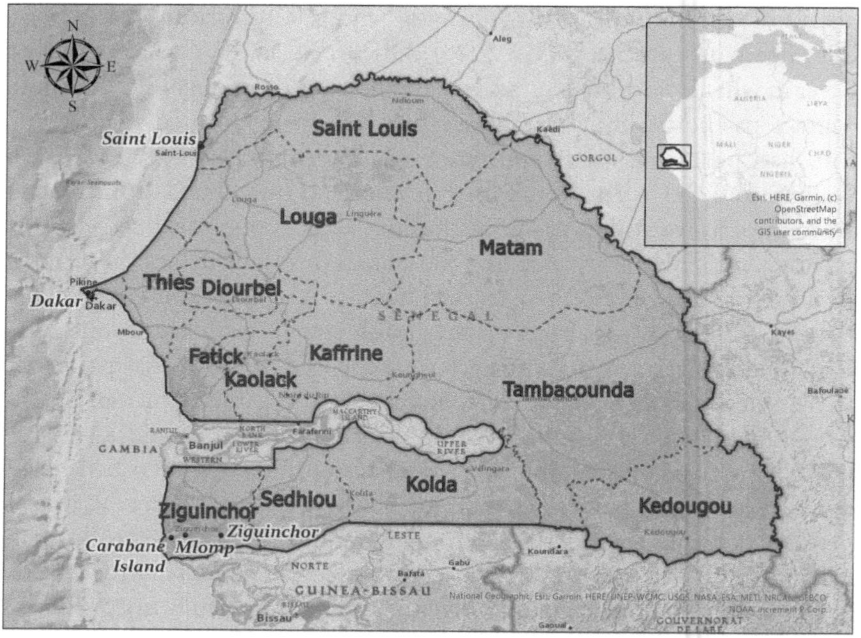

Fig. 7.2 Map of Senegal and The Gambia. (Source: Jieun Lee)

plary teams went on to train staff in other countries on proper COVID protocols (CGD 2020).

3. The rapid response system was decentralized to accommodate Senegal's districts (Fig. 7.2) so that communities from Saint Louis to Ziguinchor would have local and equitable access to tests. It's worth noting that support from the World Health Organization and Islamic Development Bank helped fund decentralized lab tests, a decision that would cut down on transportation delays and allow for speedier results. This last strategic initiative was particularly important given Senegal's haphazard geography, an artifact of French colonial rule.

Transportation between different regions of the country is made difficult due to the presence of The Gambia, a semi-enclave which cartographically slices the nation in half. The *Aline Sitoe Diatta* ferry (and before that, the *Joola*)—which runs between Dakar and Ziguinchor—has served to create new maritime linkages around The Gambia, but the pandemic led to the suspension of these onboard operations (Barton 2020a). Social distancing is near impossible aboard the ferry line due to its popularity across the region.

Senegal would soon build upon these early COVID successes by speeding up turnaround time for coronavirus tests, and by April, results were available to patients in eight hours or less. These achievements were extraordinary, given that testing was also made free to the Senegalese public and available to all, regardless of financial means (Magome 2020). By May 2020, the Pasteur Institute was actively collaborating with the UK-based company, Mologic, to manufacture diagnostic kits that could produce COVID-19 results within ten minutes for $1 USD; they estimated that 500–1000 tests could be analyzed within one day and up to four million per year (Yeung 2020). Pasteur Institute's Director, Amadou Sall, argued that for researchers at the DiaTropix infectious disease testing facility—an in-house program of Pasteur Institute—highly equipped laboratories were not actually as critical as many thought. Instead, Sall argued that decentralized systems incorporating "pocket-sized tests" which were not designed to turn a profit were the most important development for not only COVID-19 but future pandemics (Harrisburg 2020). That Dakar's Pasteur Institute was only one of two laboratories across Africa equipped to test for coronavirus early on in the pandemic surely played a role in shaping Senegal's aggressive COVID testing plan. It also did not take long before medics at Fann Hospital were able to monitor patients using cameras in order to minimize contact with them and help slow the spread (BBC 2020).

Yet while Senegal harnessed sound science and technology in developing its rapid response plan, the country was also emboldened by age-old approaches to health, a process that is rooted in Senegalese religious and community-based cultural beliefs (Honda et al. 2019). For example, health officials made a pledge early on in the pandemic to earmark a hospital or clinic bed not only for every patient but for the patients' contacts as well. Each newly diagnosed individual—no matter how mild or severe the case—was provided a hospital bed or health center where they stay isolated and observed. This was an ambitious and audacious goal, given the paucity of hospital and clinic beds as noted earlier on in this chapter

(World Bank 2020). But the strategy of a bed for every case, no matter how mild the systems, helped stop the spread of the virus in a country where most Senegalese live in large family compounds, making it impossible to self-isolate (WHO 2020). While the "one-bed" pledge was motivated by a desire to prevent diffusion of the virus, it also underscores the value that Senegalese place on individual human lives. Every time a coronavirus death is announced in Senegal, the Ministry adds a personal note to the record: "Senegal registered its 13th death from COVID-19 Tuesday, May 5, 2020. The death was a 94-year-old man. The Minister of Health and Social Action offers its condolences to his family" (NPR 2020). Senegal's response to the coronavirus, then, is notable not only for its thoroughness but for its humanity, a process that is unseen in other parts of the world where the pandemic has infiltrated. In Kuwait, for example, nearly 360,000 immigrant guest workers were shipped home in the wake of COVID, while Senegal made no plans to eject either migrants or expatriates (Dudley 2020). Instead, Senegal succeeded in staving off what could have been disastrous levels of spatial diffusion using the power of science and culture. Yet it was not alone in its ability to detect the disease quickly. By April 2020, a total of 43 countries on the African continent could diagnose COVID-19 effectively.

Young Demographic and Care for Elderly

A second argument employed to explain Africa's relatively lower COVID-19 infection rates is ascribed to the continent's youthful demography in which the median age is 18 (Desjardins 2019). By contrast, both Asia and South America boast median ages of 31, with statistics for North America and Europe shifting even higher given reduced birth rates in those regions. The World Bank estimates indicate that by 2100 Africa will contain 50% of the world's children aged zero to four years. This represents an opportunity for growth and innovation but also presents challenges given the region's limited natural resources (World Bank 2020). Senegal is likewise a youthful country and sits roughly at the population mean for Africa, at 18.5 years of age. Personal field observations in the country confirm that Senegal is young, vibrant, and dynamic; but some analysts use this singular fact to explain why Senegalese have managed to thrive despite the incursion of the most deadly, global pandemic of the century.

This section unpacks the explanatory power of Senegal's "youthfulness" as a rationale for low COVID-19 infections and death totals in line with the theoretical premise of this chapter. We argue that invoking a youthful population alone to explain lower case counts is reductionist and does not present a comprehensive analysis of the sociocultural context of events on ground in West Africa. Indeed, epidemiological research shows that the majority of COVID deaths target those 80 years and older, and youth—without preexisting conditions—are generally at a distinct advantage with lower infection rates. But it is reckless to conclude that African states *stumbled* upon their pandemic successes based solely on demographics (or even environmental circumstances, which we shall later address). Such deterministic arguments are reminiscent of Diamond's (1998) research on the success and failure of civilizations. In his hallmark analysis, he argues that certain populations were historically at a distinct advantage due to their geographical position on the planet. But in terms of COVID-19, there are other spatial and cultural processes operating in conjunction with existing population dynamics, which help elucidate Senegal's low case counts relative to developed parts of the world. Amplifying the complex cultural processes that contributed to Senegal's pandemic narrative is critical in order to fully articulate the forgotten nuances of COVID-19 histories and geographies. To accomplish that, we must focus on not only the role of the country's youth cohort but also its elderly demographic and their relative importance or "place" within larger society.

One promising argument deployed to understand Senegal's relatively lower COVID-19 rates is the country's remarkable lack of nursing homes in contrast to other parts of the world such as the United States. The Kaiser Family Foundation (2019) reported a total of 1,246,079 nursing facility residents across the United States, clustered predominantly in densely populated states such as New York, Pennsylvania, Texas, Illinois, California, and Ohio (Kaiser Family Foundation 2019). The Center for Disease Control and Prevention (2020) confirmed that the coronavirus pandemic disproportionately impacted the elderly in these nursing home facilities, where significantly higher rates of severe illness and death were reported (CDC 2021). By the end of June 2020—only three months into the pandemic—at least 54,000 residents and workers had died from COVID-19 in nursing homes and long-term care (LTC) facilities in the United States. Some 264,000 people were infected across 9912 sites, and those numbers would rise substantially in the months that followed (Hochman 2020). Hochman (2020) highlighted the ways in which nursing homes bore the brunt of the pandemic using one stunning statistic: residents of LTC facilities constitute less than 1% of the US population, yet 43% of all COVID-19 deaths occurred in those sites. Lack of adequate PPE, slow response plans, and poor social distancing were cited as key causes for the disproportionate impact on America's elderly. But these types of practical explications focus largely on material or physical manifestations of health alone while ignoring other social determinants. They overlook epistemological questions such as how geographical spaces for the elderly are constructed apart from society rather than *within* it and how, in turn, that form of spatial clustering of seniors contributes to death rates. In short, some societies "place" elderly in communities far removed from immediate families where care is outsourced, while states like Senegal regard seniors as venerable and important lifelong members of extended families and compounds. In sum, Senegal's human geography of geriatrics is as different from the United States as its physical climate, landforms, or biomes.

In fairness, Senegal's elderly population is relatively small compared to the United States and comprises approximately 4.7% of the country's predominantly younger demographic (Johns Hopkins 2021). But this does not negate the fact that state health policies combined with community-level respect for the elderly have led to unique gerontological geographies that fueled Senegal's COVID-19 triumphs (Fig. 7.3). In 2006, then President Abdoulaye Wade instituted measures to guarantee free access to health care for senior citizens as part of the "Sésame Plan" (Silver Eco 2016). The initiative ensured that not only would seniors living in urban centers (i.e., Dakar) have access to sophisticated health care but that elderly cohorts in rural sectors would be equally served. In 2006, Senegal boasted only eight geriatricians in a population of nearly 16 million, but new efforts to recognize and support so-called gray power are

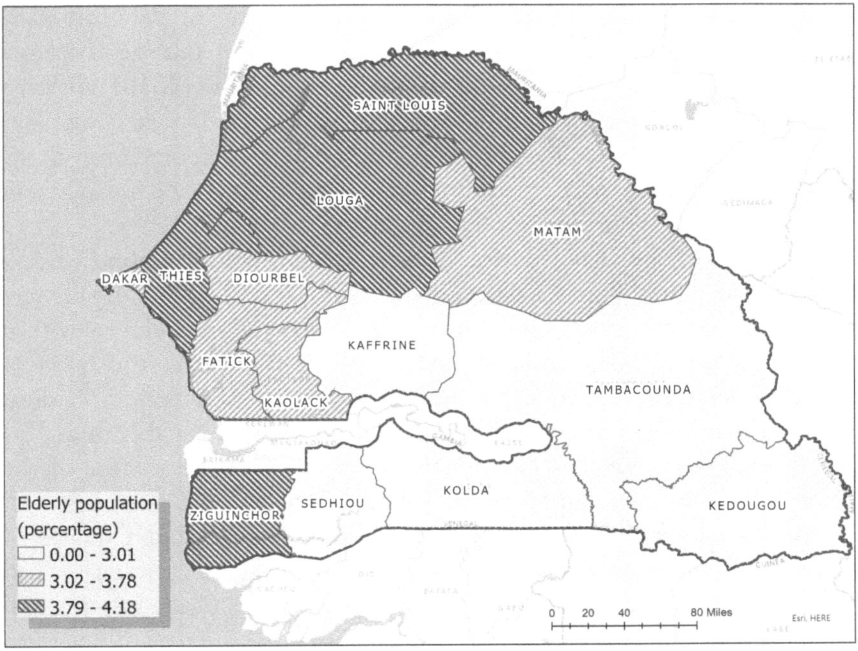

Fig. 7.3 Percentage of elderly per region (>60)

underway and are evolving (Honda et al. 2019). Yet a dominant focus on new state-of-the-art medical initiatives for the elderly overlooks the enduring cultural systems already in place to help support aging populations (Ka et al. 2019). Extended family compounds in Senegal—in contrast to traditional, Western style nursing homes—have promoted mobility, social interaction, and engagement for centuries. This is particularly important in the face of a global pandemic, where extended family compounds can serve as safe spaces for vulnerable populations, allowing seniors to social distance within their own family bubbles.

Islam has also played an important yet undervalued role in Senegal's pandemic success story, given the dominance of the faith across large parts of West Africa. Senegal is 94% Muslim, rooted in the Sunni Maliki school of jurisprudence with Sufi influences, and for a millennium, it has maintained a strong and important presence in the country (Pew Forum 2010). Religion pervades nearly every aspect of Senegalese society and is both a product and practice of everyday life; in terms of the built environment, mosques of all scales are found in both rural and urban sectors of the state. The Pew's Forum sub-Saharan Africa study (2010) confirms this fact; some 98% of those interviewed in Senegal say that religion plays a "very important" role in their lives, the highest percentage for all 19 SSA states included in Pew's comprehensive study. Mali and Tanzania, at 93%, fell closely behind in survey results (Pew Forum 2010).

Recent work by Bensaid and Grine (2014) provides a good understanding of how Islamic religious beliefs, laws, and spiritual practices shape attitudes toward not only old age but the position of elderly within society and space. The topic of the elderly is present in the body of Muslim literature, particularly in the works of Qur'anic exegesis, hadith, law, and manners in general (Ngom 2016). In his al-Adab al Mufrad, for instance, Bukhari (d. 870) devotes three chapters to the theme of the elderly; notably the Chapter of the Old Person, "bab al kabir"; Chapter of the Virtue of the Old Person, "bab fadl al-kabir"; and Chapter of Priority of the Old Person as first in both speech and question, "bab yubda' al-akbar bi al-kalam wa al-su'al" (Bensaid and Grine 2014, 142). Islam exhibits a deep appreciation for a life that is long and full of righteousness and moral goodness (16). For Sufis, old age provides the individual with the opportunity for self-purification and reform while also emphasizing the significance of the social role they occupy within the community at large. That elderly individuals were afforded critical, equitable care at the onset of the pandemic is a product of these key cultural-religious tenets of Islam. In short, these sociocultural and religious beliefs about the elderly, in particular, and humanity, in general, have also contributed to the country's resounding success in the face of COVID-19. This socioreligious dimension helps us understand that Senegal's low case count is more than an accidental by-product of its youthful population.

Widespread Support for Social Distancing

Senegal's science-driven measures to promote public health during the pandemic were met with widespread public support for mask wearing and social distancing, in contrast to what was seen in some parts of the world. To achieve such wholesale community support, the state enlisted local artists and painters to assist with national messaging or propaganda early on in the crisis. Beginning as early as April 2020, stunning graffiti was emblazoned on the walls of Cheikh Anta Diop University and the Faculty of Medicine Hospital in Dakar, reminding citizens to follow recommended health guidelines (UNAIDS 2020). This graffiti uses the power of public imagery and universal semiotics to promote community health. Organized by the RBS Crew collective, artists painted sketches of people handwashing, mask wearing, or "sleeving their sneezes" or just simple images of hand sanitizers. Religious officials, including the popular Mouride Muslim Brotherhood, also marshalled efforts to promote public health, utilizing public

displays and billboards to encourage mask usage (Fig. 7.4). This is essential given the influence that the Sufi and religious orders have across the state, whether it be in urban centers or rural locales. Clearly, Senegal was proud of its ability to harness social capital to combat coronavirus despite having limited capital resources compared to other developed states. *Le Poste*, Senegal's founding philatelic institution, would even scramble to create a COVID-19 postage stamp in 2020 to memorialize

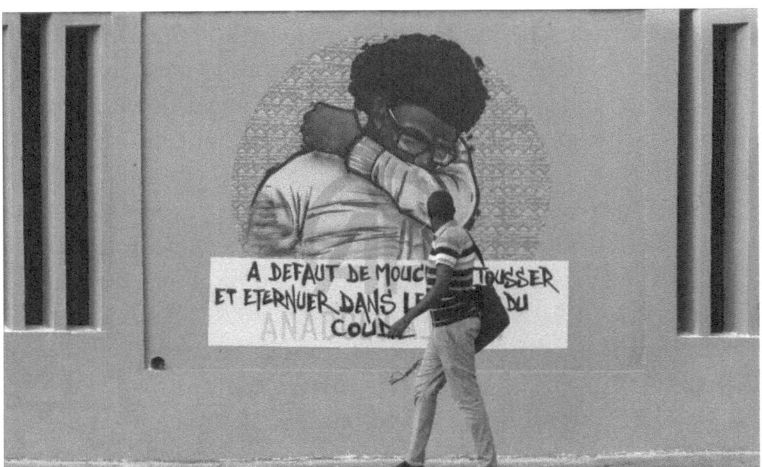

Fig. 7.4 Sleeve Your Sneeze Graffiti

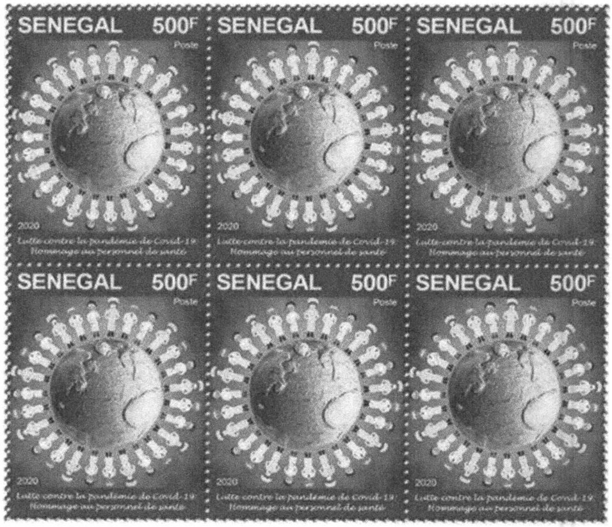

Fig. 7.5 Combat coronavirus postage stamp. (*Le Poste* 2020)

the pandemic and pay homage to those who fought valiantly to control its diffusion (Fig. 7.5). The "Combat Coronavirus" stamp series features an array of masked humans encircling the planet that at first glance resembles the virus itself. The inscription (*hommage du personnel de santé*) pays tribute to the frontline health workers toiling in villages across the state. The engraving shows how Senegal amplifies the hard work of its own health institutions while simultaneously recognizing its spatial connections with the rest of the world.

Perhaps the most important data illustrating the extent of public support for coronavirus health policies was that of Partnership for Evidence-Based COVID-19 Response, which drew on findings from a poll of 24,000 adults in 18 African countries (PERC 2020). Among other social determinants, the data revealed that Africans in general showed immense public support for COVID-19 state-mandated health measures. Most interviewees in the study reported either "completely adhering" or "mostly adhering" to washing hands, avoiding handshakes, wearing masks in public, avoiding places of worship, public gatherings, and reducing shopping trips (PERC 2020). Some 85% of Senegalese specifically complied with mask wearing in public according to the PERC study. Yet we argue that these impressive results should also be considered in the context of the cultural conditions in which such pandemic-related sacrifices are made. Avoiding handshakes or public gatherings in a state as socially and community oriented as West Africa is a remarkable achievement compared to nations where daily social interactions are not as embedded or commonplace in everyday life. The typical Senegalese greeting—in which protracted conversations or handshakes require prolonged human contact—play a critical and necessary role in society, but such protocols were largely set aside for the sake of controlling the pandemic.

Pilgrimage to Touba in 2020

The 2020 Magal religious festival—in which pilgrims across West Africa flock to the city of Touba—provides further evidence that Senegal managed the pandemic through widespread public support for COVID-19 measures. This is especially noteworthy given the intense spatial interaction of pilgrimages and the ways in which they challenge social distancing goals (Barton 2020b). Magal is a Wolof word derived from the verb "mag," which means "important" or to be old", and the Magal pilgrimage is important because of its connection to Shayk Amadou Bamba, founder of the Mouride Brotherhood, a major sect of Sufi Islam (Ngom 2016). Founded in 1887 and completed in 1963, the Great Mosque of the city shrine was constructed on Bamba's burial site, and today Touba is one of the larger metropolitan sectors of Senegal. With a capacity of 7000 people, the mosque is the destination for the Grand Magal of Touba and is one of the largest religious events in Islam (Ngom 2016). As recently as 2017, some *three million* adherents participated in this annual pilgrimage to Touba, and it was unpredictable whether pilgrims would travel to the city on October 5–6 in light of the 2020 pandemic. Magal is both a ceremony and a festival in which the faithful visit mausoleums of important Mouride leaders but also the city's marketplace, so social interactions are both frequent and intensive (Hoang et al. 2019). In short, Magal is both a religious and a spatial process, one that was neither banned nor encouraged in Senegal during the ongoing coronavirus pandemic, though some local health officials would soon advise against traveling to Touba (Gautret et al. 2020).

In October 2020, the *New York Times* article published a piece arguing, without evidence, that "most people (in Senegal) were going ahead (with Magal) despite the risk" (Maclean 2020; Gautret et al. 2020). But the truth is that only a minority of pilgrims (tens of thousands, versus millions) decided to make the journey to Touba, the vast majority choosing to celebrate Magal in their own extended family compounds or communities instead. Many West Africans spend a lifetime saving financial resources to travel to Touba, and so opting out of this religious festival was likely a difficult personal and family choice (Fisch 2020). But because of these difficult decisions across the region, new COVID-19 case counts did *not* spike in the two weeks following Magal as the global media had predicted in its hyperbolic press pieces (see Fig. 7.6). Recent research by Sokhna et al. (2021a) similarly concludes that there was no significant increase of COVID-19 case counts in Senegal following the 2020 Magal pilgrimage. While no studies have been conducted as to why potential

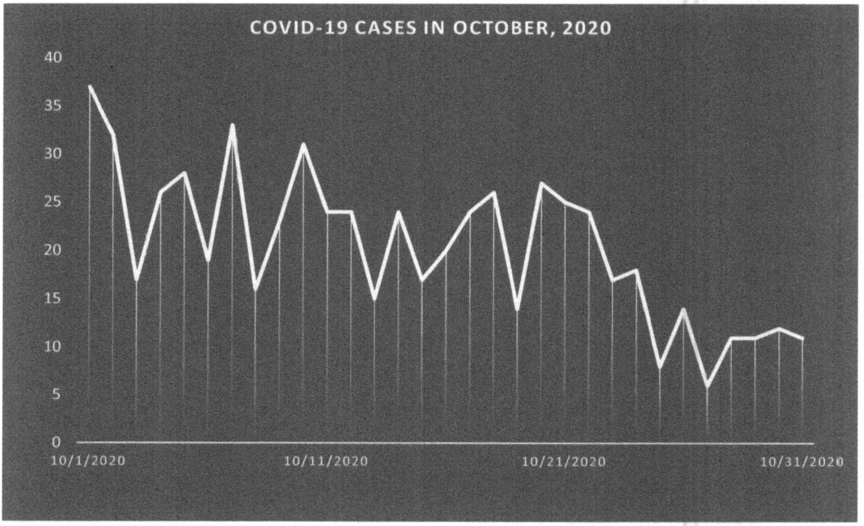

Fig. 7.6 October new case counts for Senegal post-Magal. (Source: JHU CSSE COVID-19)

pilgrims chose to worship "in place" rather than visit Touba, the substantial drop in attendance suggests the pandemic was likely the root cause. Part of this can be attributed to the principles of interdependence and collectivism which dominate Senegal in contrast to other more individualistic societies such as the United States (Gleason 2003). The Senegalese collectivist worldview is motivated primarily by opportunities to help and be helped by other people in their social networks, and this dimension is crucial for understanding how Senegal managed to excel in its management of COVID-19.

One point of contrast to Magal is that of the Sturgis, South Dakota, motorcycle rally in the United States; while not a religious pilgrimage, it drew an overwhelming 490,000 bikers during the pandemic in 2020, an attendance dip of only 7.5% from the prior year (Bonnet 2020). Thus, the largest clusters of coronavirus in Senegal were not linked to the Touba pilgrimage but instead aligned with other disease scenarios around the globe; in other words, districts with high rates of urbanization reported high incidence of the infection. Incidence maps illustrate, for example, how administrative districts such as Dakar, Thies, and Saint Louis—the most densely populated, *urbanized* regions in the country—have been hit hardest by the coronavirus (Fig. 7.7). In contrast to predictions made by global media, new COVID-19 case counts plummeted in the weeks following the Grand Magal pilgrimage, and by the end of October, the Health Ministry was reporting less than 15 new cases per day (Fig. 7.6). The *NYT* media report suggesting that religious officials would mandate that pilgrims travel to Magal in the midst of a pandemic was wholly inaccurate. Borders were proactively closed to non-nationals wishing to travel to Touba from beyond Senegal, and religious leaders formed an integral part of national health initiatives to control the spread of coronavirus (Sokhna et al. 2021b). The sky did not "fall" in Senegal, as was predicted, despite media attempts to perpetuate long-standing disease narratives related to Africa. Senegal instead took on a unique leadership role in managing the global pandemic though it was seldom included in the pantheon of states who were credited for crushing coronavirus and its diffusion.

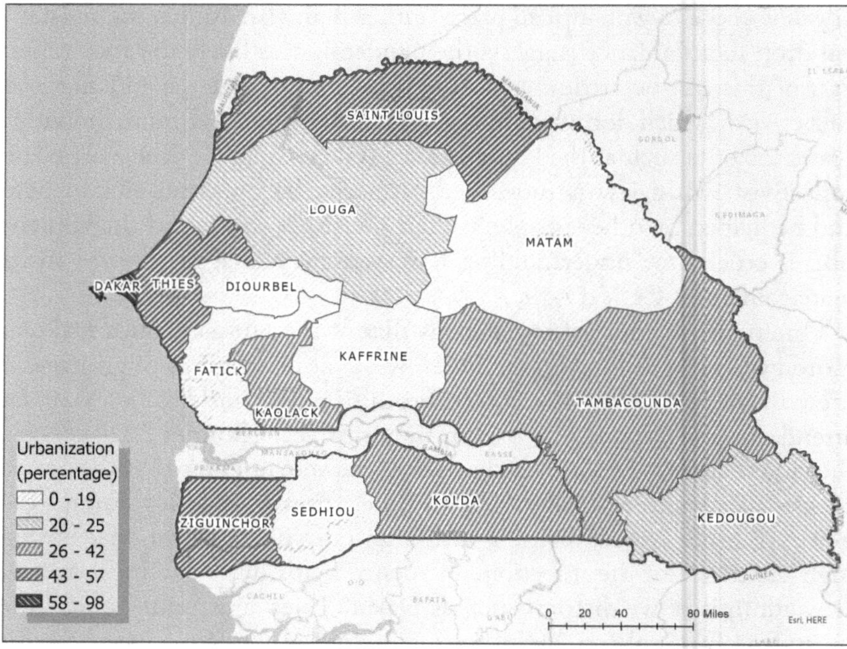

Fig. 7.7 Urbanization rates in Senegal

Environmental Conditions

One final explanation harnessed by the media to explain the low level of COVID-19 case counts across Senegal, in particular, and Africa, in general, relative to other world regions, is that of climate. Six months into the coronavirus pandemic, the BBC cited a study in which temperature, humidity, and latitude were analyzed in order to estimate potential spread and seasonality of coronavirus (Soy 2020). The study concluded that with spatial modeling it was possible to estimate an area of high risk of substantial community transmission of COVID-19 (Jamshidi et al. 2020). News outlets quickly applied this research to the African context, arguing that owing to its dominant position along the tropical belt, where temperatures and higher relative humidity are higher, COVID case counts would be significantly reduced (BBC 2020). The example of

South Africa—which contains half of the continent's coronavirus cases and straddles cooler latitudinal regimes—was employed to support this environmental argument. Yet despite its high latitudinal position, Köppen-Geiger maps reveal that South Africa actually contains a total of 13 different climate zones, from desert to humid subtropical, thus defying the BBC's environmental deterministic explanatory positions on coronavirus (BBC 2020). New data has also confirmed the ways in which warmer, more humid locales like Brazil and Florida, which fall partly within Köppen's tropical climate regime, actually showed *higher* transmission rates and case counts (Auler et al. 2020; Johns Hopkins 2021).

The truth is that the link between climate and COVID-19 is fundamentally complicated (Zaitchik et al. 2020). Weather influences the environment in which the coronavirus must survive before infecting a new host, but it also influences human behavior, which shifts the virus from one host to another. Recent research (Jamshidi et al. 2020) adds clarity to weather's role in COVID-19 infections, suggesting that temperature and humidity do *not* play a significant role in the coronavirus spread (World Meteorological Organization 2020). Taking trips and spending time away from home were the top two contributing factors to COVID-19 growth, with a relative importance of about 34% and 26%, respectively. The next two important factors were population and urban density, with a relative importance of about 23% and 13%, respectively (Jamshidi et al. 2020). That the media chose to harness environmentally deterministic arguments such as climate to explain Senegal's strong track record with COVID-19 was not surprising given the long-standing tropes about the continent. As we have shown in this chapter, however, Senegal did not *stumble* upon its success in managing this global pandemic; rather it relied upon age-old community-based structures in conjunction with rapid response systems to combat COVID's incursion into West Africa.

Moving Forward

While we have illustrated Senegal's important strides in managing COVID-19, further steps should be considered in order to ensure human safety and move toward achieving sustainable development goals. As noted earlier, early measures such as rapid response systems were critical in ensuring Senegal's pandemic successes, but bolstered screening and early detection measures can allow the country to better manage the ongoing pandemic (in World Economic Forum 2021) For example, early on in the outbreak, all of Senegal's detected cases were found following individual medical appointments at health facilities, known commonly as "passive" detection. An *active* health monitoring and diagnostic system would therefore allow Senegalese health officials to seek out disease incidence rather than stumble upon it. Furthermore, only a portion of COVID-19 recorded cases were geocoded[2] (see Figs. 7.1, 7.3, 7.7), which prevents a more nuanced understanding of the pandemic's spatial distribution across Senegal. This murky view of rural-urban disparities in Senegal can subsequently affect the efficacy of health screening, monitoring, and vaccine distribution.

That President Sall declared a State of Emergency (February 3, 2021) following pandemic's second wave underscores Senegal's need to focus on COVID-19 impacts in more populated urban centers. The map in Fig. 7.7 highlights the way in which Senegal's large urban sectors were hit hardest as evidenced by the high incidence of disease in Dakar, Thies, and Saint Louis. This disparity is a function of a long-standing urban core-rural periphery structure where high population densities continue to place pressure on existing health and community resources. Yet while the highest incidence of COVID-19 is in cities, the rural south (Casamance) still requires equitable health and medical attention, given its ongoing marginalization from the urban north. Senegalese officials should continue to collaborate with outreach workers in these rural outposts to provide necessary resources to aid them in the ongoing pandemic. This collaboration might involve an active vaccination plan that leverages global support—such as the COVAX initiative led by the WHO and CEPI Gavi Alliance—in order to ensure equal access to health resources across the country.

Despite Senegal's robust policies to eradicate poverty and inequalities, the pandemic also has threatened to reverse national efforts to reduce

[2] A description of a location—such as a pair of coordinates, an address, or a name of a place—to a location on the earth's surface.

gender equality in line with United Nations' goals. Recent reports show that rural women have long suffered economic setbacks, due in part to their participation in the informal sector and the insecure income that accompanies these activities (Diagana 2020). But with the adoption of the COVID-19 lockdown and restriction measures, women became increasingly responsible for family duties, thus exacerbating existing gender disparities (Ba 2020). A recent study (Dione et al. 2021) revealed how Senegalese women and adolescent girls have suffered from food shortages (65%) and limited spatial mobility due to basic travel restrictions (85%) in the wake of the pandemic; in fact, women in rural areas (Kolda) were impacted more than those living in urban areas (Kaolack). Therefore, while the government has provided pandemic assistance to disadvantaged households across Senegal, more policies are needed to protect rural women and girls from economic insecurity and disproportionate care burdens.

Conclusion

The main conclusion we glean from this work is that Africa's problems require African solutions, or solutions designed with Africans in mind. This is particularly applicable in the case example of Senegal's management of COVID-19 from its outset in 2020 (World Health Organization 2019, 2020; Magome 2020). We suggest that developed world regions can borrow from health initiatives generated in emerging African states like Senegal, where officials aggressively quashed the diffusion of the coronavirus pathogen by harnessing sound science, technology, respect for elderly, and repurposing rapid response teams from earlier pandemics like the Ebola (Akindele et al. 2020). Senegal has clearly made impressive strides in pandemic management—with a total of 561 deaths despite a national population of 16 million—yet it has been largely downplayed by media institutions that tend to amplify coronavirus narratives in developed states over that of developing ones. We argue that this oversight is fundamentally rooted in widespread characterizations of Africa, the "diseased continent" in which areas south of the Sahara are seen as breeding grounds for new pathogens rather than hearths for health-based innovations (World Meteorological Organization 2020). When Senegal's COVID-related successes are in fact acknowledged by the media, they are often justified by demographic or deterministic variables such as climate and environment. The subtext of this dominant discourse is that African states somehow *stumbled upon* their successes rather than self-generated their solutions. The reality is that Senegal authored its unique, community-based approach in managing the coronavirus pathogen by heavily prioritizing people over profit. Their achievements should be amplified along with other states like New Zealand in the pantheon of countries that effectively managed the COVID-19 crisis in 2020. Coronavirus continues to be an emerging, rapidly evolving situation, but regardless of what unfolds, this will not negate the fact that we have much to learn from Senegal's early management of the pandemic.

References

Akindele, Abidemi, et al. 2020. COVID-19 Pandemic: A Case for Phytomedicines.". *Natural Product Communications* 15 (8). https://doi.org/10.1177/1934578X20945086.

Al Jazeera. 2020. A Timeline of the Trump Administration's Coronavirus Actions. April 23, 2020.

Auler, A.C., F. Cassaro, V. da Silva, and L. Pires. 2020. Evidence That High Temperatures and Intermediate Relative Humidity Might Favor the Spread of COVID-19 in Tropical Climate: A Case Study for the Most Affected Brazilian Cities. *Science of the Total Environment* 729: 139090. https://doi.org/10.1016/j.scitotenv.2020.139090.

Ba, Selly. 2020. COVID-19: What Will Be the Impact on Gender Inequality in Senegal? Gunda Werner Institute.

Barton, Karen. 2020a. *Africa's Joola Shipwreck: Causes and Consequences of a Humanitarian Disaster*. Lanham: Lexington (Imprint of Rowman and Littlefield).

———. 2020b. Geography, Islam, and Africa. Chapter 8 in *The Palgrave Handbook of Islam in Africa*, ed. Fallou Ngom, Mustapha Kuri, and Toin Falola, Kuri. Switzerland: Palgrave Macmillan.

BBC News. 2020. Coronavirus in Senegal: Keeping COVID at Bay. October 4, 2020.

Bensaid, Benaouda, and Fadila Grine. 2014. Old Age and Elderly Care: An Islamic Perspective. *Cultura, International Journal of Philosophy of Culture and Axiology* 11 (1): 141–163. https://doi.org/10.5840/cultura20141119.

Bonnet, Siandhara. 2020. Attendance Down, but Spending up at 80th Sturgis Motorcycle Rally. August 15, 2020. *Rapid City Journal.*

Campbell, John. 2020. The Potential for the Coronavirus in Africa. February 12, 2020. *Council on Foreign Relations.*

Center for Disease Control. 2021. Rates of COVID-19 Among Residents and Staff Members in Nursing Homes—United States, May 25–November 22, 2020.

Center for Global Development. 2020. Senegal's Response to COVID-19. May 29, 2020.

Desjardins, Jeff. 2019. Mapped: The Median Age of the Population on Every Continent. February 15, 2019. *Visual Capitalist.*

Diagana, Ousmane. 2020. *The Silent Epidemic.* World Bank, December 10, 2020.

Diamond, Jared. 1998. *Guns, Germs and Steel.* New York: WW Norton.

Dione, Malick, Codé Lo, Moustapha Seye, Abdou Salam Fall, Melissa Hidrobo, Agnès Le Port, Jessica Heckert, and Amber Peterman. 2021. *Women and Adolescent Girls' Experience with COVID-19 in Rural Senegal.* Policy Note, February 2021. Washington, DC: International Food Policy Research Institute (IFPRI).

Dudley, Dominic. 2020. Kuwait Deports 360,00 Foreigners as Gulf's Expat Exodus Continues. August 11, 2020. *Forbes.*

Fink, Sheri. 2020. As Virus Resurges in Africa, Doctors Fear Worst to Come. December 26, 2020. *New York Times.*

Fisch, Yesica. 2020. Tens of Thousands Attend Senegalese Pilgrimage Despite COVID-19. October 10, 2020. *Taiwan News.*

Foley, Erin. 2001. No Money, No Care: Women and Health Sector Reform in Senegal. *Health Policy, and Health Care Delivery in Africa*, Spring 2001: 1–50.

Gautret, Phillipe, Ndiaw Goumballa, Van Thuan Hoang, and Cheik Sokhna. 2020. The 2020 Grand Magal of Touba, Senegal in the Time of the COVID-19 Pandemic. *Travel Med Infectious Diseases* November–December, Published Online 2020 September 17. https://doi.org/10.1016/j.tmaid.2020.101880.

GIS Lounge. 2020. The Johns Hopkins Coronavirus Map Dashboard Receives a Billion Hits a Day. April 7, 2020.

Gleason, Michael. 2003. *Cultural Models of Individualism and Collectivism in a Context of Development: Self-Efficacy Versus Interdependency in Rural Senegal.* Doctoral Dissertation, University of Georgia.

Harrisburg, Kim. 2020. Here's How Africans are Using Tech to Combat the Coronavirus Pandemic. April 5, 2020. World Economic Forum.

Hoang, V.T., N. Goumballa, T.L. Dao, T.D.A. Ly, L. Ninove, and S. Ranque. 2019. Respiratory and Gastrointestinal Infections at the 2017 Grand Magal de Touba, Senegal: A Prospective Cohort Survey. *Travel Medicine* and *Infectious Disease.* 32.

Hochman, David. 2020. Four Months That Left 54,000 Dead From COVID in Long-Term Care. December 3, 2020. Association of American Retired Persons.

Honda, Ayako, Nicolas Krucien, Mandy Ryan, Ibrahama Diouf, Malick Salla, Mari Nagai, and Fujito Noriko. 2019. For More Than Money: Willingness of Health Professionals to Stay in Remote Senegal. *Human Resources for Health* 17 (28). https://doi.org/10.1186/s12960-019-0363-7

Ihekweazu, Chickwu, and Emmanuel Agogo. 2020. Africa's Response to COVID-19. *BMC Medicine* 18: 151.

Jamshidi, Sajad, Maryam Aniasad, and Dev Niyogi. 2020. Global to USA County Scale Analysis of Weather, Urban Density, Mobility, Homestay, and Mask Use on COVID-19. *International Journal of Environmental Research and Public Health* 17 (21): 7847. https://doi.org/10.3390/ijerph17217847.

Johns Hopkins University. 2021. COVID-19 Data Repository by the Center for Systems Science and Engineering (CSSE). https://github.com/CSSEGISandData/COVID-19.

Ka, Ousseynou, Boris Arthur Aboua Ghebi, Abdoul Aziz Ndiaye, Mamadou Makhtar Mbacke Leye, Mamadou Diallo, and Souhaibou Ndongo. 2019. The Determinants of Fall in the Elderly at the Geriatric Center of Ouakam (Senegal). *World Journal of Public Health* 4 (1): 24–29.

Kaiser Family Foundation. 2019. Total Number of Residents in Certified Nursing Facilities.

Lemière, Christope, Vincent Turbat, and Juliette Puret. 2012. *A Tale of Excessive Hospital Autonomy: An Evaluation of the Hospital Reform in Senegal.* World Bank, HNP Discussion Paper.

Maclean, Ruth. 2020. The Pilgrimage Must Go On: Senegal Holds Festival That Could Draw Millions. October 6, 2020. *New York Times.*

Magome, Mogotsi. 2020. Several African Nations Roll out Measures to Fight Virus. March 15, 2020. *American Broadcasting Corporation News.*

Monmonmeier, Mark. 1991. *How to Lie With Maps.* Chicago: University of Chicago Press.

National Public Radio. 2020. *Senegal Pledges a Bed For Every Patient.* Goats and Soda Series, May 17, 2020.

Ngom, Fallou. 2016. *Muslims Beyond the Arab World: The Odyssey of Ajami and the Muriddya.* New York: Oxford University Press.

Ojeda, Glenn. 2012. Understanding Senegalese Exceptionalism and Religious Tolerance. October 5, 2012. Berkeley Center.

Partnership for Evidenced-Based COVID Response (PERC). 2020. Using Data to Find a Balance: Part 2.

Paul, Elisabeth, Youssoupha Ndiaye, Farba Sall, Fabienne Fecher, and Denis Porignon. 2020. An Assessment of the Core Capacities of the Senegalese Health System to Deliver Universal Health Coverage. *Health Policy Open.* https://doi.org/10.1016/j.hpopen.2020.100012.

Pew Forum. 2010. *Tolerance and Tension: Islam and Christianity in Sub-Saharan Africa.* New York: Pew Forum on Religion and Public Life.

Seydi, Moussa. 2018. Personal Communication, Ngaparou, Senegal.

Silver Eco. 2016. Senegal Takes Steps Toward Ensuring the Well-Being of Elders. September 9, 2016. silvereco.org/en/senegal-takes-steps-towards-ensuring-the-wellbeing-of-elders/.

Sokhna, Cheikh, et al. 2021a. The Grand Magal of Touba was Spared by the COVID-19 Pandemic. *International Journal of Infectious Diseases,* Published Online January 9, 2021. https://doi.org/10.1016/j.ijid.2021.01.006.

Sokhna, C., N. Goumballa, and P. Gautret. 2021b. The Grand Magal of Touba in the Time of a Dengue Outbreak in Senegal. *Travel Medicine and Infectious Disease* 28: 107–108.

Soy, Anna. 2020. Coronavirus in Africa: Five Reasons Why COVID-19 Has Been Less Deadly Than Elsewhere. *BBC News,* October 7, 2020.

UNAIDS. 2020. Lessons Learned from HIV for COVID-19 in Senegal. June 3, 2020.

US Embassy in Senegal. 2020. The Contribution of the United States to Senegal's Response to COVID-19. April 2, 2020.

World Bank. 2020. Hospital Beds (per 1000). World Bank Indicators.

World Economic Forum. 2021. Go Early, Go Hard and Keep It Simple: How Senegal Is Staying Ahead of the COVID-19 Pandemic. February 3, 2021.

World Health Organization. 2019. *WHO Global Report on Traditional and Complementary Medicine.* Geneva: World Health Organization.

———. 2020. WHO Supports Scientifically-Proven Traditional Medicine. May 4 2020.
World Meteorological Organization. 2020. Health? Correlations: Busting the Myths.
Yeung, Peter. 2020. Cheap and Easy $1 Coronavirus Test to Undergo Trials in Senegal. May 13, 2020. *New Scientist.*
Zaitchik, Benjamin, et al. 2020. A Framework for Research Linking Weather, Climate, and COVID-19. *Nature Communications* 11 (1): 5730.

8

Ẹnulẹbọ: Ethical Imperative of Yorùbá Thought on Eating for COVID-19-Related Crises

Adewale O. Owoseni

Introduction

The ongoing COVID-19 pandemic around the world reiterates again the downside of the human-Other relationship. This is due to the insensitive subjugation of the *Other* in vulnerable position or status, including non-human animals. These animals are oftentimes the subject of indiscriminate objectification as mere utility/tools in the course of human engagement with them. And this results in far-reaching consequences that demand expedient resolution; otherwise, the threat of human extinction looms. We speak here of the stark reality of indiscriminate engagement of animals as source of food, experimental tool for laboratory tests, and object of use in industrial and agricultural complex, among others, which have led to certain consequences like extinction of rare species/

A. O. Owoseni (✉)
Department of Philosophy, University of Ibadan, Ibadan, Nigeria

Center for the Advancement of Scholarship (CAS), University of Pretoria, Pretoria, South Africa

F. Egbokhare, A. Afolayan (eds.), *Global Health, Humanity and the COVID-19 Pandemic*, https://doi.org/10.1007/978-3-031-17429-2_8

habitat, eco-biodiversity crises, and changes that demand practical initiative as well as management.

The pervasive reality of the COVID-19 pandemic emerged out of the pursuit of human survival through feeding on pangolins, a situation that seems, in recent times, to have earned China (where the practice of eating pangolins is prominent) the label of a "contagious" nation. The extent of the widespread of COVID-19 infection has also implicated the charge of conspiracy from China to the far-reaching ends of the USA, WHO, and other prominent international agencies (Wang X et al. 2021b). This has fueled the prevalence of distrust, suspicion of ill intention, unreliability, as well as blame game along the corridors of international polity. While strategic efforts and literature have been generated to re-humanize the world through various strategies to mitigate the wide spread of COVID-19 to ensure the safety of the human race, ethical reflections from indigenous contexts that could also proffer complementary efforts are yet to be given critical consideration. Leveraging on this gap, this discourse gestures in that direction through a critical analysis of the Yorùbá indigenous conception of eating to further mitigate the far-reaching effects of COVID-19-related crises in terms of suspicion, distrust, unreliability, and blame game, among others.

In light of this, the chapter is divided into three sections. The first section examines the polemics of human and animal relations in lieu of COVID-19, with specific reference to the philosophical debate surrounding the idea of eating as a pattern of human relations with animals. The second section extends this background of philosophical debate to the context of eating as an ordinary and extraordinary norm of sacrifice within Yorùbá thought. Also, it explores other Yorùbá beliefs about the significance of "eating" (as sacrifice) to enhance a balanced and harmonious existential state of affairs. Section three focuses on the ethical implication of indigenous Yorùbá thought on eating to the ongoing COVID-19 pandemic; also, the need to incorporate its heuristic value within the global order toward the mitigation of the undesirable consequences of COVID-19-related crises is thus emphasized.

The Goat as a Scapegoat: COVID-19 and the Phenomenon of Eating

Ewúrẹ́ jẹ́ ẹran-ilé tó máa ń ji ìyà púpọ̀ nítorí àìgbọràn rẹ̀.
(The goat is a domestic animal that deserves beating due to its disobedient nature.)

The foregoing expression is an opening line of a popular Yorùbá nursery rhyme that is often deployed to teach little children about the consequences of disobedience and recalcitrance. While the heuristic essence of deploying the metaphor of the goat as a scapegoat is commendable for the enhancement of good behavioral tendency in children, its devise of animals (through the significance of the goat) as the embodied victim of disobedience legitimizes the trend of indiscriminate humans' attitudinal disposition that shapes human engagement with animals. In other words, human framing of animals as object for enacting the moral significance of human sociality extends to biological, physical, and metaphysical rationale of human relationship with animals. In this sense, the sociocultural conferment of entitlement to beat the goat (since it embodies some attributes, subject to human standards) similarly foregrounds the reason for framing animals as veritable source of food or nutrients, tools for experimentation, and vector of diseases, among other possible range of human engagement with animals.

Such situation seems to suggest that the valuation of animals and their essence is subject to human discretion and for the purpose of furthering human existence and well-being. This position is exclusively anthropocentric and hence toxic for its non-consideration of nonhuman well-being within the environment. And this is even despite the fact that it could be projected through the prism of weak anthropocentrism[1] in mainstream Western philosophy (Norton 1982). In Christos Lynteris (2019), we find a significant argument corroborating the human framing of animals as "epidemic villains," especially within the context of the global incidence of the COVID-19 pandemic. Lynteris's argument turns

[1] Weak anthropocentrism expounds the idea that human values are the foundation of nonhuman and environmental values.

critical attention to the implication of the biopolitics of blaming nonhuman animals as vectors or host of the disease through which the human race is confronted with the threat of extinction. Besides the undercurrent of bio-political dynamics of the global pandemic, the socioeconomic factor of global contestations of states like the USA and China as well as international agencies like WHO cannot be underrated (NYtimes 2020; World Health 2020; Brooking Institutions 2020).

Lynteris's contention further demonstrates the need to re-consider the bio-political blame game charge against animals in light of their subdued agency as object of consumption for the satiation of human nutritional needs as well. It follows that the process of consumption or eating becomes a value-based phenomenon that demands critical engagement in lieu of the consequences of humans' will to survive. This implies that it is not enough to reduce the cause of the COVID-19 pandemic to the animal vector of the viral disease without antecedently reflecting on the point of entanglement between the agency of human and animal. It is difficult to deny that the agency of animals becomes subdued at the moment they are commodified as source of food or nutrient for human consumption, while the agency of human lives becomes active through the process of consuming or eating the animals. Generally, it is believed that pangolins, consumed in Wuhan, China (the source of the spread of the disease) is one of the major reservoirs of COVID-19. Eating, within this context, therefore raises the philosophical issue around the moral justification of humans feeding on the nonhuman *Other*, especially animals and plants. Alastair Norcross's (2004: 229–245) narrates the experience of Fred who, because of the loss of his taste buds due to a terrible accident, set up a basement laboratory that enabled him to process the cocanemone present in brains of piglets in ways that allowed him to regain his taste for mousse chocolate.

This story provides the justification for the human legitimization of eating (in order to attain a pleasurable gustatory experience) that involves horrific inflictions of pains on animals. This justification for eating drives the practice of factory farming and industrial production of animals as utility "patients" for the satiation of human desires, needs, and ultimately survival. While human need to eat in order to survive is not underrated by Norcross, overreliance on feeding on animals over other sources of nutrient is contended. This implies that the nullification of the human practice of eating animals is not tantamount to the privation of human well-being. Within the field of animal ethics, such reasoning is strengthened by the arguments that disapprove human treatment of animals as marginal objects due to certain criteria of capacities. Such arguments are referred to as argument from marginal cases.

Arguments from marginal cases spur the controversy of whether it is equally reasonable or otherwise, to indiscriminately instrumentalize humans, especially those in persistent vegetative state, the senile, or the infants, in similar ways that animals are used. This is because the senile, vegetative, and infant are lacking in moral responsibility, obligations, rationality, and consciousness. In other words, if the argument for the consumption of animals is founded on human exceptionalism justified by their capacities for rationality, functional cognitive capacity, moral responsibility, or agency, among others, over animals, then it follows that the consumption of humans in marginal conditions also makes moral sense. Scholars like Carl Cohen (1986), Mary Anne Warren (1987), and David Schmidtz (1998) disapprove of this analogous justification of treating humans (in this context, eating humans) in marginal conditions the same way we would treat or relate with animals. Warren (1987: 483) opines that there are indeed "powerful practical and emotional reasons for protecting non-rational human being, reasons which are absent in the case of nonhuman animals." For Cohen, the failure of the arguments from marginal cases lies in the fact that:

> It mistakenly treats an essential feature of humanity as though it were a screen for sorting humans. The capacity for moral judgement that distinguishes humans from animals is not a test to be admonished to human beings one by one. Persons who are unable, because of some disability to perform the full moral functions natural to human beings, are certainly not for that reason rejected from the moral community. ... What humans retain when disabled, animals have never had. (Cohen 1986: 461)

Thus, for Cohen, Warren, and others, being a human in marginal states or condition is not a sufficient reason for advancing the argument for eating humans in the same way we eat animals. In other words, according to

Schmidtz (1998: 61), humans and animals are "relevantly different types." For Jeremy Bentham (2000) and Peter Singer (1975), acknowledging the capacity commonly shared by humans and animals is cogent for gauging human treatment of animals prior to the consideration of the relevant differences between them. Both scholars argued that the shared experience of sentiency or capacity to feel pain is a sufficient criterion for the moral consideration of humans and animals. If this argument holds, then we have what it takes to mitigate the indiscriminate abuse and killing of animals for food, as well as subjection of animals to intense harm situation of factory farming, experimental laboratory, and other forms of engagement, which objectify animals.

Bentham and Singer's radical argument for elevating the status of animal to that of subject has received serious critical attention in environmental ethics and critical animal studies. But this will not detain us here. The crucial point that brought us to this discourse is worth reiterating. This is the point that human consumption or eating of animals is a pattern of human relationship (as *Self*) with animals (as an inclusive *Other*), and there are extant arguments in Western philosophical discourse that proffer arguments for or against the moral justification of eating animals. It takes little reflection to argue that the incidence of COVID-19 becomes inevitable given the logic of the human-centered understanding of eating the *Other*. This eating dynamics must contend, inevitably again, with the fact that the *Other* sometimes serve as hosts to various viruses waiting to find more suitable hosts. The viral occupation of the body or the environment of the hosts, in most cases, poses a threat to the host's survival. The instance of the mortality rate of human persons due to COVID-19 has manifested such threat. Such situation demands aggregating plausible insights from diverse epistemologies and ethics for mitigating the various crises generated by the pandemic. Given this understanding, since the debate regarding the moral justification of human utility of animals is indeed prominent and inexhaustible in Western philosophy, it seems not out of place to counteract with alternative readings deriving from "subaltern" indigenous worldviews regarding the phenomenon of eating (as one of the way in which human utilizes animals), which has far-reaching implication for the realization of harmonious human well-being and state of co-existence. In light of this, the next section considers the example of Yorùbá indigenous notion of eating as an alternative reading to moderate COVID-19-related crises.

Ẹnulẹbọ: "Eating" in Yorùbá Thought

Literature on the cultural phenomenon of eating among the Yorùbá is very rare. The available materials that are proximate to the discourse are concerned with food culture, food taboos, and food taxonomy, among others (Oso 1977; Ogundele 2007; Allen 2014). While intellectual reflection on these proximate issues is prominent, critical consideration of the dialectics of eating within the same culture is less advanced. The expediency of subjecting eating to critical attention stems fundamentally from its general manifestation as a human-centered activity that often commodifies nonhuman entities (plants and animals) as target-object to be eaten. The indigenous Yorùbá of Southwest Nigeria, like most people across the world, are also conditioned by the universal human necessity of eating to enhance the integrity of their health and survival. Literature exists pertaining to what the Yorùbá eat, their culinary practices, and preferences that are subject to many factors which include sociocultural, geographical, topographical, and climatic conditions.[2]

A philosophical reflection derives from a meta-ethical conceptual analysis of the popular indigenous Yorùbá notion of *Ẹnulẹbọ*. Taken from two root words—ẹ*nu* (mouth) and ẹ*bọ* (sacrifice)—*Ẹnulẹbọ* becomes a conceptual assemblage that literally translates as the "mouth is sacrifice." *Ifá*, the Yorùbá divinatory and literary corpus, provides a further understanding of the cultural perception of the relationship between eating, the mouth, and sacrifice that *Ẹnulẹbọ* signifies. According to the fifth verse of *Ọwọ́nrín Méjì* in Odù Ifá (a chapter in *Ifa*):

[2] See Ogunsanya, A. O. 2015. "Changing Pattern in Feeding, Dressing and naming among Yoruba of South-Western Nigeria since 1960. *Nigerian Journal of Social Studies* Vol. XVIII (2).

Ẹnu nií jẹ́ Olúbọ̀bọ̀tiribọ̀ baba ẹbọ	The mouth is Olubobotiribo, father of sacrifice
Ǹjẹ́ kín là mbọ ní' Fẹ̀	What do we worship in Ife?
Ẹnuu wọn	Their mouth
Ẹnuu wọn la mbọ ní' Fẹ̀	It is their mouth we worship at Ife
Ẹnuu wọn	Their mouth.
Mo fún gbá	I did this
Mo fáwo	I did that
Enuu won	Their mouth
Ẹnu wọn kó mọ le rí mi bájà	Their mouth cannot embattle me
Ẹnuu wọn	Their mouth
Mo wálé	I arrived home
Mo wánà	I sojourned
Ẹnuu wọn	Their mouth
Ènuu wọn kó má le rí mi bájà	Their mouth cannot embattle me
Ẹnuu wọn	Their mouth

From the Odù, there are two conceivable senses of *Ẹnulẹbọ*—the literal and the meta-literal. Literally, *Ẹnulẹbọ* refers to the activity of the mouth as the major channel of consumption which determines the human state of health. This also implies that since the mouth is the recipient of food contents, then the latter invariably becomes "the sacrifice ingredient" for the mouth. And, the quotidian necessity of eating to survive implies not only that the mouth accepts food as its daily sacrifice but also that there is an obligation to be mindful of what to offer the mouth as sacrifice in the survival equation. The expression ẹ*nuu wọn là mbọ ní'Fẹ̀* (it is their mouth we worship at Ifẹ̀) in the Odù aptly reiterates this Yorùbá point of view. This also means that in this perspective, the mouth becomes a center of "worship" since it accepts food as daily sacrifice. Such conception also seems to foreground a meta-literal interpretation of the mouth.

At the meta-literal level, the representation of the mouth extends to the moderation of utterances. Thus, the invocation of ẹ*nuu wọn là mbọ ní'Fẹ̀* speaks to the prudential instinct to exercise moderation in utterances that could otherwise undermine peaceful coexistence or generate disharmony in interpersonal relationships. The belief is that anyone who takes this invocation serious and moderate the mouth in interpersonal interaction or engagement receives certitude of safety from ill intentions from vicious forces or persons. The assurance of such safety is what the Odù conveyed in the line *ẹnu wọn ò lè rí mi bájà, mo wálé, mo wánà … ẹnu wọn* (their mouth cannot embattle me, I arrived home, I sojourned … their mouth). The virulence of an untamed mouth therefore becomes the harbinger of chaos in social bonding that should be tamed. Both the literal and the meta-literal conception of the mouth therefore converge around the significance of human well-being and the role of the mouth in mediating it.

However, there is another correlative conception of *ẹnulẹbọ* in Yorùbá thought that is not limited to the heuristic value of eating as an avenue to individual, relational, and social well-being. In this sense, *ẹnulẹbọ* signifies a convergent point of interdependent relationship among humans and between humans and extra-human forces. This point of interdependent relationship is signaled through that act of invitation to eat by a host/supplicant and the acceptance of such invitation by the "target" recipient, which may be humans or extra-human forces. This implies that the practice of invitation and acceptance to eat constitutes a continuum from the realms of humans (i.e., human-to-human relations) to the realm beyond the humans. In this context, eating becomes a communion or what Ann Allen refers to as "communal eating."[3] This is aptly captured in the Yorùbá lyrical chant:

A gbé orí ilẹ̀ a jẹ eku o	We lived on the land, and ate rat together
A gbé orí ilẹ̀, a jẹ ẹja	We lived on the land, and ate fish together
A gbé orí ilẹ̀, a jẹ ìgbín	We lived on the land, and ate snail together
Àṣẹ di ọwọ́ ilẹ̀	The force of our witness is the Land
A jọọ mu[4]	On which we communed together.

[3] See Allen, A. 2015. "Food and Culture: Continuity and Change in the Yoruba of West Africa and their Diasporas." In S. Magliveras and C. Gallin (eds) *Odysseys of Plates and Palates: Food, Society and Sociality*. Oxford, United Kingdom: Inter-Disciplinary Press.

[4] This is culled from Personal Communication with Ifa Priest Olaleye, October 22, 2021. Olaleye is a researcher and scholar of Yoruba religious studies at the Department of Religious Study, University of Ibadan, Nigeria.

As communion, eating generates vertical (human and gods/deities realm) and horizontal (human realm) bonding. When the Yorùbá say, *ẹyẹlé kìí bóníléjẹ, kó bá oníilé mu, kó wá di ọjọ́ ikú, kó yẹrí*—"the dove never dine and wine with the owner of the house and then on the day of death, attempt to flee/escape"—they gesture at a sense of fidelity to care about one another within the context of the shared eating qua communion. This shared sense of fidelity to care for one another yields the state of a balanced self or group/communal fulfilment. The notion of *Akẹ́bọdọ́run* (the conveyor of sacrificial offerings to "heaven") aptly captures the Yorùbá understanding of such balanced sense of self or communal fulfilment. *Akẹ́bọdọ́run* in Yorùbá thought is the frame of reference for the interdependency of all agents (human/nonhuman, host/receiver) involved in the shared eating (i.e., the process of invitation and acceptance to eat), which is propelled by fidelity to care for one another that results into bonding toward a common goal/survival (symbolized by "heaven"). The Odù Ifá about *Alásán, Orí,* and *Òrìsà* recounts the implication of the non-acknowledgement of the implicit sense of fidelity derived from bonding through eating together:

Ifá ní 'ta ni ó tó bá Alásán r'òkun	Ifa asked who will sojourn with Alásán
Ògún ní òun bá' Alásán r'òkun	*Ogun* answered he would sojourn with Alásán
Wọ́n ní ìwọ Ògún, to bá d'elere	They said 'You Ogun, when you arrive at Elere
Níbi wọ́n gbé bí ọ lọ́mọ	The place of your birth
Tí wọ́n bá fún ní akọ ajá,	If you are offered a male dog
Tí wọ́n fún ẹ ní obì tó gbó	If you are offered a ripe kola-nut
Tí wọ́n fún ẹ ní olagbalagba epo	If you are offered sweet and tasty palm oil
Tí wọ́n fún ẹ íi gbogbo ohun tí òun jẹ	If you are offered all your favorite meals
Ògún ní, tí òun bá ti yó tán	Ogun said that after he is well fed
Ó ní ìjálá ni òun máa sun lọ ilé tontonton	He would chant *Ijala* all the way home

Wọ́n ní ìwọ Ògún,	They said 'You, Ogun
O tó Alásán bá r'òkun	You are not qualified to sojourn with Alásán
Òòsà ńlá dìde,	Oosa nla stood up
Ó ní òun bá Alásán r'òkun	He said he would sojourn with Alásán
Wọ́n ní ìwọ Òòsà ńlá	They said, 'You Oosa nla,
Tí wọ́n ba fún ẹ	If they offer you
Ní gbogbo ohun tó ńjẹ	Everything you enjoy to eat'
Ó ní tóun bá yó tán	He said that once he feeds well
Ó ní òun ó padà sílé òun ni	He would return to his home
Wọ́n ní kò tó bá' Alásán r'òkun	They said, he is not qualified to sojourn with Alásán
Gbogbo àwọn Òrìsà ni wọ́n dìde	All the deities stood up
L'ọ́kọ̀ọ̀kan	One after the other
Kálùkù wọn wí pé tí wọ́n bá ti fún àwọn	Each one of them said once they were offered
Ni ohun tí àwọn mọ̀ ọ́n jẹ	Their favorite meal
Oníkálùkù wọn a padà sílé	They would return to their home.
Nii Orí bá dìde	Then, Ori stood up
Ó ní òun ó bá Alásán r'òkun	And said he would sojourn with Alásán
Wọ́n ní ìwọ Orí	They said 'You, Ori
Tí wọ́n bá fún ẹ ní adìẹ okoko	If you're offered a chicken meal
Tí wọ́n fún nígbà, tí wọ́n fun lawo	And if they offered you this and that
Tí wọ́n fún ni gbogbo ohun tó mọ̀ ọ́n jẹ	And all that are your favorite meals
Ó ní, òun ó bá Alásán r'òkun	He said, he would still sojourn with Alásán
Ni Ifá bá ní	Then, Ifa said
Orí nìkan nii kí Alásán bá r'òkun[5]	It is only Ori that Alásán should sojourn with

[5] Personal Communication with Ifa Priest Olaleye, October 22, 2021

The significance of the role of Ori in the Odù, which generates diverse perspectives about the nature of human destiny in the search for a meaningful life, is reenacted through the invitation of the deities to a sojourn that involves feasting or eating their favorite meals. The verse emphasizes Alásán's expectation of virtuous display of reliability, trust, and forbearance from each of the deities who is expected to complete the sojourn with him, especially after being offered their favorite meals as inducement. To Alásán's dismay, none of the deities were willing to complete the sojourn with him except Ori. The point stressed in the Ifá verse is that there is an expedient need to prioritize the relational virtues of reliability, trust, and forbearance over self-aggrandizement, self-centeredness, and self-interest in the course of interpersonal relationship derived from the acceptance to eat and accompany Alásán on the journey. In the final analysis, the meta-ethical core of the intent to converge to eat primes up a situation of reliable and balanced relationship between the *self* and the *Other*, which is fostered through the possibility of looking up to one another for solidarity, support, and assistances that are capable of mediating blame games or self-propelled interests.

In the Yorùbá worldview, eating configures a dialectical relationship between human and extra-terrestrial forces consisting of deities and divinities, gods and goddesses, and ancestors. Eating in this context is essentialized as sacrifice (*ẹbọ*) to the supernatural forces. The Yorùbá concept of *eeru* refers to the ingredients offered to the forces as food in Yorùbá belief. In other words, *eeru* is the food content brought forward by a client or supplicant as the appropriate and prescribed sacrificial offering to the supernatural forces. It is believed that this food content is inclusive of welfare provisions or gifts (similar to a kind of usury/tithe) from the gods/deities to the Ifá priest. This is so since the priest also have to be well sustained to perform his role effectively, even though his role is perceived as a service to humanity. The procession of such food offering as rites of appeasement is also foregrounded by the metaphysical acknowledgement of the hierarchy and potency of the gods, goddesses, or deities.

According to Olaleye, Ifá is the one who sends invitation to the gods and goddesses to come and feast on sacrificial offerings. And a special portion of the sacrifice is always separated for Èṣù, the trickster god, who is believed to have huge appetite to consume indiscriminately and who also serves as witness of the supplicant's promise to offer the sacrifice. To breach this promise ultimately evokes Èṣù's wrath on the non-complying supplicant. In other words, Èṣù sanctions any sort of default that disrupts the process or rites of food offerings to the gods, which is occasioned by the supplicant's failure to fulfil the promise to make such provisions. In Yorùbá belief, disruption in the process of eating is further consolidated in the rationale for food taboos, or *èèwò* (Thorpe 1967). *Èèwò* refers to things or actions that constitute aversion to the appetitive preferences, desires, nature, or dispositions of persons and gods/deities in Yorùbá belief. In this sense, offering food contents or ingredients that are counter to the preferences of gods/deities constitute *èèwò*, which is accompanied by inevitable consequences of the wrath of such gods. Since the Yorùbá believe that offering *èèwò* angers the gods/deities, its repercussion for a fettered or unpalatable state of human and environment well-being is granted as inevitable. Such fettered state may be manifested as famine, drought, diseases outbreak, and oftentimes death within the community among other undesirable crises.

This also extends to the cultural conception of the association of these forces with nonhuman entities like trees, animals, groves, and so on that are often conceived as the symbolic totems or accomplices of the gods. Existing research recount some of the fundamental beliefs that underscore human and beyond human relationship in terms of the appropriateness of sacrificial contents that are religiously certified as proper and befitting for the forces to eat. For instance, in the situation where the sacrifice involves the use of animals for incurring healing, good/favorable destiny, and so on, Olusola Ajibade (2006) notes that Ògún prefers dogs, snail, tortoise, and ram; Ṣàngó prefers ram; and Òrúnmìlà likes rats and mudfish. The act of presenting food ingredients that do not suit the appetitive preferences of these gods amounts to a taboo (*èèwò*) and is tantamount to offering the gods *iwọọ* (poison). *Èèwò* and *iwọọ* in this context become interconnected, in lieu of the perception of what qualifies as edible for the consumption or acceptance of the gods/deities. Given that the food content or ingredients of such offering to the gods is inclusive of welfare provisions (*eeru*) for the priests involved as well, it follows that the avoidance of *èèwò* and *iwọọ* extends to human persons.

In other words, ensuring the attainment of a balanced state of human well-being, which is devoid of crises such as infections/diseases outbreak, demands a cautious consideration of what is befitting and proper also for human consumption, even though in Yorùbá context, such inclusive welfare provisions for persons involved constitute some portion of what is due for feeding/appeasing the gods. Eating/sacrifice at this point is a continuum of a balanced state of well-being from human persons to the nonhuman forces and deities. While it may be difficult to assert that the specificities of this Yorùbá cultural tradition of food taboo belief is universal across varying cultural contexts, its significant hint about the need to disapprove of eating just anything that seems edible and may trigger crises (by virtue of disregard of such beliefs) is nuanced. To this extent, Yorùbá notions of *èèwò* and *iwọ̀ọ̀* deter indiscriminate eating, a situation that could avert undesirable consequences of large-scale pandemic. Persons found guilty of non-compliance of such cultural restriction of indiscriminate consumption are believed to be reprimanded and sanctioned by the wrath of the forces on the offenders, which may include affliction or infliction (sickness, mental instability, infections, and so on). In situation like this, the Yorùbá believes in pacifying the deities to avert such sanctions. In the following, Ṣàngó is pacified to avert his wrath on offenders who commit such taboo:

Olójú Orógbó, ẹlẹ́kẹ̀ẹ́ Obì oo	The one with eyes for bitter kola, cheeks for kolanut
Eégún tí yọ iná lẹ́nu	The masquerade that spits fire
Òòsà tí ba ológbò lẹ́rù	The deity that scares the cat
Ajísayégbẹ̀gẹ̀ ọkọ iya olórógbó	*Ajisayegbege*, husband of 'iya olorogbo;
Ẹni fojú di ọ́, Sàngó o gbé[6]	Whoever underrates Ṣàngó, would be doomed.

The emphasis on "bitter kola" in the above reiterates the significance of the role the kola plays in entreating him to forgive an offender. The popular saying that *Ṣàngó ki'je obi, afi orogbo*—"Ṣàngó does not eat kola-nut except bitter kola"—further corroborates this. It is important to note that

[6] This rendition is a popular cognomen of *Sango* (god of thunder) in Yoruba belief.

Yorùbá conception of "extra-human" or nonhuman forces reflect an anthropomorphic understanding in order to convey meaningful ethical guidelines for human relationship through the symbolic totems and spatial affinities of the forces. This is implicitly reiterated through the appetitive disposition of the forces (undergirded by taboo beliefs) to allay indiscriminate consumption of almost anything in the name of "food" or sacrifice to the gods. Again, this reiterates the previous hint that "eating" as a process in Yorùbá thought constitutes a continuum among humans and between human and nonhuman forces. It signals the call for a common convergence between humans and nonhuman beings to enhance a harmonious balance, from which fidelity of interdependent relationship unfolds, which results into bonding.

It further implies that for human-to-human relationship, "eating" as a process elicits the ideal of giving and receiving, tolerating each other, and fostering a sort of solidarity to attain a balance of co-existence (as previously hinted in the concept of *Akẹ́ẹ̀bọdọ́run*). For human and nonhuman relationships, "eating" initiates the call for well-being or harmony from realms beyond the physical through obeisance of moderated relationship with the gods, underscored by beliefs that deter indiscriminate consumption of almost anything. We will now draw the larger implication of this indigenous notion of eating on COVID-19 and its related crises.

Imperative of Yorùbá Thought of *Eating* for COVID-19 Crisis

The essential question remains: How does this indigenous conception address the crisis spurred by COVID-19? The emergence of COVID-19 constitutes not only a public health concern but also an existential challenge that demands more than a singular approach that goes beyond just vaccine production and circulation to mitigate its far-reaching effects. Leveraging on health insights and the relational worldview that derive from indigenous thought system of the Yorùbá provides a glocal perspective in the search for an urgent resolution. The Yorùbá cultural perspective takes the relationship between humans and animals and the idea of eating that derives from the perception of the latter by the former, seriously. The Yorùbá understanding of eating as bonding/communion inscribes the values of solidarity, interdependency, tolerance/forbearance, and the vitiation of a self-centered worldview. These values, we have been arguing, have the potentials to neutralize the far-reaching effect of the disruptive interactions that have characterized the incidence of COVID-19 among nations.

For the Yorùbá, the contents of any acceptable sacrifice are determined by the appetitive preference of the deities demanding the sacrifice (Awolalu 1973). The framework of culinary taboos (*èèwò*) also concretize the disapproval of indiscriminate eating, undergirded by the possibility of instigating the deities' wrath because of the possible imbalance or disharmony of human and environmental well-being. Beyond this appeal of the avoidance of supernatural wrath, the projection of the disapproval of indiscriminate eating to an extent spurs the need to prioritize re-modification of cultured culinary habits, as evidenced in the incidence of the COVID-19 outbreak (Huremovic 2019), which involved overt human exploitation and hunting of pangolins for the purposes of trade and food (Wang Y et al. 2021a). Emphasis on such re-modification is due to the global rate of casualty as a result of COVID-19. Within the Yorùbá understanding of eating, indiscriminate or excessive consumption speaks to the possibility of *iwọ̀ọ̀* (poisoning), which induces ill health and could even lead to death. *Iwọ̀ọ̀* substantiates the scientific connection between eating and infection, one fundamental link that plays a significant role in the provenance and epidemiology of COVID-19.

Furthermore, eating as a process (as implied in Yorùbá thought) initiates an extended conception of eating as a schema of interdependent social interaction and relationship that is aimed toward the accomplishment of harmony, reliability, friendship, and solidarity. As an act of extending invitation and acceptance of invitation to feed, it implies a collaborative network of relationship, where each and every one ought to relate with one another with "true and fair" intention as host/supplicant and invited guests. In such situation where the ethical virtues of eating (i.e., truthfulness, fairness due to communing or bonding together) underscore the physical act of eating either meat or other edibles, the potency of *Iwọ̀ọ̀* would become neutralized (since people who possess such intent to bond would not attune to the vicious agenda of poisoning one another). The common interest or intention to commune (as symbolized in the course of converging to eat) together culminates into the idea of *Akẹ́bọdọ́run*, which has been previously clarified.

A veritable way to situate the heuristic value of *Akẹ́bọdọ́run* is to examine its import on the dynamics of global power contestation. The blame game attributed to China as the cause of the global predicament of public health challenge of COVID-19 spurs discriminatory outburst in feasible dimensions, such that China is almost synonymously perceived as the "contagious race," who intends to blemish the entire human race for the sake of techno-scientific advancement and global political economy gains (Wang et al. 2021b; Nyika et al. 2021). While normative judgment regarding the veracity or otherwise of the reading of conspiracy theories of blame game conferred on the positionality of China in the scheme of things is suspended in this discourse, the point granted is that in whichever way the blame game turns, the human race becomes polarized by identity of differences, which ultimately triggers the struggle of the *Self* (China, in this case) against the *Other* (USA, WHO, developing/underdeveloping nations). In simple terms, such identity of difference reflects in the manifest strategies of production of various COVID-19 vaccines and media propaganda of its source/cause (inclusive of the trend of infodemic) by various contesting nations that implicitly involve in "comparative competition" for world acknowledgment. Persistent struggle of *Self* over the *Other* or vice versa trumps the realization of a harmonious or flourishing condition for the attainment of a common goal or survival, which is the point of emphasis in the notion of *Akẹ́bọdọ́run*.

Alluding to the interactive model of eating as a process of bonding/communing, as explicated in Yorùbá thought, could possibly purge the contesting powers/nations of suspicious intent and tussle for recognition of the *Self* over the *Other* or vice versa. When the notion of eating as communion is embraced as a framework for international or intercontinental diplomatic relations, all diplomats, agencies, and collaborators involved would hardly imagine the deployment of conspiracy, inspired by ill intent (*Iwọ̀ọ̀*—poisoning or corrupting) as strategy of interaction or relationship. Optimistically, this would engender strong bonding that would be shared through solidarity with one another for the attainment of common good, sustainable survival, and balanced well-being that is devoid of schisms of interest in the course to mitigate the crisis spurred by the incidence of COVID-19. This means that such philosophy of eating would aid forbearance and tolerance with/of one another within the international polity, and it would also get rid of suspicion and blame game syndrome. In other words, all international stakeholders or agencies implicated in the COVID-19 pandemic would dare to converge together and commune with one another to earn a common trust and reliability to seek indivisible human well-being and existential state of balance. They would all become collaborators toward mitigating COVID-19, and in Yorùbá coinage, they would earn the honor of being *Akẹ́bọdọ́run*. Needless to say, in the absence of such common ethical understanding of model of interaction or interdependency (instantiated through Yorùbá thought of eating as a process of bonding or communion), the flip-side predicament of nationalistic rivalry and vindication from blame game through purposeful continental and intercontinental media propaganda and wide-scale production or "aids" of efficacious vaccines, especially by super power states, as well as the political economy of annexing reliance and trust from the so-called dependent developing and underdeveloped states of the world would continually abound. This simply means that the fruition of the imperative of bonding or communion suggested in Yorùbá thought of eating for COVID-19-related crises would remain a utopia.

Concluding Remarks

This discourse attempted to inquire the extent to which the plausible ethical motifs of bonding/communion, trust, reliability, tolerance, and forbearance that are derived from indigenous Yorùbá conception of "eating" can foster an alternative resolution strategy to douse the far-reaching effect of COVID-19-related crises of suspicion, conspiracy, distrust, and unreliability within the context of international polity that is suffused with blame game. It asserts an optimistic view about leaping from a glocalized context of understanding the complication of the crisis spurred by the incidence of the global pandemic. The heuristic value of some Yorùbá notions regarding the phenomenon of eating like *Enulebo* and relevant *Ifa* citations among other beliefs were thus conceptually framed for concretizing the optimistic view of the discourse. The discourse submits that while the value of eating as bonding in Yorùbá thought projects a progressive ideal for realizing common trust within international/intercontinental diplomatic corridors, relegating its heuristic value as a mere ethno-national appendage would readily obviate its universal appeal, hence rendering it as a utopia.

References

Ajibade, G.O. 2006. Animals in the Traditional Worldview of the Yorùbá. *Folklore* 10 (30): 161.

Allen, A. 2014. Food and Culture: Continuity and Change in the Yorùbá of West Africa and Their Diasporas. In *Odysseys of Plates and Palates: Food, Society and Sociality*. Netherland: Brill.

Awolalu, J.O. 1973. Yorùbá Sacrificial Practice. *Brill Journal of Religion in Africa* 5: Fasc.2.

Bentham, J. 2000 (Reprint). *An Introduction to the Principles of Morals and Legislation*. Kitchener: Batoche Books.

Brooking Institutions. 2020. A Modern Tragedy? Covid-19 and US-China Relations. 10 July 2020. https://www.brookings.edu a-….

Cohen, C. 1986. The Case for the Use of Animals in Biomedical Research. *The New England Journal of Medicine* 315: 865–870.

Huremovic, D. 2019. Brief History of Pandemics (Pandemics throughout History). In *Psychiatry of Pandemics*. Switzerland: Springer Nature.

Lynteris, C. 2019. *Framing Animals as Epidemic Villains: Histories of Non-human Disease Vector*. Palgrave Macmillan.

Norcross, A. 2004. Puppies, Pigs and People: Eating Meat and Marginal Cases. *Philosophical Perspectives, 18, Ethics* 8: 230–245.

Norton, B.G. 1982. Environmental Ethics and Non-Human Rights. *Environmental Ethics* 4 (1): 17–36.

Nyika, A., G.T. Nyika, J.T. Nyika, et al. 2021. Covid-19 Pandemic: Questioning Conspiracy Theories, Beliefs or Claims that Have Potential Negative Impact on Public Health Interventions and Proposal for Integrated Communication and Information Dissemination Strategies (ICIDS). *Journal of Development and Communication Studies* 8 (1). https://doi.org/10.4314/jdcs.v8i1.1.

NYTimes. 2020. US.-China Feud over Coronavirus Erupts at World Health Assembly. 10 July 2020. www.nytimes.com 2020/05/18.

Ogundele, S.O. 2007. Understanding Aspects of Yorùbá Gastronomic Culture. *Indian Journal of Traditional Knowledge* 6 (1): 50–56.

Oso, B.A. 1977. Mushrooms in Yorùbá Mythology and Medicinal Practices. *Copié de Economic Botany* 31: 367–371.

Schmidtz, A. 1998. Are All Species Equal? *Journal of Applied Philosophy* 15 (1): 57–67.

Singer, P. 1975. *Animal Liberation*. New York: New York Review.

Thorpe, C.O. 1967. *Awon Eewo Ile Yorùbá*. Ibadan: Onibon-Oje.

Wang, Y., N. Leader-Williams, and S.T. Turvey. 2021a. Exploitation Histories of Pangolins and Endemic Pheasants on Hainan Island, China: Baselines and Shifting Social Norms. *Frontiers in Ecology and Evolution* 9: Article 608057.

Wang, X., S. Zuo, H. Chan, et al. 2021b. Covid-19-Related Conspiracy Theories in China: The Role of Secure versus Defensive In-Camp Positivity and Responsibility Attributions. *Journal of Pacific Rim, Psychology*. https://doi.org/10.1177/18344909211034928.

Warren, M.A. 1987. Difficulties with the Strong Animal Rights Position. *Between the Species* 2 (4). Nedlands, Australia.

World Health Organization. 2020. *Novel Coronavirus (2019-nCOV) Situation Report-13*. Geneva. 10 July 2020. https://www.who.int/docs/default-source/coronaviruse/situation-reports/20200202-sitrep-13-ncov-v3.pdf.

9

Epidemiology and an Epistemic Evaluation of the Management of COVID-19 in Nigeria

Anselm K. Jimoh and Francis Ikhianosime

Introduction

Although pandemics are issues for epidemiological discussions, the way and manner they are managed by countries that are affected have socio-economic and political undertones, which necessarily come with epistemic transactions. By epistemic transactions, we mean the transfer of information between a testifier and a hearer and all that inform and/or dispose the hearer to believe and accept the testimony of the testifier. These can have negative or positive impact on how effectively the pandemic is managed. It also calls to question some moral and ethical issues. In the wake of the first index case of COVID-19 in Nigeria on February 27, 2020, the Nigerian government got generous monetary donations from well-meaning individuals and institutions to assist with the

A. K. Jimoh (✉)
Department of Philosophy, SS. Peter and Paul Major Seminary, Ibadan, Nigeria

F. Ikhianosime
Department of Philosophy, Seminary of All Saints, Ekpoma, Nigeria

F. Egbokhare, A. Afolayan (eds.), *Global Health, Humanity and the COVID-19 Pandemic*, https://doi.org/10.1007/978-3-031-17429-2_9

management and control of the spread of the virus. Ever since, daily statistics on the spread indicate that it geometrically increased, spreading from one state of the federation to another. Practically almost all the states in Nigeria have at least some cases, with Lagos State being the epicentre and worst hit. The Nigerian government seems to have delayed its response, adopting reactive measures rather than being proactive, in restraining the spread of the virus. Controversies trailed the use of the billions of Naira from donations by individuals and institutions towards the management of the virus. The lack of availability of test kits; the lip service of the government to control the spread, which is visible in the lack of aggressive public awareness strategies; the politicisation of the truth and palliatives to aid compliance with the stay-at-home recommendation and ensure effective lockdown—all these, coupled with the various conspiracy theories easily accessible on social media, cast aspersions on the epistemic transactions regarding the management of COVID-19 in Nigeria. Consequently, the lack of trust evoked by the government's lack of commitment and sincerity induced apathy on the part of the public and increased the rate of crimes all over the nation.

The present chapter is a critical analysis and evaluation of the Nigerian government's response to the management of the spread and control of the COVID-19 pandemic. First, we analyse COVID-19 within the context of the philosophy of epidemiology espoused by Alex Broadbent. Second, we interrogate the Nigerian government's response to COVID-19, with special attention to the epistemic transactions and control measures adopted. Thereafter, we evaluate the efforts aimed at managing COVID-19 in Nigeria. We conclude that for the effective management of pandemics in Nigeria, there is the need for commitment to the truth about the actual situation at hand, unity of efforts to deal with it and transparency in the epistemic transactions about the pandemic.

COVID-19 as a Global Pandemic

The coronavirus disease (COVID-19), initially called (2019-nCoV), is one of the greatest public health challenges for our time. It belongs to the zoonotic diseases in animals and humans. These are respiratory diseases common to bats, cats, and birds, which mimic pneumonia and often manifests with clinical symptoms such as fever, cough, shortness of breath, muscle pain, exhaustion, etc., in humans. Among the different coronaviruses that threaten humans, five have been identified in the twenty-first century, namely: HCoV-NL63, HCoV-HKU1, HCoV-SARS, HCoV-MERS, and SARS-CoV-2 (Dzieciatkowski, et al. 2020). In 2003, there was an outbreak of a strain of coronavirus, Severe Acute Respiratory Syndrome (SARS) also known as HCoV-SARS, which was responsible for more than 8000 deaths. The new coronavirus, COVID-19, symptomatologically resembles that of SARS; hence, it is regarded as SARS-CoV-2 but commonly called COVID-19.

COVID-19 is highly contagious. It is mainly transmitted through respiratory droplets and aerosols when infected persons sneeze, cough, or interact with other persons at close proximity of less than two metres. Between December 12, 2019 when the first case was reported in Wuhan, China, and February 23, 2021, the number of recorded cases worldwide has reached 112,102,423 million, with 2,480,696 deaths (www.worldmeters.info/coronavirus). Having taken a global dimension, spreading rapidly across six continents, World Health Organisation (WHO) declared the coronavirus a pandemic on March 11, 2020. Given the daily linear rise of cases and resulting deaths, it is difficult to trace the Case Fatality Ratio (CFR) because of the fluctuating figures of contraction and deaths in different regions. CFR is determined by the number of reported deaths per number of reported cases. In Nigeria, the total confirmed cases stand at 152,616 with 1862 deaths as at February 23, 2021 (www.worldmeters.info/country). Our interest in this chapter is the fact that COVID-19 poses both an epidemiological and epistemological crisis.

COVID-19 as an Epidemiological Crisis

Epidemiology is a field of scientific inquiry that studies "the distribution and determinants of disease and other health states in the human population through group comparisons to improve population health" (Broadbent 2013: 1). This definition implies that epidemiology induces answers or solutions from an inferential analysis. It assembles and analyses statistics and details of groups, and makes inferences from them. As a field of scientific inquiry, epidemiology and philosophy are closely connected in the sense that philosophy interrogates epidemiology. In this wise, Broadbent explains six features that make epidemiology philosophically exciting. One, epidemiology engages questions of causation; it investigates the causes or determinants of diseases. Two, it is nonconformant to standard philosophical images of science. Three, it uses observational methods and does not necessarily involve controlled experiments. Four, it counts things and draws up conclusions from comparisons of different counting. Five, it involves population thinking; the idea that population may be thought to bear health-related properties. Six, it has high stakes that raise moral and epistemic implications about values (Broadbent 2013: 1–10).

Epidemiology advances diverse reasons about the causes of COVID-19, some of which conflict because of the application of different epidemiological models. The latter are usually grounded in population thinking, and the projection from a particular population may not apply to another population. For instance, the epidemiological projection from Italy may not be applicable as a prediction for Madagascar. The implication here is that population thinking in a place can generate fear and anxiety in another population, thereby creating an epidemiological crisis. In relation to COVID-19 that seems to have defied successful control so far, the predictions about its effects and containment have remained woeful.

The principle of causation, which is common to epidemiological and philosophical inquiries, further outlines why COVID-19 is an epidemiological crisis. Epidemiology has vested interest in causation because of "its goal of identifying the causes of diseases (both modifiable and non-modifiable) so that the disease or its consequences might be prevented" (Mcgwin 2010: 599). This vested interest is premised on the fact that the measure of the "strength of association are also used as measures of causal strength" (Broadbent 2013: 26). Consequently, strong grounds to establish an association imply the strength of its causation. Even though epidemiology lacks an integrated notion of causation, it is nevertheless the basis upon which prediction, control, and theses are made. Therefore, it is left with the burden of justifying why a particular cause is linked with a particular effect.

The rate at which particular diseases are contracted provide evaluative paradigms for epidemiological concerns with diseases. Therefore, to understand the value of rate in epidemiology would enrich our understanding of the scope of COVID-19 because the rates of its contraction would help us to measure the appropriate (or inappropriate) level of intervention required to contain its spread. Generally, rates in epidemiology are evaluated either as (i) case-specific mortality or (ii) case-specific fatality. Case-specific mortality measures the death from a specific condition in the overall population. Thus, to determine the case-specific mortality rate of COVID-19 within a particular country, we divide the total population of the country by the total cases of death recorded. On the other hand, case-specific fatality measures the death from a specific condition in the limited population of infected cases. This is not that straightforward with COVID-19 because it is difficult to ascertain all those who have died from it, given that there are equally other underlining health conditions that may be responsible for the particular deaths. For instance, when a COVID-19 patient who has underlying conditions of asthma, HIV, and tuberculosis dies, it is not easy to adjudge that the patient died of COVID-19 and not asthma or tuberculosis. Epidemiologists describe this challenge as the "true rates" of case specificity.

The fact that a COVID-19 patient with other underlying conditions dies can be a case-specific for either or both COVID-19, and the other underlying conditions. This creates an epidemiological challenge with COVID-19. Arguably also is the truth that fatality rates are not restrictive to either COVID-19 and/or other underlying conditions. They are equally dependent on several other factors like poor health care system, inappropriate drug administration, the political situation at a time, and/or the counting practices of a particular system, etc. (Canali 2020). This increases the epidemiological complexity in analysing fatality rates, especially for COVID-19.

Cases of COVID-19 can only be ascertained with medical diagnosis. Thus, if a country or system lacks the capacity to engage in testing a large number of patients, its resulting number of recorded cases would be low, which does not necessarily imply a low rate of prevalence in the country. Almost across the board, we seem to be dealing with a situation of artificially low cases of COVID-19 because of undertesting. This is complicated with the fact that carriers of the virus can be both symptomatic and asymptomatic, yet they are equally dangerous to public health. In Nigeria, for instance, when the first 1000 cases were recorded, the number of those tested was below 25,000. In this case, getting the true rates and making proper epidemiological computation becomes difficult.

COVID-19 as an Epistemological Crisis

Following from the analysis above, COVID-19 is not just an epidemiological crisis; it is also an epistemological crisis. According to Francis Beer and Robert Hariman, we can understand COVID-19 as an epistemological crisis from four perspectives: (i) description, (ii) explanation, (iii) prediction, and (iv) control (2020: 19–28). In addition to these four, we may add the social or moral aspect. The descriptive aspect involves not having an accurate aggregate of the measures of this pandemic, that is, the inability to correctly represent the situation of the pandemic as it is, as well as some deliberate aspects of hiding the truth about the accurate situation of the pandemic. Truth is a fundamental element for epistemology and for pursuing any knowledge claim. Interpretations in epidemiology cannot be imaginary; they must be based on available statistics. Even if a prediction is to be made based on a counterfactual analysis, it must be a leap from what is available or correct. The strength of inference is that the particulars must be true, before making a general claim. However, as Beer and Hariman argue, the descriptive dilemma is in the obscurity of truth. For instance, "in some cases, like China, governments hide the truth; in other cases like deaths in homes or nursing facilities, or from pre-existing conditions, the numbers are simply not included in the totals" (Beer and Hariman 2020: 20). This obstruction of truth can only lead to a predictive framework with a misleading forecast, which weakens the foundation for any authentic analysis, and comes with a lot of epistemological implications. For instance: Can science always tell us the truth? Can we rely on scientific investigations as the basis for arriving at the truth always or must we subject them to further interrogation? The question of representing the situation accurately or the disruption of data for analysis makes the issue a grave concern. Fareed Zakaria argues that the figure of contraction coming out of some countries like Brazil, Nigeria, and Indonesia is "artificially low" (2020). This indicates that statistics are tampered with, if that is the case—obstructing the truth, then it would definitely create an epistemological problem.

Explanation as an epistemological casualty of COVID-19 arises from using different epidemiological models, based on several assumptions, to explain the situation. If there are just a few valid resources to confirm or falsify the assumptions, it would ultimately implicate the overall dynamics of predictions and theorisations from such scientific models. Karl Popper argues in his falsification thesis that what makes science distinct from pseudo-science is the ability to be falsified. According to him,

> A theoretical system is to be considered as scientific only if it makes assertions that may clash with observations; and a system is, in fact, tested by attempts to produce such clashes, that is to say by attempts to refute it. Thus, testability is the same as refutability, and can therefore likewise be taken as a criterion of demarcation. (1963: 256)

If Popper is correct, a claim is not scientific merely because its observational account is supported; rather, a claim's scientificness is predicated on its falsifiability. Although, Imre Lakatos (1970) and Thomas Kuhn (1970) repudiate Popper's claim, the strength of the falsification thesis for our present consideration is that we do not have sufficient resources to verify or falsify most of the epidemiological claims. An instance is the claim that COVID-19 is more fatal in regions with colder temperatures. This cannot be easily falsified because of contradictory shreds of evidence. Also, there is the fact that the phenomena—all the variables that are analysed to advance an explanation for a particular epidemiological position on COVID-19—are increasingly paradoxical. For instance, Neil Ferguson's epidemiological model, which is strongly favoured, predicts that lockdowns can overturn the primary infection peak, whereas John Ioannidis' model criticises lockdown measures and makes dire predictions, like economic downturns, from it (see Roy 2020; Stegenga 2020). The plurality of epidemiological postulations and predictions, which sometimes have sharp contradictions, makes the issues of COVID-19 a subject of epistemological concern. The non-linearity of predictions and models is probably responsible for the various conspiracy theories about COVID-19, and this has counterproductive consequences.

Predictions function in the epistemological crises because, coming from the different epidemiological models, they constitute modes of knowing. The interest of epistemology here is about the reliability of such predictions, if they work, and how they can be used to improve social learning. Epidemiological predictions about COVID-19 depend largely on inductive logic and probability, which is a function or product of a Bayesian model. A Bayesian model is a statistical model which deploys probability to represent all uncertainties. Bayesian epistemology in particular, and the epistemology of science in general, deals with questions of what counts as evidence in favour of a hypothesis and how probability can be raised to the level of positive evidence for a theory. This is the dilemma which predictions from COVID-19, like any other scientific prediction, faces. According to Alex Rosenberg, the problem is "whether the fact that some data raise the probability of a hypothesis makes the data positive evidence for it" (2000: 117). It is not always clear how some claims raise the probability of a hypothesis, thereby constituting a piece of positive evidence for it. The case that certain facts make a situation highly probable does not make it a conclusive positive evidence for a given claim. Yet, science moves from this level of probability to a given. Furthermore, given that this becomes a basis for theorisation, prediction of future events resting on such claims as well as being a source of knowledge becomes epistemologically problematic since it does not rest on warranted grounds. Such a claim is fallible. This is why science too is regarded as fallible. The problems associated with probabilism as an epistemic subject weaken scientific predictions on COVID-19 and this makes such predictions liable to fallibility.

The concern with control as one of the epistemological crises of COVID-19 arises from the deficits in description, explanation, and prediction. Beer and Hariman regard it as the chaotic medical and public health response to the pandemic (2020: 22). For them, the poor management of the pandemic by the public health systems due to poor health facilities, insufficient testing, poor tracking mechanisms of contact tracing, etc., makes it less predictable and more difficult to forecast the end of COVID-19. It also reveals the decay caused by the politicisation of the health sectors of many countries, Nigeria inclusive. While some countries were proactive, many others were ill-prepared to handle health emergencies and the geometric rise of new cases. The poor control mechanism directly affects the quality of information on COVID-19 as well as making it less extrapolative.

These epistemological crises about COVID-19 come with a social and/or a moral dimension. They create social dysfunctions like biased media reportage on COVID-19 cases. This can arise from either an inflated estimation of the cases, perhaps for political reasons, as it is alleged in Nigeria for instance, or a deflated analysis of the cases to diminish fear and anxiety among the population. This implies what Miranda Fricker (2007) describes as testimonial deficits. Testimonial deficit or excess leads to epistemic injustice, hence, the issue arising thereof is regarded as a social and/or moral problem. Epistemic injustice is a grave concern for virtue epistemology. Within the network of epistemic transactions about COVID-19, there are palpable situations of deficits, either: (i) because there is no wholesome system that can accurately capture the records of cases, (ii) no comprehensive medium to report the exact situations, or (iii) because the information is deliberately warped to suit some ends. COVID-19 remains a complex health situation because of its checkered mutation patterns, which makes it difficult to ascertain some issues about it conclusively. This social or moral aspect makes the perspectives of understanding, interpretation, prediction, and control of epistemological crises. Against this framework, we proceed to analyse the management of COVID-19 in Nigeria.

Management of COVID-19 in Nigeria: Mirroring the Crises in Context

COVID-19 has overwhelmed many countries in the world, including countries with robust health sectors. Nigeria is not an exemption; her case is even worse because of her penurious health sector. Upon identification of the first recorded case of COVID-19 in Nigeria, an Italian citizen, the National Emergency Operations Centre began contact tracing of suspected cases linked to the Italian. By March 9, 2020, two more index cases were identified from 27 suspected cases spread across Edo, Lagos, Ogun, and Kano states and the Federal Capital Territory (NCDC 2020). Since then, the official recorded cases of COVID-19 have risen on a daily basis all around the country.

The management of COVID-19 in Nigeria is believed to draw upon the success recorded in the control of other epidemics like Polio and Ebola. However, and unfortunately too, unlike Ebola and Polio, which have vaccines, there was no known immediate vaccine for COVID-19. Recently though, Pfizer-BioNtech, Moderna's mRNA-1273, AstraZeneca, Janssen, and Novavax's COVID-19 vaccines have been developed. Regardless of this development, the management and administration of COVID-19 seems to have overwhelmed many African countries, unlike other deadly epidemics in the past. Based on a modelling study to examine the preparedness of African countries and their vulnerability to COVID-19, Marius Gilbert et al. (2020: 871–877) claim that even though Nigeria and Ethiopia have the second highest importation risk from China, they are highly vulnerable to the virus. Egypt, Algeria, and South Africa are most vulnerable to COVID-19 because they have the highest importation risk from China. The study further argues that with early detection and prevention, flight bans, and travel restrictions, future risks may be altered. Given her population and health facilities, Nigeria has a moderate capacity to control the outbreak. The claims of this study notwithstanding, and regardless of some successes recorded in curtailing the spread of the virus, there are some grave worries in the way Nigeria is managing COVID-19.

In the wake of the pandemic, the Nigerian Government set up a Presidential Task Force (PTF) on COVID-19 in collaboration with the Nigeria Centre for Disease Control (NCDC) under the auspices of the Ministry of Health. The PTF was to ensure and monitor the adherence to the precautionary and safety measures to be adopted in control of the spread of the virus. One of the earliest measures was to strengthen surveillance at five international airports in Nigeria—Enugu, Lagos, Rivers, Kano, and the Federal Capital Territory (FCT) international airports. Subsequently, the NCDC reportedly set up a "Coronavirus Preparedness Group" that involved various stakeholders, including the Port Health

Services of the Federal Ministry of Health. Screening was heightened at the point of entry into the country, particularly for those coming from China, and public health awareness was increased for Nigerians across the country through the NCDC (see Ihekweazu 2020).

Despite the already existing facilities provided for molecular diagnosis for all epidemic-prone diseases by the National Reference Laboratory established to fight against Ebola, Nigeria was faced with the initial challenge of specific testing equipment and technical expertise on COVID-19. To combat this initial challenge, the Ministry of Health sought advice from WHO on how to deal with the new virus. However, not until the second index case was announced on March 8, 2020, did more concrete steps in the management of COVID-19 commenced. At this point, there were already 219 primary and secondary contacts of the two index cases being monitored (NCDC 2020). Some of the concrete steps taken were the cancellation and/or postponement of some events that would warrant public gatherings, like the National Sports Festival initially scheduled for Benin City from March 18, 2020 and the suspension of the National Orientation Camp of the National Youth Service Corp already ongoing across the country. Nigeria subsequently placed a travel ban on 13 countries with high cases of the virus, including the United States, the United Kingdom, Germany, and France (see Ogundele 2020). With 226 new cases and a total of 6401 index cases, the Federal Government had to close all institutions of learning on March 19, 2020 (see Olaleye 2020).

As the index cases continued to soar, more precautionary measures were taken to control the spread of the virus. For instance, land and sea borders of many states were closed, movements were restricted, compulsory wearing of nose masks, and compulsory provision of running taps and hand sanitizers at open places were announced. On March 23, 2020, the Lagos and Abuja international airports were closed. Given that these were two epicentres with a total index profile of 7526 cases of the virus, many saw this move as belated. The Federal Government of Nigeria (FGN) subsequently officially banned interstate travels and enforced a complete lockdown for the states of Lagos, Ogun, and the Federal Capital Territory, Abuja because of the preponderance of index cases. By the end of March, almost all states in the country have prohibited public gatherings, including churches, mosques, hotels, pubs, and markets, except for the sale of food and essential commodities. Other measures taken included the prescription of the observance of social distance based on WHO's recommendations. Isolation centres were opened to keep COVID-19 patients away from others, and contact tracing of suspected cases was initiated. Basically, the Nigeria Government applied what can be regarded as a general approach adopted by many Western nations in dealing with the same crisis. For Franklin Obeng-Odoom, this is "conventional wisdom" (2020: 20), and for Charles Soludo (2020), it is a "trial-and-error template of Western nations" and "copy and paste response."

To ameliorate the effects of the ravaging pandemic and the measures taken to control its symmetrical spread in Nigeria, both the private and public sectors, individuals and corporate institutions made several interventions in terms of magnanimous contributions. For example, under the auspices of the Coalition against COVID-19, private sector leaders in Nigeria donated a whooping sum of 21. 5 billion Naira, while the Central Bank of Nigeria (CBN) announced a one trillion Naira stimulus package. Also, the FGN asked the National Assembly to approve a 500 billion Naira intervention fund, and also withdrew $150 million from the Sovereign National Fund and indicated it would borrow $6.9 billion; all purportedly to manage the effects of COVID-19 (see Fasan 2020). These huge sums of donation generated and appropriated were used to acquire palliatives for distribution as relief materials for the populace.

Regardless of what appears to be a robust management plan by the Nigerian Government in fighting the COVID-19 pandemic, there are palpable lapses and gaps in the enforcement of the plan and possible recovery options. This is even made worse with the second wave of the virus, and its mutations. These have consequently affected compliance with some of the prescribed health norms. On the one hand, there is a situation of distrust by Nigerians in the Government's efforts to fight the pandemic. On the other hand, the people are sceptical about the entire records and reports on COVID-19 in Nigeria, reasoning that it has been politicised. It is interesting to note that distrust and scepticism are epistemic vices that seem to truncate the management of COVID-19 in the country.

Epistemic Evaluation of COVID-19 in Nigeria

COVID-19 has generated an epistemic community for conversation in Nigeria, between the government and the governed both with agential powers. While the government has the capacity for enforcing control, the people serve as the epistemic interlocutors. The information transfer between the government and the governed, which we describe as epistemic transaction here is a conversational situation involving knowledge transfer. It entails the transmission of testimonial knowledge by the government as the speaker to the governed as the hearers. According to John Greco, knowledge transmission as we have in epistemic transactions involves a cooperation between the speaker and hearer—a joint agency—that requires trust (2019: 93). And Shannon Brick argues that "In most testimonial transactions between adults, the hearer's obligation is to accord the speaker a level of credibility that matches the evidence that what she is saying is true" (2020: 490). Where the hearer cannot accord the speaker the required level of credibility because the available evidence does not match the speaker's claim, the hearer is not obliged to believe the speaker. Therefore, the hearer is justified not to believe the speaker. The absence of the speaker's credibility and/or a disparity between the speaker's testimony and the available evidence warrants the lack of belief in the hearer in the testimony of the speaker. If it is the case that the speaker deliberately exaggerates or distorts her information, and therefore, misinforms the hearer, then the speaker (in this case the Nigerian government) would be epistemically culpable in her information purveyance. Epistemic culpability implies that the agent is guilty of negligence, misrepresentation and distortion of facts. According to Fricker, there are two kinds of dysfunctions in epistemic transactions: (i) credibility excess and/or (ii) credibility deficit (2007: 17). Credibility excess results when a speaker receives more credibility than is otherwise due to her, and credibility deficit occurs when a speaker receives less credibility than is otherwise due to her. In the management of COVID-19 in Nigeria, the credibility economy suffers deficit occasioned by the mismanagement of the process, and the culpable dysfunctions in the administration of the process.

The mismanagement is due to the many irreconcilable paradoxes with COVID-19 in Nigeria. For instance, there is no apparent corresponding effects of the use of the billions of Naira raised, even in the health sectors. In allusion to this, Peter Adeyemi (2020) avers that,

> The standards obtainable in, and the number of isolation-centres nationwide are controversial. In Nigeria, those in isolation centres are not on ventilators, but they have the energy to walk around and protest a lack of care and are even able to escape from treatment centres. The palliatives provided at all levels of government are parlous and ridiculous.

Some have even argued that while COVID-19 is a killer disease in Europe and America, it is a business disease that has been highly politicised in Nigeria. Some individuals and groups are believed to be feeding fat on the donations, while some of the index cases appear merely nominal. Some records show that in some isolation centres in Nigeria, rather than seeing sick people, it looks like an entertainment centre and some even protest that they are not properly taken care of. In almost a year (February 27, 2020 to February 23, 2021) of COVID-19 rage in Nigeria, we have about 1862 deaths from 152,616 total confirmed cases. This compounds the credibility deficit given the poor hygienic context, poor social distancing culture, poor consulting clinics, poor use of nose masks, which sometimes has become dust-carriers and chin masks rather than a virus-protective shield, and etc. This scenario makes many suspicious of the authenticity of the daily official statistics provided by NCDC.

Another paradoxical situation derives from shutting religious worship centres to avoid overcrowding while markets are allowed to function without proper observance of the health prescriptions. While schools were shut, Sadiya Umar-Farouq, the Minister of Humanitarian Affairs, Disaster Management and Social Development, announced the continuation of the feeding of school children under the Nigeria Home Grown School Feeding Programme (NHGSFP). There were also reports of huge sums of money spent on palliatives which only very few Nigerians benefitted from.[1] It became public knowledge during the #EndSARS nationwide protests that corrupt politicians and government officials hoarded these palliatives for selfish and future personal gains. This further strengthens the allegation of the politicisation of the pandemic. In the face of the fight against COVID-19, the Nigerian Association of Resident Doctors complained about poor working conditions and lack of provision of Personal Protective Equipment (PPE). They even threatened industrial action if their working conditions do not improve (Bakam 2020).

The case of Mrs. Suzan Idoko-Okpe, a Nigerian-British citizen in Benue State, is a specimen case of the flaws and mismanagement of COVID-19 in Nigeria. Having returned from London and fatigued from the trip, she decided to see a doctor on March 22, 2020, two days after her journey. She was later declared a COVID-19 case and quarantined. She raised an alarm that the entire process has been stage-managed, and there was misplacement of information. Thereafter, she sued the FGN. She cried out to the public in a recording that went viral:

> This is Susan Idoko Okpe, nee Lawani. I am pleading with everybody to please tell the Nigerian government to let me go. This is my 16th day of incarceration. What have I done? What have I done? Benue State lied to me that I have COVID-19. I just got the result yesterday after 15 days and the result is a stage play with different dates, birthdays, different recordings which they know, and trying to put right. (see Etakibuebu 2020)

There are many other such cases of discrepancies among the identified index cases which gives credibility to Dr. Saka Haruna, the Kogi State commissioner for health's complaint that they are under pressure to announce false COVID-19 cases (Odogun 2020).

The mismanagement of information about the coronavirus in Nigeria has grave consequences and implications for the control of its spread in the country. Some of these consequences include a sharp economic downturn, which would imply massive retrenchment of workers in many establishments; the rise in crime—for example, the emergence of "the

[1] It was very interesting to discover, during the looting of warehouses containing palliatives that followed the hijacked #EndSars notionwide protests, that it may be true that such reported huge amounts were actually spent on palliatives.

one million boys," who terrorised many communities in Lagos during the lockdown; etc. All these make the management of COVID-19 in Nigeria epistemically culpable. Also, the poor network of epistemic transaction oftentimes results to misinformation, and provides basis for conspiracy theories. Although the NCDC tries to disseminate information to the public through text messages and periodic information jingles on radios and televisions, these have proven to be grossly inefficient, given the wide pool of information, misinformation, and even disinformation on COVID-19, especially those available on social media.

The battle against COVID-19 has created a global infodemic—overbearance of information with deliberate attempts to misinform the public in order to undermine public health. This makes trustworthy sources of information and reliable guidance difficult (WHO 2020, also see Ball and Maxmen 2020). Misinformation and conspiracy theories have stifled some progressive and scientific efforts in the proper management of COVID-19 in Nigeria. Since the dawn of the pandemic, several unfounded interpretations about the cause, spread, and treatment of the disease have surfaced—from pseudo-scientific elucidations to apocalyptic explanations. Arguably, some of the reasons misinformation have stifled the management of COVID-19 in Nigeria include low literacy level in Nigeria, the politicisation of information dissemination, absence of a unified epidemiological model, fear and anxiety factors, and religious fanaticism. Some analysts have unscientifically labelled COVID-19 as a spiritual problem that can be solved or cured by fasting and praying, while some have sought spiritual assistance from marabouts, spiritual healers, diviners, and other ritual processes.

Concerning the conspiracy theories, Philip Ball and Amy Maxmen noted that "on March 19, 2020, a website www.Biohackinfo.com falsely claimed that Bill Gates planned to use a coronavirus vaccine as a ploy to monitor people through an injected microchip or quantum-dot spy software." Again, on April 8, 2020, Pastor Chris Oyakhilome linked the emergence of 5G technology to the spread of the virus in a YouTube sermon. These and similar conspiracy theories have received several backlashes and refutations. They have, however, distorted the belief system concerning COVID-19 in Nigeria, causing a disconnection between scientific consensus and analytic thinking in curbing the virus. A distorted belief-system would weaken analytic thinking regarding how to best control the virus because it breeds epistemic vices like distrust, gullibility, prejudice, close-mindedness, and insouciance. These challenge genuine knowledge and truth about COVID-19 at the least, and make its management more complicated at the most.

Given a variety of factors, for instance: (i) the capacity of the coronavirus to mutate, (ii) the limitedness of the knowledge of the scientific community about COVID-19, and (iii) the manipulation of information about the pandemic by the political class, it is tricky to refer to "truth about COVID-19." Truth as an epistemic concept is immutable; thus, it is epistemically challenging to apply such a concept that is immutable to a mutating virus because what is known about the virus today may turn out not to be the case in a future date. This would further imply (ii) above, namely that the scientific community's knowledge of the virus at any given point in time may not be all that needs to be known at that given point in time since a mutated variant of the virus may present a yet to be known information about the virus. This scenario is further complicated by the tendency of the political class to manipulate the uncertainties about the pandemic posed by (i) and (ii) above. Therefore, when we refer to "truth about COVID-19" we mean what is already, and correctly known, irrespective of what is yet to be known, about COVID-19. Truth here is epistemic success resulting from a reliable process and coheres with existing facts.

Concerning misinformation and conspiracy theories which are very infectious and influential particularly in the adoption of curative options for COVID-19 in Nigeria, several probable curative remedies have been unscientifically explored. These range from the use of chloroquine to different herbal combinations, some of which have led to medical complications among the users. The conflict between different epidemiological analysis and projections, and the absence of any prescribed pharmacological option(s) in Nigeria exacerbates the COVID-19 quandary. Even though some herbal practitioners have advanced different herbal cures, of which Cugzin by the Benedictine Monks in Ewu, Edo State is foremost, none has received pharmacological validation or government support. Not even the herbal option from Madagascar, which is alleged to have helped the country combat COVID-19, has received formal validation.

The lack of validation and support for local medications is part of the epistemological crisis that challenges the management of COVID-19 in Nigeria. It is a reflection of an ideological structure of epistemic inferiorisation; an epistemic dysfunction in which an agent considers what she believes or knows as inferior to other beliefs and claims by other agents. Epistemic inferiorisation is also a part of epistemic transaction in the sense that it involves how the hearer appropriates credibility to a speaker's testimony. In a situation where an agent S considers herself inferior to another agent X, S has the tendency of attributing excess credibility to X whom S considers as an epistemic superior. This is the scenario that has played out so far, such that the herbal options from Africa, Nigeria inclusive, are largely considered unacceptable because they lack Western validation, and not necessarily because they failed pharmacological tests. This is an epistemic inferiorisation that is itself, an extension of Western superiority complex and imperialism. Obeng-Odoom (2019) and Helen Lauer (2006) have plausibly explicated this as a form of intellectual marginalisation in which Africa, African scientists, and African systems are considered backward; victims of primitive traditions and superstitions. Consequently, "Africa is written out of serious rethinking, as others arrogate unto themselves the power to think for Africa" (Obeng-Odoom 2020: 9).

In the light of the above, we agree with Björn Freter that Africa needs a desuperiorisation of thought (2020: 121). Africa hegemonically depends too much on Western models and thought, which sadly blinds her from her rich heritage and values. In the case of COVID-19, Nigeria's approach is wholesale a Western approach to the problem—the lockdowns, travel restrictions, use of Western medications, social distancing, etc. While we do not disagree with the positivity of some of these prescriptions, however, we firmly maintain, as Soludo (2020) argues, that some of them are practically unsuitable for Africa. In combating COVID-19, Nigeria is waiting *entirely* on Western-approved solutions rather than explore her veritable trado-medical options, which may be complemented with Western solutions. This is a typical case of epistemic inferiorisation, which has not allowed our management options to thrive.

A Management Paradigm for COVID-19 in Nigeria

Even though the mutating nature of the coronavirus makes it difficult to be understood, the greed of Nigerian political elites coupled with epistemic inferiorisation shows that our leadership is epistemically vicious rather than virtuous. The government's infidelity with information transfer has resulted in the poor management of COVID-19 in Nigeria. To this end, we propose a management approach that is based on the unity of our efforts which is only possible if there is transparency and authenticity of information transfer and a commitment to the truth about the actual situation of the pandemic in Nigeria. Our proposal derives its theoretical strength from some aspects of the monadology of Gottfried Leibniz which sees substance as unity.

According to Leibniz, monads are unique, with each having its own spiritual individuality. They are, however, united in such a way that no external cause, except an internal principle, can influence their inner being (Leibniz 2003: n. 11). This implies that the development and actualisation of monads is caused by some internal mechanism. Monads are, in no way, isolated entities; they can interact with other monads, but they do not exert principal or existential influence on each other's being. For Leibniz, reality entirely consists of monads.

One aspect of Leibniz's monadology that interests us is the idea of self-actualisation; the notion that monads develop from within. If the fight against COVID-19 is to be won in Nigeria, the leadership should regard Nigeria as a compound monad, in which case, we must explore internal mechanism to fight COVID-19 from within. Efforts to manage and control the spread of the virus should be advanced from internal analysis and available local options, while at the same time, we take note of global best practices and apply them where and when applicable. By this we mean that the measures we adopt to check the spread of the coronavirus must take cognizance of the particularities of the Nigerian society, we should not just copy measures adopted elsewhere, which may not be applicable here. When we apply measures that are not indigenous to us, they should be with due regard to tackle the problem from within than from without.

Epidemiological models must duly recognise and respect the local environment and population, and recommendations, proposals and predictions ensuing thereof must not be alien to us. Therefore, the first management option concerning COVID-19 that Leibnizian monadology offers us is the need to study the crisis internally—explore internally available options, pharmacological possibilities, and taking precautionary measures that comply with our peculiar setting.

We opine that some of the precautionary measures in the current management of COVID-19 in Nigeria are not immediately realisable. For instance, the effects of lockdown measures would have been ameliorated by exploring virtual possibilities. In Nigeria, the use of Information and Communication Technology (ICT), particularly in the education sector, is relatively very low; teaching-learning processes are still mostly traditional. Many tertiary institutions (not to talk about secondary and primary) lack standard and functional e-library and online Learning Management System (LMS). Yet, it was the immediate option (based on what was obtaining in many more developed nations), recommended by the Ministry of Education to all schools that the closure of schools during the lockdown would not significantly disrupt academic activities. Such an option is bound to fail when learners are not Internet-savvy or compliant.

Adopting an internal approach option would encourage the exploration of local medications without necessarily jettisoning global medical and health options since both would complement each other for the good of the populace. If we do not explore local herbs in the cure of COVID-19, we would be stalling the possible development of our local remedies, some of which have proven helpful with some sickness and past epidemics. The philosophy of "herd immunity"—when more people have become immune to a particular disease, provides a philosophical backing here. For instance, even though malaria is still prevalent in Africa and Nigeria, it is not so much of a killer disease anymore because more people have developed herd immunity to it. Herd immunity occurs when, over some time, people use a particular common treatment procedure or adopt domestic forms of treatment that has helped to boost their immunity. Given our proposed paradigm option, exploring herbal alternatives that we are used to would be a plausible way to go. If vigorously and clinically pursued, it can lead to a locally developed remedy that would boost our national integrity, which would in turn weaken the superiorisation idea from the West. This calls for an epidemiological model that can correctly project the situation in Nigeria, and be a scientific basis for prediction and projections.

We can again draw on Leibniz's monadology to tackle the problem of testimonial deficit or excess in the epistemic transactions towards a better management of COVID-19 in Nigeria. According to Leibniz, while some monads can clearly reflect the world, others do not. A proper act of perception (reflection) of the world consists in consciousness, which only a rational soul or mind is capable of. Leibniz puts it thus: "I think it right that the general name of Monads or Entelechies should suffice for *simple* substances which have *perception* only, and that the name *Souls* should be given only to those in which perception is more distinct, and is more accompanied by memory" (2003: n.19). Apart from consciousness, the rational soul as a created monad has the ability to know *necessary* and eternal truth. Therefore, Leibniz argues that all our reasoning should be grounded on two principles: (i) the principle of contradiction and (ii) the principle of sufficient reasoning. By (i), we judge what is false by what involves contradiction and what is true by what is opposed to contradiction, and by (ii), "we hold that there can be no fact real or existing, no statement true, unless there be a sufficient reason" (Leibniz 2003: nos. 31–32).

Based on Leibniz's analysis, epistemic claims should be interrogated using the principles of contradiction and sufficient reasoning. Prior to putting out any information, they should be diligently analysed against the backdrop of these principles. Conspiracy theories thrive when they are not properly interrogated, and this is the case with the cacophony of paradoxical information on COVID-19 in Nigeria. Many people either doubt the information they receive, or approach them with some apprehension. The absence of a proper epistemic filter of information on COVID-19 in Nigeria is obscuring the truth about the pandemic. In his analysis of perception, Leibniz describes two kinds of truth: (i) necessary and (ii) contingent truths. Necessary truths are discovered through analysis and resolved into simpler ideas and truths. Contingent truths are based on facts (Leibniz 2003: n. 33). If information on COVID-19 go through the filter of analysis and they are based on facts, they would be both belief-worthy and truth-worthy. This would in turn increase compliance with precautionary health directives on COVID-19. Sincerity is an epistemic virtue that can increase trust and diminish insouciance, and other epistemic vices. Therefore, if the Nigerian government is sincere and transparent, and stop politicising the information transfer regarding the virus, it would improve the management of its spread. Also, a proper analysis of issues about the virus would diminish the ember of epistemic incongruity that beclouds it as both an epistemological and epidemiological crisis. We therefore, insist that until we subject epistemic transactions on COVID-19 to atomic analysis and facts, we would continue to face issues of testimonial excess or deficit in the epistemic economy and obstructions with its proper management in Nigeria.

Furthermore, given that monads are simple or atomic substances and atoms are the smallest indivisible units of a substance, if we atomise the management process of COVID-19, we can detect the missing links and gaps in the epistemic transactions. For instance, rather than provide index cases according to binary value, they should be arrived at based on proper atomic analysis. The point here is that we should decentralise the management system and allow particular tracing and analysis. This would make for easy break down and identification of details and facts, and eliminate the allegations of ghost cases. It will also ensure transparency in the entire management process.

Leibniz's monadology provides us the basis to argue for an inward look in dealing with the coronavirus pandemic in Nigeria. This does not imply that we discard global best practices; not in today's global world of critical interdependence, rather, it is an insistence on domestication. It is a proposal that we work with a management paradigm within the context of the Nigerian experience, which would include exploring local pharmacological options, ensuring proper epistemic transactions based on analysis and facts. If this is done, it has the possibility of dispelling the present apathy and improve compliance with safety measures.

Conclusion

In this chapter, we examined how COVID-19 is being managed in Nigeria. First, we situated it within the global crisis of a pandemic and noted that it has posed both an epidemiological and an epistemological crisis. As an epistemological crisis, the authenticity and truth about what we know concerning the virus and its spread in Nigeria is beclouded, and therefore, impedes its proper and effective management. Given the deficits in the epistemic transactions about the virus in Nigeria, we argue that there is need for transparency and commitment to truth; that the government should stop politicising the known facts about the actual situation of the pandemic. This would generate the required trust in the people who would in turn unite in collaboration with the government in the efforts to stem the tide of the virus. If, however, the government continues to allow some of our leaders make a business out of it, the present apathy on the part of the people would remain since the people would continue to lack trust in the government's sincerity of purpose. Upon our analysis and examination of the situation as it obtains presently in Nigeria, we submit that for the effective management of the COVID-19 pandemic in Nigeria, commitment to truth on the part of the government, unity of efforts and transparency in the epistemic transactions about the pandemic is imperative.

References

Adeyemi, Peter. 2020. COVID-19 Grandstanding Over Religion. *The Nigerian Tribune*. Accessed June 6, 2020. www.tribuneonline.com.

Bakam, Armstrong. 2020. Resident Doctors Threaten Strike, Issue FG 14-day Ultimatum. *The Punch* (May 30, 2020). Accessed June 6, 2020. www.punchng.com.

Ball, Philip, and Amy Maxmen. 2020. The Epic Battle Against Coronavirus Misinformation and Conspiracy Theories. Accessed May 27, 2020. www.nature.com.

Beer, Francis, and Robert Hariman. 2020. Learning from the Pandemic: Catastrophic Epistemology. *Social Epistemology Review and Reply Collective* 9 (5): 19–28.

Brick, Shannon. 2020. Epistemic Neglect. *A Journal of Knowledge, Culture and Policy* 34 (5): 490–500. https://doi.org/10.1080/02691728.2020.1737748.

Broadbent, Alex. 2013. *Philosophy of Epidemiology*. New York: Palgrave Macmillan.

Canali, Stefano. 2020. Further Philosophical Consideration about COVID-19: Why we Need Transparency. Accessed May 12, 2020. https://dailynous.com/2020/03/13/.

Dzieciatkowski, Tomasz, Lukasz Szarpak, et al. 2020. COVID-19 Challenge for Modern Medicine. *Cardiology Journal* 27 (2): 175–183. https://doi.org/10.5603/CJ.a2020.0055.

Etakibuebu, Godwin. 2020. Mismanagement of COVID-19 by Nigerian Authority: Case Study of Mrs Suzan Idoko-Okpe. *The News Guru* (June 3, 2020). Accessed June 6, 2020. www.thenewsguru.com.

Fasan, Olu. 2020. COVID-19 Funds: Nigeria's Private Sector Shouldn't Donate to Government. In *Business Day* (April 20, 2020). Accessed May 28, 2020. www.businessday.ng/Columnists.

Freter, Björn. 2020. Decolonisation of the West, Desuperiorisation of Thought, and Elative Ethics. In *Handbook of African Philosophy of Difference*, ed. Elvis Imafidon, 105–127. Cham: Springer. https://doi.org/10.1007/978-3-030-14835-5_5.

Fricker, Miranda. 2007. *Epistemic Injustice, Power and the Ethics of Knowing*. Oxford: Oxford University Press.

Gilbert, Marius, Giulla Pullano, Francesco Pinotti, et al. 2020. Preparedness and Vulnerability of African Countries Against Importations of COVID-19: A Modelling Study. *Lancet 2020* (395): 871–877. https://doi.org/10.1016/S0140-6736(20)30411-6.

Greco, John. 2019. The Role of Trust in Testimonial Knowledge. In *Trust in Epistemology*, ed. Katherine Dormandy, 91–113. London: Routledge. https://doi.org/10.4324/9781351264884-4.

Ihekweazu, Chikwe. 2020. Steps Nigeria Is Taking to Prepare for Cases of Coronavirus. In *The Conversation*. Accessed May 28, 2020. www.theconversation.com-deli.

Kuhn, Thomas. 1970. Logic of Discovery or Psychology of Research? In *Criticism and the Growth of Knowledge: Proceedings of the International Colloquium in the Philosophy of Science*, ed. Imre Lakatos and Alan Musgrave, vol. 4, 1–24.

Cambridge: Cambridge University Press. https://doi.org/10.1017/CBO9781139171434.003.

Lakatos, Imre. 1970. Falsification and the Methodology of Scientific Research Programmes. In *Criticism and the Growth of Knowledge: Proceedings of the International Colloquium in the Philosophy of Science*, ed. Imre Lakatos and Alan Musgrave, vol. 4, 91–196. Cambridge: Cambridge University Press. https://doi.org/10.1017/CBO9781139171434.009.

Lauer, Helen. 2006. Cashing in on Shame: How the Popular 'Tradition vs. Modernity' Dualism Contributes to the 'HIV/AIDS Crisis' in Africa. *Review of Radical Political Economics* 38 (1): 90–138.

Leibniz, Gottfried W. 2003. *Monadology. In Classics of Philosophy, ed. Louis Pojman*. 2nd ed. New York: Oxford University Press.

Mcgwin, Gerald, Jr. 2010. Causation in Epidemiology. *American Journal of Opthamology* 150 (5): 299–601. https://doi.org/10.1016/j.ajo.2010.06.031.

NCDC—Nigeria Centre for Disease Control. 2020. COVID-19 Outbreak in Nigeria: Situation Report. March 9, 2020. Accessed May 27, 2020. https://ncdc.gov.ng/diseases/sitreps/.

Obeng-Odoom, Franklin. 2019. The Intellectual Marginalisation of Africa. *African Identities* 17 (3–4): 211–224.

———. 2020. COVID-19, Inequality, and Social Stratification in Africa. *African Review of Economics and Finance* 12 (1): 3–37.

Odogun, Gbenga. 2020. We Are Under Pressure to Announce False COVID-19 Cases—Kogi. *The Punch Newspaper*. (May 8, 2020). Accessed June 6, 2020. www.punchng.com.

Ogundele, Kamarudeen. 2020. Update: FG Places Travel Ban on China, Italy, US, UK, Nine Others. *The Punch Newspaper.* Accessed March 18, 2020. www.punchng.com/featured.

Olaleye, Aluko. 2020. [UPDATE] Coronavirus: FG Orders Closure of Varsities, Schools Nationwide. *The Punch Newspaper*. Accessed May 19, 2020. www.punchng.com/news.

Popper, Karl. 1963. *Conjectures and Refutations: The Growth of Scientific Growth.* New York: Harper and Row.

Rosenberg, Alex. 2000. *Philosophy of Science: A Contemporary Introduction.* London and New York: Routledge Taylor and Francis Group.

Roy, Shovonlay. 2020. COVID-19 Pandemic: Impact of Lockdown, Contact and Non-contact Transmissions on Infection Dynamics. (Preprint) www.medRxiv.org. (April). https://doi.org/10.1101/2020.04.04.20050328.

Soludo, Charles C. 2020. COVID-19: Can Africa Afford Lockdowns? In *Business Day* (April 24, 2020). Accessed May 29, 2020. www.businessday.ng/article/covid-19.

Stegenga, Jacob. 2020. Fast Science and the Philosophy of Science. https://dailynous.com/2020/05/13/.

WHO: World Health Organization. 2020. Novel Coronavirus (2019–nCoV), Situation Report–13, (February 2, 2020).

Zakaria, Fareed. 2020. This Is Just the First of a Cascading Crises. *The Washington Post*, April 3rd. Online Edition. https://www.washingtonpost.com.

10

Borders, Boundaries, and Identities: Navigating the Barriers to Solidarity and Cohesion in a Pandemic

Adeolu Oluwaseyi Oyekan
and Wasiu Abiodun Balogun

Introduction and Background

The COVID-19 pandemic represents fundamental challenges to public health, human security, and economies across the globe. COVID-19 is also reconfiguring social fabrics in societies and resetting social relations among people with accelerated amplification of existing sociocultural fault lines. Across borders and boundaries, and within national entities, social identities and class relations are forged in different forms as COVID-19 ravages. Across borders, COVID-19 is reshaping solidaristic behaviors as states evolve nationalistic measures in the fight against what

A. O. Oyekan (✉)
Identities and Social Cohesion in Africa (ISCIA), Nelson Mandela University, Port Elizabeth, South Africa

W. A. Balogun
Department of History and International Studies, Lagos State University, Ojo, Lagos, Nigeria
e-mail: wasiu.balogun@lasu.edu.ng

F. Egbokhare, A. Afolayan (eds.), *Global Health, Humanity and the COVID-19 Pandemic*, https://doi.org/10.1007/978-3-031-17429-2_10

is clearly a social scourge. While COVID-19 may have heightened social disconnectedness among geographical entities, communities, and people, it has yet, undoubtedly, created the need for the global community to foster a common agenda and act in solidarity against the pandemic. The paradoxical reality of the COVID-19 pandemic, where the world is expected to act "together-apart" in combating a health emergency, highlights the uniqueness of the problem at hand and the urgent need for a shared agenda against it.

From the start of COVID-19, political leaders across the globe have intensified the call for solidarity; propagating the message that "we are in this together," in the fight against the pandemic. Such calls have echoed the need for behavioral change, sacrifices, and collective being. Hence, as part of a globally coordinated multipronged approach to combating COVID-19, several states have adopted extreme social measures, such as lockdown, social distancing, and isolation, which have significantly reinforced segregation and identity formations in some states and among a good number of people, and group solidarity in several others.

Whereas the idea of "shared threat" offers a compelling justification for building solidarity, differing risk management capacities and deep-rooted socioeconomic cleavages undermine the quest for building and sustaining such solidarity particularly in a pandemic. This should however not deny the centrality of solidarity in combating the ravaging scourge given its many social challenges and dynamics. Therefore, the challenge for global and national leaderships across different borders and boundaries is forging a sense of "us" rather than "I's" in the fight against a pandemic whose antidote thus far has been social segregation and national isolation. Social solidarity may not offer a magic bullet, but the critical role it plays in rolling back a pandemic of social division cannot be overemphasized; hence, it remains a key component of public campaign strategy against the coronavirus.

The focus of this chapter is to explore the different dimensions of the need for solidarity in pandemic management, drawing from diverse experiences around the coronavirus. These dimensions include those between citizens in nation-states to one another, the people and the government, as well as governments and peoples across nation-states. Divided into five main parts, we explain briefly in the first the emergence of COVID-19, while in the second and third parts, we examine the strains on solidarity during the pandemic at both the local and global levels. The fourth part is an explication of the idea of solidarity, while in the last, we explore how the notion of solidarity within closed polities and transnational solidarity at the global level can help in mitigating some of the challenges that have either been created or aggravated by the pandemic.

Coronavirus: Emergence and Impact

Pneumonia-like symptoms in a cluster of patients on December 8, 2019, in Hubei Province of Wuhan City, China, had woken up the world to the reality of a pandemic that would reshape social settings and social formations and reinforce age-old identity crises while creating a new sociopolitical order of social distancing and national isolationism. Society's ready bulwarks against health emergencies, solidarity, and cohesion come under significant pressure as national boundaries and borders are closed, social identity fostered, and social distancing normalized. Wuhan had gifted the world a social pandemic.

Coronavirus (Covs) belongs to the virus family of *Coronaviridae* pleomorphic RNA virus. At present, though efforts are being intensified by global pharmaceutical giants and research institutes to develop coronavirus vaccines, information gap and age-long sociocultural biases, misconceptions, and misinformation about possible adverse side effects of available vaccines constitute a clog in the wheel of progress of COVID-19 vaccination. Twelve months from when the first coronavirus fatality was reported on January 9, 2020, the emergent fatalities evidenced across the world has created a high-risk health emergency in COVID-19. On January 7, 2020, the Chinese Center for Disease Control and Prevention recorded the first case of the coronavirus, and on March 11, the World Health Organization (WHO) declared COVID-19 as a pandemic. As we write this chapter, in slightly over one year, global deaths on account of the virus have gone past the two-million mark (*Johns Hopkins University*, 2021).

Though a health crisis, COVID-19 has created a "2020 emergency" in all spheres of human endeavors, and for several years to come, the global community will continually seek measures to deal with its aftermaths. Coronavirus has visited on the global population a devastation of unparalleled magnitude. Global COVID-19 deaths jumped to 2,501,626, with over 112.7 million cases globally as of 17:24 GMT on Thursday, February 25, 2021 (Johns Hopkins University, 2021). But that number has a social component that offers insights into the social dynamics of the pandemic.

Millions of businesses across the globe are confronted with existential threat. The impact of the pandemic on jobs and livelihoods is already being felt especially in Third World countries of Africa, Asia, and Latin America. The most affected belong in the informal economies where there is an obvious lack of social security safeguards against emergencies. According to the International Labour Organization (ILO), lost labor income will heighten relative poverty for informal workers and their dependents to 56% points in lower- and low-income countries, compared to 52% points in high-income countries (ILO 2020). With many struggling to earn a living during lockdowns, the challenge of survival becomes dire, and there is heightened propensity for criminality. It is apparent that the different dimensions of the impact of coronavirus speak to the social elements of the pandemic. Job losses, criminality, and lack of access to capital and health needs manifest heightened social stratification within societies and across borders. And for societies where extreme socioeconomic divisions are already entrenched, such cleavages will further be accentuated by the pandemic. In the United States, where the consequences of the pandemic have been uneven, reflecting age-long socioeconomic cleavages in American societies, millions of people have lost their jobs, with black and Hispanic communities recording higher unemployment rates compared with white. Yet, the risk of contracting COVID-19 and dying of the virus is higher among minorities and persons of color (Wadhera, et al., 2020). By the end of the first quarter in 2020, among the 36 million jobs lost, households of less than $40,000 annual income had recorded about 40% share of pandemic-induced job losses, with unemployment rates among white standing at 14.2% compared to 16.7% among black and 18.9% among Latinx (Spievack, et al. 2020). The precarious socioeconomic conditions of the Almajiris in northern Nigeria would be accentuated by the pandemic, widening further social stratification gaps and entrenching endemic poverty among a people perpetually confined to the social pyramid base in Nigeria.

Coronavirus and the Manifestation of Differences within States

With the exception of a few countries—North Korea, Turkmenistan, Samoa, Solomon Islands, Tuvalu, Vanuatu, Tonga, Palau, Marshall Islands, Micronesia, Nauru, and Kiribati—with no reported cases, COVID-19, in terms of reach, spread, and rapidity, is the first truly "global" pandemic (Aljazeera, 2020). As the pandemic unfolds, countries adopted measures in line with WHO guidelines, with the global multilateral health agency leading the fight against the virus. However, there existed marked differences in local responses to the pandemic as seen in the cases of the United States, United Kingdom, and Nigeria. As it turned out, such differences were shaped by national leadership, risk and emergency management capacity, level of national awareness, and economic and technological development, among others.

The United States' response to the pandemic offers an interesting case in leadership capacity and policy initiation in times of crisis. The first case of COVID-19 was reported in Washington on January 20, but a new report of the Centers for Disease Control and Prevention (CDC) has found that there were COVID-19 infections in the United States as far back as December 2019 (Basavaraju, et al., 2020). While the report reignites controversies surrounding the origin of the virus, it highlights a fundamental challenge of national awareness in America's response to the pandemic.

The United States' approach demonstrates a clear lack of an overall national response and a failure of leadership and policy. United States' federalist and constitutional structure places the responsibility for public health on the shoulders of the states, and cities and counties could act in that regard with delegated authority. In effect, in ordinary times, states could exercise sweeping powers to protect their citizens' health, with due consideration for individual rights as contained in the constitution.

Expectedly, the federal government's public health authority is limited to ensuring that measures are put in place to prevent interstate or international spread of diseases. However, in emergency and extraordinary times, the two tiers of government have the legal authority to activate emergency powers to guarantee public health and safety and protection of human life (Altman, 2020). As it turned out, after his initial self-description as a wartime president, President Donald Trump announced to the American people that the federal government would only provide the necessary "backup" to states which are expected to have primary responsibility in containing the pandemic. Though in line with conservative principle of devolution of powers in relations to public health emergencies, the president's decentralized and fragmented approach resulted in extreme variation in the national response to coronavirus (Rebecca, et al., 2020). The lack of an overall national response highlights a major weakness in the country's federalist arrangement regarding public health management structure, which shared public health governance powers among the three tiers of government.

The structural weakness in the US public health governance framework is reinforced by President Trump's rhetorical buckshot on coronavirus. After several weeks of denial of the existentiality of the virus, President Trump conceded to the reality of the pandemic by describing it as a "Chinese virus," an obvious reference to the origin of the virus but a social profiling strategy using the pandemic to prejudice China. For most part going forward, the national leadership in the United States was more preoccupied with projecting the image of a nation in charge of the health crisis by justifying America's responses against those of China than coordinating national response measures. It is therefore not surprising that the United States, as of Thursday, February 25, 2021 (1724 GMT), had recorded 28,348,259 cases and 506,500 deaths, 20% of global death toll, the highest by any country (Johns Hopkins University, 2021).

The US COVID-19 experience is as much a case of historic neglect and underfunding of state and local public health systems as it is that of social stratification and national cohesion impact. This is highlighted by disproportionate impact of COVID-19 on racial and ethnic minorities in the United States. Systemic social and economic challenges to health create institutionalized health inequalities among racial minorities and further foster structural racism. In the United States, prudential evidence suggest that African Americans have a higher rate of COVID-19 infections and higher death rates from the disease than whites (Wadhera, et al., 2020; Keating, et al., 2020). This is also the case with Hispanics and Latinos across US cities and counties (Keating, et al., 2020). lCO-VID-19 pandemic, beyond being a health problem, is a fundamental social crisis amplified by inherent challenges of social justice. So, at the heart of inequalities in access to healthcare in the United States are genuine concerns about social justice, and without addressing fundamental social justice challenges in education, housing, healthcare, and administration of criminal justice-issues that foster pervasive, pronounced, and persistent racial discrimination, health disparities highlighted by US COVID-19 experience will continue to exist. Navigating the challenges of the pandemic would require social justice, social inclusion, national solidarity, and cohesion as much as science-based policy interventions and programs.

Unlike the United States, the United Kingdom maintains a centrally planned and coordinated national response to COVID-19. At the start of the pandemic, the United Kingdom held a cautious approach to containing the virus by holding back drastic changes and measures which would have shut down the economy and put families in lockdown. The United Kingdom had started with a "wait and see" approach, which allowed for a trend analysis of the pandemic, but the government soon realized the futility of indifference and national lethargy. From a clear lack of strategic plan and publicly stated goal for combating the virus, the government quickly fraternized with the herd immunity option by ensuring a high enough number of infections thereby reducing non-immune potential hosts for the virus. However, from February 21, when the first case of coronavirus was reported in a 75-year-old woman in Nottinghamshire, the United Kingdom witnessed a steady rise in COVID-19 cases, a development which forced the government to put the country on a 3-month lockdown with aggressive "hfs"—hand, face, space—public enlightenment campaigns (Solomon, 2020). A second lockdown was announced on November 5 as a response to the second wave of the pandemic which peaked at the start of August 2020. The first wave had ravaged the United

Kingdom between March and April, characterized by a high infection rate, followed by a steep and a steady decline in new cases.

And like the United States, the UK coronavirus experience is a true test of national leadership in times of health emergency. Though their approaches differ, very little separates the two countries especially on preparedness, awareness, and national leadership needed in a time of global emergency. The social dimensions of the pandemic offer significant similarities especially on the issue of social justice and health disparities. In the United Kingdom, people of color, especially blacks and South Asians, have a higher risk of COVID-19 death compared with whites (BBC News, 2021). This gap may have closed during the second wave of the pandemic especially with blacks, and Bangladeshi and Pakistani people still experience three times the risk (ibid). Minority populations also have higher number of multigenerational households, predisposing older individuals and aged parents living with grandchildren to increased risks of COVID-19 infection.

Nigeria offers an exciting case study not so much for her status as a Third World but for her unique socioeconomic attributes which reflected in the country's COVID-19 strategy. COVID-19 highlights deep-rooted socioeconomic and security challenges bedeviling Nigeria. The first case of COVID-19 in Nigeria was reported on February 27, 2020, and on March 29, the president gave his first COVID-19 address that also rolled out strategies to combat the virus. Like the United Kingdom, Nigeria's approach, initially, was cautious and lethargic, but the Federal government and Lagos state, the epicenter of the pandemic, soon swung into action as the pandemic ravages. The government adopted a cocktail of health, economic, security, and social measures in combating the virus. For several months, starting from March 2020, the Federal government of Nigeria introduced extreme measures; borders were shut, lockdowns imposed, and interstate travels suspended (Amzat, et al., 2020). These measures were reinforced by social measures and guidelines, such as social distancing, compulsory mask wearing, and handwashing. A Presidential Task Force (PTF) on COVID-19 was set up to provide leadership on policy initiatives and coordinate activities of government agencies involved in the fight against the virus. While the Nigerian Centre for Disease Control (NCDC) was charged with developing capacity for testing, developing public health protocols and guidelines, and facilitating training, the Ministry of Humanitarian Affairs, Disaster Management and Social Development was saddled with the task of addressing socioeconomic challenges of the pandemic across the country through palliative measures (Ibid).

Nigeria's institutional approach to combating the virus is not markedly different from that of the United States. For instance, Nigeria's PTF has functional similarities with the US Task Force on COVID-19 chaired by Vice President Mike Pence. There are also similarities in terms of protocols, guidelines, and policy measures against the virus. Beyond the approaches, the social ramifications of coronavirus across the three countries profoundly influence existing socioeconomic fault lines and cleavages and are sustained by social justice challenges of access to healthcare, job opportunities, housing, and education. In the case of Nigeria, COVID-19, though a leveler in so many ways, also reinforces existing prejudices and social cohesion challenges in the country. While this may be true for both the United Kingdom and the United States, the difference lies in the degree of impact. In a country where access to basic health is a function of social status and economic class, Nigeria's COVID-19 experience vividly shows that there is a strong link between income and health, a development suggestive of a linear relationship between policies that promote economic equity and justice and health outcomes.

The COVID-19 Pandemic and the Strains on Global Solidarity

Prior to the pandemic, global politics had been at its most divisive. The repudiation of multilateralism by the United States in addressing issues related to climate change, the Iran nuclear deal, and unilateral withdrawal from the Syrian war, made complex by the involvement of ISIS across Syria and Iraq, were all complicated by rising populism in parts of Europe, with a lack of coherent plan to address worsening refugee crisis. What the pandemic did therefore was not to create global divisions but to worsen them in manifestly different ways. The management of the pandemic rather than bring the global powers together became an opportunity to continue their antagonistic politics.

The United States, for instance, began by blaming China for concealing information about the virus, and this blame escalated further when China was accused of masterminding the pandemic (The Guardian 2020). To drive home the point, the United States went further to accuse the World Health Organization (WHO) of connivance with China and followed up by cutting its funding to the Organization in the process, before finally serving a notice to pull out (New York Times 2020). The withdrawal of the United States from the WHO at such a critical time made it difficult to develop a unified global response for managing the virus. Efforts to use the platform of the G7 to muster a global response failed at the first meeting over differences about what name to call the virus in the communiqué (WSJ 2020). To put it succinctly: attempts at a coherent global response to the pandemic have been overshadowed by hegemonic tussles, especially between China and the United States.

Without a coherent global response, there began a scramble for control and monopolization of critical resources such as ventilators, masks, and other protective gears. There were widespread reports of hostile interceptions of supplies heading for some countries by others who exercised greater bargaining power. With the exception of Cuba that sent medical personnel and other resources to Italy, and China's offers of assistance to a number of countries in Europe and Nigeria, collaborative efforts have been very limited. Even at that, China's pandemic diplomacy has come under severe criticisms as largely ineffective interventions designed more for political leverage and influence than for the management of the virus (Drezner 2020).

China's domestic response to the virus has been described as ruthless but effective, with reports of lockdowns and massive surveillance operations to monitor infections and spread. However, allegations of discriminatory implementation of the measures surfaced, with black people reportedly being targets of draconian, racist measures that bear no direct semblance with the facts of the pandemic. While some were prematurely thrown out of their accommodations, others were denied use of public spaces such as restaurants, eateries, and pharmacies, with signs boldly indicating that "blacks are not allowed" (HRW 2020). The targeting of "the other" since the outbreak of the pandemic is however not limited to China, as people of Asian descent have been frequently targeted and intimidated for causing the pandemic and its spread (UNESCO 2020), in a manner reminiscent of past pandemic discriminations during the outbreak of Ebola, Zika virus, and Asiatic flu, among others (Ransing et al. 2020).

The pandemic has also brought to the fore, more than before, the increasing inequalities between countries in the West and those in the global South. While there is no doubt that the global economy has been massively impacted negatively, the implications have been severe in places riddled by endemic poverty than developed nations. In countries like Nigeria, South Africa, and across Central America, lockdown measures were difficult to enforce on account of the inability of the various governments to adequately provide palliatives (Maffioli 2020). The varied success in demonstrating economic resilience, resource mobilization, as well as economic sustenance has shown that COVID-19 is not an equal opportunity pandemic in many respects (Stiglitz 2020).

There are numerous efforts ongoing in different parts of the world to find a vaccine for the virus, with varying degrees of progress. The efforts however are uncoordinated, largely on account of the polarized nature of global politics. The discovery of a vaccine, or many variants of it, does not appear designed to benefit people from the developing parts of the world. Using the global scramble for ventilators and masks as metric, developed countries appear better positioned to prioritize their citizens in a way that makes those in the global south appear as afterthoughts. There are pointers to the fact that equitable access to vaccines will be constrained in part by various measures being put in place by developed countries, which essentially amount to acts of vaccine nationalism (Fidler 2020). Thus, questions on how COVID-19 vaccines are to be best distributed have focused on equitable distribution within countries, such as targeting vulnerable populations and healthcare and essential workers (Phelan et al. 2020), with less focus on equitable distribution between different countries. Infrastructural limitations needed for vaccine preservation have also added to the obstacles faced by many Third World countries, especially in Africa.

The question at this juncture is what type of response is best in managing the pandemic. Should individuals prioritize their autonomy over collective action and interests? Ought nations to manage it as self-sustaining, sovereign polities with limited obligations to members with clearly defined attributes of belongingness, obligations, and benefits? What are the advantages of an ethics of solidarity in the curtailment and management of the pandemic, as well as its fallouts? Are there motivations for transnational efforts toward eradication and recovery? A country may, for instance, decide to leverage on the notion of solidarity for managing the pandemic within its own borders without feeling motivated to join hands with other countries in an act of transnational solidarity. It may also be deemed useful to solidarize in combating the pandemic, without the feeling of a need for extended solidarity post-pandemic. Political solidarity, in terms of domestic or foreign policy choices, is equally separable from civic solidarity, wherein the people voluntarily take actions that promote the eradication of the virus while avoiding those that spread it. We shall attempt to answer these questions shortly. Before then, however, the next section will be a synoptic conceptualization of solidarity.

The Concept of Solidarity

Solidarity simply means a feeling of unity between people who have the same interests or goals or a unity that produces or is based on community of interests, objectives, and standards. The term, however, assumes a different meaning when it is being deployed in the context of state welfare systems or in discussions in political philosophy. As Christian Arnsperger and Yanis Varoufakis (2003) opine, when politicians, philosophers, and political activists use the term "solidarity," it simply refers to a generous disposition, a propensity to sacrifice something such as values on behalf of some targeted group of people (e.g., refugees) whose welfare one deems important. For them, the essence of solidarity lies in the hypothesis that people are capable of responding sympathetically to (or empathizing with) a condition afflicting "others," irrespective of who those others are or whether one cares for them personally. From this explanation, we can glean two important impressions. First, the term "solidarity" is used in respect to the "other," and not the "self/individual," and second, "solidarity" is independent of the relationship that exists between the individual and the other. That is, it does not matter whether the "other" is a friend, family, or stranger; what matters is the "condition" that is afflicting the "other" which the individual identifies or sympathizes with.

According to David Miller (2017), to understand the concept of solidarity, there is a need to make a distinction between solidarity *among* a group of people and solidarity *with* a group of people. Miller argues that solidarity with a group of people—for instance, a group that is suffering hardship at the hands of an oppressive regime—means identifying with them emotionally, trying to imagine what it must be like to be in their place, and then taking symbolic or practical steps to help them.

Solidarity among a group of people, on the other hand, presupposes the following: there is a sufficiently precise and shared sense in which a people constitute a group, that is, there must be some feature or set of features that binds a people together; there is a relationship that is reciprocal in the sense that each member recognizes and is recognized by the others as belonging to the group; the attitude adopted toward fellow members of the group is one of concern and support; and more importantly, the group accepts collective responsibility for what its members do (Miller, 2017: 64–65). Miller further explains that solidarity (among a people) is very instrumental within the human society for it advocates protection for members of a group in the sense that other members can be expected to come to one's aid when one gets into difficulties. Also, it provides a check on inequality and also implies social trust in the sense that groups are able to solve collective action problems, since members can usually be relied upon to comply voluntarily with rules that benefit the group as a whole, and so, it reduces the need for coercive measures to ensure that agreements and contracts are carried out (Miller, 2017: 66).

The concept of solidarity, however, has been described by political theorists, philosophers, and sociologists as an enduring challenge in almost all liberal democratic societies because of the view that solidarity requires individuals to tolerate views and practices they dislike, to accept democratic decisions that go against their beliefs or interests, and to moderate the pursuit of their own economic self-interest to help the disadvantaged. This challenge brings us to question whether there is a need for solidarity between citizens and whether we can achieve solidarity within and between diverse social groups. In response to this, Keith Banting and Will Kymlicka (2017) argue that "solidarity" is a social concept which applies at the level of a modern, culturally diverse, democratic society as a whole and refers to attitudes of mutual acceptance, cooperation, and mutual support in time of need such that if citizens are to maintain a good society, especially in the context of growing diversity, they must have, if not virtue or altruism, then some degree of solidarity. This means that citizens must at times be motivated by attitudes of mutual concern and mutual obligation toward their fellow co-citizens.

They distinguished three different dimensions of solidarity that can (and should) exist in contemporary democratic societies, namely, civic, democratic, and redistributive solidarity. *Civic solidarity* is a relationship that is characterized by mutual tolerance; acceptance of people of diverse ethnicities, languages, and religions as legitimate members of the community; and openness to newcomers from diverse parts of the world. *Democratic solidarity* entails support for basic human rights and equalities, such as the equality of men and women, tolerance for the political expression of diverse cultural views consistent with basic rights and equalities, and acceptance of compromises among legitimate contending interests. *Redistributive solidarity* involves support for redistribution toward the poor and vulnerable groups, support for the full access of people of all backgrounds to core social programs, and support for those that recognize and accommodate the distinctive needs and identities of different ethno-cultural groups (Banting & Kymlicka, 2017: 4).

Furthermore, Banting and Kymlicka argue that the concept of solidarity within a democratic culturally diverse society helps motivate people to accept the strains of commitment involved in building and maintaining a decent, good, or just society, particularly in contexts of diversity. Solidarity, they opine, is important within diverse social groups, maybe not so much for its intrinsic value but for its functional role in motivating compliance with the demands of justice. Thus, solidarity is a necessary (though not sufficient) condition for a just or fair society

(Banting & Kymlicka 2017). In contrast, however, Jacob Levy (2017) argues that the aspiration to ground democratic politics on the concept of solidarity is a futile attempt because it rests on philosophical mistakes, ideological illusions, and empirical misunderstandings.

Levy argues that the inhabitants of a political community are not a particular subset of humanity united by allegiance to some particular political ideal, and neither are they demarcated set of persons who share in a common inheritance of advantages and disadvantages, resources, and relationships. Rather, fellow citizens are, in a fundamental sense, moral strangers to each other, united only by the shared circumstances of inhabiting a common political jurisdiction, and not by any prior relationship that legitimizes, grounds, underlies, or stands outside of those circumstances. He posits that the concept of solidarity especially within liberal democratic and culturally diverse societies creates an imaginary line between "us" and "them" such that those who fall outside the line or those who do not share solidarity tendencies with other citizens are regarded as "enemies." He, therefore, submits that there is a need for contemporary democratic societies to explore the possibility of having a political life among strangers, that is, a kind of civil arm's-length relationship with fellow citizens who are neither friends nor enemies and who are living with disagreement and managing it with no real hope of reconstituting as based on some deeper agreement or a social bond that trumps all others (Levy, 2017, 107–110).

Miller argues, however, that solidarity does not necessarily advocate general consensus on values because political cultures, especially democratic ones are multifaceted, and so, one does not have to sign up for everything in order to be included as part of the "we." For him, therefore, solidarity permits and even encourages loyal opposition, so long as it is clear that one's loyalty to the political community itself is not compromised (Miller, 2017, 68).

Managing the COVID-19 Pandemic: The Case for an Ethics of Solidarity

Given the nature of the pandemic, and the massive disruption it has brought upon day-to-day living as well as patterns of social organization across the world, there is very little doubt that returning to normal, or finding a new normal, will require enormous resources and planning. The question then is whether it is useful to proceed within and between different countries on the basis of solidarity or find solutions separately and individually. Yet, putting the matter this way is not so straightforward. At the local level, the case for solidarity, grounded on the notion of belongingness, appears a bit more straightforward than at the global level, though numerous challenges abound.

One of the challenges many countries have faced is how to balance public safety with assertions of individual or group autonomy and identity, with which many of the measures introduced appear to be in conflict. Social distancing rules, for instance, have been breached in defense of cultural, social, and religious rights and rites in South Korea (BBC 2020), the United States, and Nigeria among other places, leading in some cases to violent confrontations with law enforcement agents (Corbin, 2020; Agusi et al., 2020). While in the case of Korea and Nigeria, religious worship was deemed more important than safety rules provided by the governments and experts, in the United States, super-spreader events, such as the campaigns of former President Trump, have been hinged on the liberties guaranteed in the First Amendment of the constitution. There have also been clashes between authorities and groups who assert their rights not to wear face masks. There is an increasing number of anti-vaxxers, who are committed to declining vaccination eventually when they are ready (The New York Times, 2020).

Concerns about the powers of the state at a time of rising totalitarianism across the world have also fueled suspicions that some of the containment measures are at best deliberately exaggerated to increase surveillance, strengthen the powers of the state, curtail people's rights, and roll back democratic freedoms. This view has been reinforced by suggestions that pandemic management requires greater state efficiency and competence and has little or nothing to do with democracy. At a more extreme level, it would appear that the demands of democracy are perceived as an impediment to the state's capacity to effectively respond to the pandemic (Roberts 2020; Fukuyama 2020). In more than 60 countries, elections were put off or rescheduled in the larger interest of "public safety" (IDEA 2020). In South Africa, the perceived high-handedness of the security agencies in enforcing lockdown rules has generated serious debates (Labuschaigne 2020; Seekings & Nattrass 2020). These polarizing situations have the implications of deepening the impact of the pandemic, with the attendant cost on lives and resources. The challenge then lies at least partly in building support, or better still, consensus, around genuine measures targeted at the pandemic in a way that reassures the people that such measures are necessary and, in the main, temporary.

The nature of the pandemic as a public health issue creates a plausible basis for solidarity within local boundaries. By its very nature, solidarity is relevant to public health, because in contrast to personal healthcare, whose primary focus is the individual patient, public health aims for the longevity and functioning of populations through collective action (Karako-Eyal 2018). Further, the successful implementation of public health measures on the one hand, and the extent to which they gain normative legitimacy on the other, largely depends on the extent of the cultural sense of solidarity and cooperation among the people (Jennings 2015).

Thus, while there may be arguments that a pandemic, no matter how serious, should not upend rights that are taken as givens under normal situations. But then, it can as well be argued that in a pandemic, obligations of solidarity are bigger than the claims of autonomy, especially when such obligations do not constitute greater harm to the individual than it benefits the public. Wearing face masks, maintaining social distancing, and observing lockdown rules (save for situations in which people are left with no means of survival and sustenance) constitute little or no risk to the people, whereas flouting these rules, depending on the severity of the virus, is capable of spreading it, thereby endangering the lives of many other citizens. This is even more so when the carrier is asymptomatic and spreads the virus, especially to those who are vulnerable. It may be reasonable for the state to enforce the observation of non-harmful regulations that may safeguard public health. Similarly, group activities such as religious worships and ceremonies capable of exacerbating the impacts of the virus require modifications that prioritize both the safety of members of such groups as well as others who may be negatively affected by their own exposure.

Conversely, governments have the responsibility to make preventive measures as clear as possible and provide cushions to minimize the negative impact its considered measures may have. Additionally, building confidence and trust in the citizenry requires imposing measures which, though may be tough in a few cases, are not themselves more harmful than the virus. For instance, contact tracing, screening, and tracking through facial screening apps generate apprehensions about the possibly draconian use of such powers without assurance that the measures are indeed temporary and that the measures are more scientific than political. If people are required to stay indoors for indefinite periods, socially distanced, deploy their skills on the frontline, or to accept a vaccine despite a barrage of hostile internet propaganda, they need a sense that such demands are coming from trustworthy sources, are given for good reasons, and are geared toward plausible, public goals (Roberts 2020).

Also, preexisting inequalities that exposed the poor and groups like BAME (blacks and minority ethnic groups) to the ravaging effects of the virus in the United States and the United Kingdom have contributed to its spread and casualty figures in the affected countries. In South Africa, there exists significant inequalities in the distribution of ill health and disability, with the implication that the need for health services to diagnose and treat these illnesses becomes greater among lower socioeconomic groups. There is a strong correlation between these inequalities in illness and a host of socioeconomic factors, such as inequitable access to portable water, housing, sanitation, education, employment, and income (Gopalan & Vasconcellos 2019). These challenges, left unattended, have the capacity to undermine even the best of responses to a pandemic, now and in the future. Managing the pandemic and preventing possible recurrence transcend its mere curtailment and require more lasting measures to address social imbalances not caused by the virus, but nonetheless exposed and amplified by it.

At the global level, solidarity requires that different countries work together at a multilayered level of containing, eradicating, and recovering from the virus. So far however, not much seems to have been achieved collectively at the first stage of containment. Divergent interests between global powers, especially the United States and China, have made mutual cooperation difficult and rendered multilateral platforms such as the World Health Organization (WHO), the G-7, and the G-20 largely ineffective. The implication of this is that different countries have had to battle the pandemic within their limited resources and interest. One notable instance was the scramble for personal protective equipment (PPEs) and the reported hijacks of supplies, as a result of fierce bidding wars. Also, discussions on vaccines have focused more on their distribution and usage within national boundaries, without much reference to developing countries.

In coping with the economic and social effects of the pandemic, there have also been interesting policy options, as different countries plan to overcome the ruinous impacts of the virus on economic growth. For instance, the EU has agreed to a union-wide economic stimulus, but the agreed package has been caught up in right-wing politics that stalls implementation. Many of the affected countries in the developing world are therefore more seriously confronted with the management of the pandemic in the immediate and its consequences in the near future.

As earlier alluded to, the motivation for transnational solidarity differs from Durkheim's (1997) idea of mechanical solidarity. Philosophically, questions as to whether we have obligations toward strangers have generated diverse views, even as globalization has deepened integration between states (Appiah 2007). Defenders of cosmopolitanism, for instance, argue that solidarity is extendable to all humans, irrespective of the particular group to which they belong. On the contrary, some argue that nationality limits the scope and reach of the norm of solidarity to nation-state citizens and/or the population occupying a state territory (Nowicka et al. 2019).

One question about the possible source of motivation for transnational solidarity in the face of global inequality has continued to generate debates. Solidarity, as we have earlier averred, finds easier expression within the bounds of political communities where the people have a sense of shared identity. Conversely, the motivation to solidarize with the distant other appears to be much weaker. In managing the pandemic then, it is important to identify the possible source(s) of commitment to collective actions that benefits all.

The case for global solidarity we believe, can be hinged on the notion of broadening regard for others as being worthy of equal moral consideration. This consideration helps simultaneously hold attachments to particular identities, such as members of one's political community, while acknowledging the fact of shared humanity with others. Attachment, couched in universalist terms as we have done, is admittedly weaker than particular ones, and it is easy to see that the salience of particular attachments is reinforced in many ways by facts of shared experiences and close affinity. Building global solidarity on this type of commitment therefore, and complementing the notion of shared humanity, requires an appreciation of the increasing interdependence of the world we live in. This interdependence has increased the scale and scope of the risks and burdens that constitute significant threats to people across the world, such as the coronavirus pandemic.

Working toward the curtailment of global challenges makes a demand on people across diverse cultural and political communities for a broader sense of shared responsibility for the preservation and sustenance of humans and the environment. The ethics of solidarity as we espouse here, then, rests on the twin notions of shared humanity, which is an inherent moral worthiness and equality of all persons, and prudence, which propels an instrumental appreciation of the need for cooperation for the survival and flourishing of all. Seen this way, the apparent contradictions between the demands of particularistic, in-group solidarity and the impulses of universal solidarity can be reconciled and mutually acknowledged.

The notion of shared humanity, while fundamental, has a limitation of practical nature. The acknowledgment of the moral worthiness of others may encourage us to avoid discriminatory actions against them but does not motivate us in very strong ways to cooperate with them or act in ways that enhance their interests. On the other hand, prudential appreciation of current global challenges and the threats they pose provides a strong basis for action, but on an ad hoc basis. Proceeding from an approach which combines the inherent equality of all with instrumental, self-interested sense of prudence addresses the weaknesses of each, taken in isolation.

For the foreseeable future, the threats of pandemics, environmental crises, and terrorism, among others, suggest strongly that there will be a need for sustained interdependence and solidarity across the globe. What this suggests is that whereas the commitments that come from prudential considerations may be situational and instrumental, the scale and dimensions of the challenges are likely to motivate a prolonged period of cooperation for collective survival. What this implies is that global challenges may serve as catalyst for the deepening of interdependence and the deepening of commitments between groups whose motivation for solidarity was hitherto weak, on account of limited binding factors. Importantly too, while particular attachments remain strong and continue to enjoy primacy, the increasing emergence of different sites of identification and self-definition, cutting across religious, sexual, and gender persuasions among others, continue to make the boundaries of solidarity less rigid than they used to be.

It is therefore possible to imagine a form of solidarity that transcends sameness to accommodate those who are neither like us nor members of our political community (Nowicka 2017). This recognition of the obligations owed to those who, by voluntary or imposed categorization, appear as different defends the possibility of a form of global solidarity that complements rather than override internal solidarity engendered by the group or nation-state (Habermas 2004). This type of solidarity can either be specifically universal in its universality, by applying to all persons across different states, or particular yet universal, by transcending boundaries to apply to specific groups that are for instance defined by gender, occupation, age, or religion (Duyvendak et al. 2016). Transnational solidarity therefore becomes possible when we accept the possibility of multiple belongings, and the logic of simultaneity that at once incorporates people into an expanded conception of the community at the level of the global, while acknowledging their commitment and belongingness to the nation-state (Levitt & Glick Schiller 2004; Nowicka et al. 2019).

With respect to the pandemic, the imperative of global solidarity becomes obvious once we note that beyond being a public health issue for the individually affected countries, it is also a global health issue with social, economic, and political implications. Historically, pandemics have played significant roles in transforming societies, whether in the moderation or widening of influence; the decline of a given civilization, as it was in the case of Rome; or redistributing power (McNeil 2020; Drezner 2020). Historically too, multilateral institutions, to make the World Health Organization (WHO) a specific example, have arisen in times of crisis of global proportions (Fidler 1999). In recent time however, right-wing populism and resurgent nationalism have eroded the recourse to multilateral, interstate agencies as vehicles of shared solutions to common challenges, in a way that not only undermines the capacity for their effective functions but also questions their relevance. The pattern in which the pandemic has spread, and the way it has affected the global economy, however, suggests that it won't be fully controlled anywhere until it is controlled everywhere, and the economic downturn won't be reversed until there is sustainable, equal global recovery (Stiglitz 2020).

There is a need then for a global approach to the pandemic that focuses on its immediate and future threats, as opposed to the gridlock occasioned by the tussle for domination among the big, powerful countries. In developing the mechanisms for managing the pandemic at the global level, one of the issues arising is the need to manage the closure of borders and the attendant restriction on migration in a way that does not reinforce isolationism. While a pandemic like COVID-19, by its nature, necessitates measures that severely curtailed cross-border movement, there is a fear that it has the tendency to feed into populist inclination to blame foreigners as the source of all ills (Muller 2017).

The closure of borders is, however, beneficial in the sense of preventing further spread of the virus through migration from and into particular countries. In this way, restricting border movements becomes an approach that ought to reinforce a mutual sense of obligation to help others stay well because their well-being at the time requires that we maintain safe distancing rather than deepening an "us" against "them" perception. In this way, distancing becomes a way of reinforcing cohesion and exhibiting solidarity with others (Metz 2020). Divisive and discriminatory rhetoric has not been proven helpful in managing the pandemic. It is therefore important to enhance mechanisms that deepen transnational engagement and solidarity even as physical borders assume greater importance for the moment.

Strengthening global solidarity will require the reforms of multilateral agencies so that they are better positioned to coordinate responses to the big challenges for which they were created. It is important as well to strengthen multilateral agencies for a more effective management of global challenges in a way that complements national efforts. It is also important to focus on equitable distribution of resources such as kits and vaccines, in a way that helps countries that are ravaged by the virus but are relatively ill-prepared in managing it. Attempts to focus mainly on national needs, especially by the developed countries, are likely to delay the global eradication of the virus for much longer, effectively allowing it to remain a threat to the world at large.

Post-pandemic recovery efforts will also be needed to revive the economies of weak nations in a way that will stimulate global growth and engender sustainable development. Not only will this impact positively on overall global recovery and economic outlook, but it will also likely enhance the capacities of such countries to prepare and cope better with future pandemics, should they arise. Widening global inequality, it can be argued, has contributed to the inability of many countries in the global south to adequately respond to the pandemic. Acting in solidarity therefore requires more than immediate assistance to ameliorate the direct impacts of the pandemic. More important is the reorganization of the international economic structures to be fairer and more equal.

Conclusion

In this chapter, we have examined the challenges posed by the coronavirus pandemic within societies and indeed across the world. It is apparent that beyond the immediate health ramifications, it has impacted negatively on social and economic spheres in different countries with disruptions that may prove extremely difficult to surmount. Managing the pandemic therefore requires an attitude of solidarity within and between states. Hegemonic tussles between global superpowers have made it nearly impossible for coordinated confrontation of a common problem, with its attendant tolls. Similarly, societies that have left some groups economically and socially vulnerable have experienced serious difficulties in managing the pandemic. It is therefore important that the vertical structures that perpetuate inequality within and between states require a reassessment and reorganization, if the world is to beat the coronavirus and be better prepared for the next pandemic.

Acknowledgments The contribution of Adeolu Oyekan to this work is based on the research supported by the National Research Foundation of South Africa (Grant Number 99188, SARChI Chair in Identities and Social Cohesion in Africa, Nelson Mandela University). Opinions, findings, conclusions, and recommendations expressed in this work are those of the authors' alone, and the NRF accepts no liability whatsoever in this regard.

References

Agusi, Ebere Roseann, Sandra Ifynneke Ijoma, Chizuruoke Stephen Nnochin, Nnaemeka Onyekachi Njoku-Achu, Chika Ignatius Nwosuh, and Clement Adebajo Meseko. 2020. The COVID-19 Pandemic and Social Distancing in Nigeria: Ignorance or Defiance. *The Pan African Medical Journal* 35 (52): 1.

Altman, Drew. 2020. Understanding the US Failure on Coronavirus—an Essay by Drew Altman. *BMJ* 370: 1.

Amzat, J., K. Aminu, V.I. Kolo, A.A. Akinyele, J.A. Ogundairo, and M.C. Danjibo. 2020. Coronavirus Outbreak in Nigeria: Burden and Socio-medical Response During the First 100 Days. *International Journal of Infectious Diseases* 98: 218–224. https://doi.org/10.1016/j.ijid.2020.06.067.

Appiah, Kwame Anthony. 2007. *Cosmopolitanism: Ethics in a World of Strangers*. New York: W.W. Norton & Co. Inc.

Sridhar V. Basavaraju, et al. 2020. Serologic Testing of U.S. Blood Donations to Identify SARS-CoV-2-reactive Antibodies: December 2019-January 2020, *Clinical Infectious Diseases*. doi:https://doi.org/10.1093/cid/ciaa1785

BBC. 2020. Shincheonji and Coronavirus: The Mysterious 'Cult' Church Blamed for S Korea's Outbreak. https://www.bbc.com/news/av/world-asia-51851250

BBC News. 2021. Covid: South Asian Death Rates Still 'alarming' in Second Wave. Covid: South Asian death rates still 'alarming' in second wave - BBC News. February 9.

Corbin, Caroline Mala. 2020. Religious Liberty in a Pandemic. *Duke LJ Online* 70 (1): 1–28.

Durkheim, E. 1997. *The Division of Labor in Society*. New York: The Free Press.

Duyvendak, J.W., et al. 2016. *The Culturalization of Citizenship: Belonging and Polarization in a Globalizing World*. London: Palgrave Macmillan.

Fidler, P. David. 1999. *International Law and Infectious Diseases*. New York: Oxford University Press.

———. 2020. Vaccine Nationalism's Politics. *Science* 369 (6505): 749. https://doi.org/10.1126/science.abe2275.

Fukuyama, Francis. 2020. The Pandemic and Political Order. *Foreign Affairs* 99: 26.

Gopalan, P.D., and K. De Vasconcellos. 2019. Factors Influencing Decisions to Admit or Refuse Patients Entry to a South African Tertiary Intensive Care Unit. *SAMJ: South African Medical Journal* 109 (9): 645–651.

Human Rights Watch. 2020. China: COVID-19 Discriminations against Africans. https://www.hrw.org/news/2020/05/05/china-covid-19-discrimination-against-africans.

International Labour Organisation (ILO). 2020. As Job Losses Escalate, Nearly Half of Global Workforce at Risk of Losing Livelihoods. https://www.ilo.org/global/about-the-ilo/newsroom/news/WCMS_743036/lang%2D%2Den/index.htm

Jennings, B. 2015. Relational Liberty Revisited: Membership, Solidarity and a Public Health Ethics of Place. *Public Health Ethics* 8 (7): 7.

John Hopkins University. 2021. Coronavirus Resource Centre. COVID-19 Map - Johns Hopkins Coronavirus Resource Center (jhu.edu).

Karako-Eyal, Nili. 2018. Beyond the Ethical Boundaries of Solidarity: Increasing Vaccination Rates through Mandatory Education to Solidarity. *Tex. A&M L. Rev* 6: 345.

Keating, D., Eunjung Cha, A. Florit, G. 2020. 'I just pray God will help me': Racial, ethnic minorities reel from higher covid-19 death rates'. The Washington Post. Nov. 20.

Maffioli, Elisa M. 2020. Consider Inequality: Another Consequence of the Coronavirus Epidemic. *Journal of Global Health* 10 (1): 1.

McNeil Jr, D. G. 2020. Trump says US is leaving WHO, but experts aren't so sure. *The New York Times*, May 30. https://www.nytimes.com.

Metz, T. 2020. What Does An African Ethic of Social Cohesion Entail for Social Distancing? *Developing World Bioethics* 1: 1–10.

Nowicka, Magdalena, et al. 2019. Transnational Solidarity, the Refugees and Open Societies in Europe. *Current Sociology* 67 (3): 383–400.

Phelan, Alexandra L., Mark Eccleston-Turner, Michelle Rourke Allan Maleche, and Chenguang Wang. 2020. Legal Agreements: Barriers and Enablers to Global Equitable COVID-19 Vaccine Access. *The Lancet* 396 (10254): 800–802.

Ransing, Ramdas, et al. 2020. Infectious Disease Outbreak Related Stigma and Discrimination During the COVID-19 Pandemic: Drivers, Facilitators, Manifestations, and Outcomes Across the World. *Brain Behavior, and Immunity* 1: 555–558.

Rebecca, L., Haffajee, J. and Michelle M. 2020. Thinking Globally, Acting Locally — The U.S. Response to Covid-19. https://www.nejm.org/doi/full/10.1056/NEJMp2006740#article_citing_articles

Roberts, Adam. 2020. Pandemics and Politics. *Survival* 62 (5): 7–40.

Solomon, T., 2020. Coronavirus: The UK Approach Explained. The Conversation https://theconversation.com/coronavirus-the-uk-approach-explained-133672

Spievack, N., J. Gonzalez, and S. Brown. 2020. Latinx Unemployment Is Highest of All Racial and Ethnic Groups for the First Time on Record. *Urban Wire* blog. May 8. https://www.urban.org/urban-wire/latinx-unemployment-highest-all-racial-and-ethnic-groups-first-time-record

Stiglitz, Joseph. 2020. Conquering the Great Divide *Finance and Development* 1: 17–19.

The Guardian. 2020. Trump Says China Could Have Stopped Covid-19 and Suggest US Will Seek Damages. April 28. https://www.theguardian.com/world/2020/apr/28/trump-says-chinacould-have-stopped-Covid-19-and-suggests-us-will-seek-damages.

UNESCO. 2020. "COVID-19-related discrimination and stigma: a global phenomenon?". *https://en.unesco.org/news/covid-19-related-discrimination-and-stigma-global-phenomenon*

Wadhera, R.K., P. Wadhera, P. Gaba, J.F. Figueroa, K.E.J. Maddox, R.W. Yeh, and C. Shen. 2020. Variation in COVID-19 Hospitalizations and Deaths Across New York City Boroughs. *JAMA 323* (21): 2192–2195.

Wall Street Journal. 2020. G-7 Meeting Ends in Disagreement Over Coronavirus Name.

11

Discourses of the Wandering *Almajiri* Child as Representation of the (Post-) COVID Generation

Malami Buba and Mikailu Ibrahim

"The world is on the brink of a catastrophic moral failure and the price of this failure will be paid with lives and livelihoods in the world's poorest countries."
—Tedros Adhanom Ghebreyesus (Director-General, WHO)

Introduction

There seems to be no better words to describe the role of the humanities in global health than the "moral" case advanced by the Director-General of the World Health Organization (WHO), Tedros Adhanom Ghebreyesus, reported in the *Guardian* UK (January 19, 2021). He was

M. Buba (✉)
Division of African Studies, Hankuk University of Foreign Studies, Global Campus, Yongin, South Korea

M. Ibrahim
Department of English and Literary Studies, Usmanu Danfodiyo University, Sokoto, Nigeria

F. Egbokhare, A. Afolayan (eds.), *Global Health, Humanity and the COVID-19 Pandemic*, https://doi.org/10.1007/978-3-031-17429-2_11

referring to the vaccine nationalism that saw only 25 vaccines administered in any low-income country as against the 39 million given in high-income countries. In the same report, the Director-General argued that: "It's not right that younger healthier adults in rich countries are vaccinated before health workers and older people in poorer countries." There are other "moral failures" even in these developed economies, as when the United Kingdom was forced to reconsider the withdrawal of free school meals to disadvantaged children during school holidays (*Guardian* UK, January 20, 2021) or when thousands of dollars are sent to millions of individuals who have lost their livelihood during the COVID-19 pandemic. At the same time, it saw the greatest rise in the wealth of the world's richest individuals, with one estimate noting that the $540 billion made by the ten richest individuals is "enough to vaccinate everyone in the world" (*Guardian* UK, January 26, 2021). Even low-income countries, such as Nigeria, are being forced to address the pandemic's economic challenges by opening a social safety net register to support petty traders in distress, as reported in *Premium Times* of January 19, 2021. Humanity has been blighted not only by the actual disease but perhaps more insidiously by the continuing mental and psychological disorders as a result of the absence of a "human touch.". As Falola (2016: 86) pointed out: "Humanity itself (as a being, in the individual and collective sense) becomes totally diminished without the humanities." And herein lies the role that the humanities can play in, at the very least, uncovering the nature both of local and global iniquitous practices that often hit the "most vulnerable of the vulnerables" hardest. The wandering child, such as the Nigerian *almajiri* child, is undoubtedly one of the most vulnerable members of humanity.

The wandering child has been a feature of the global south since the beginning of the scourge of globalization. Images and representation of the child as a scavenging menace to public morality abound in major cities of Africa and the Americas. They come in many "colors": as street children, as beggars, as hawkers, and as the domestic help. As the force of the law is being unleashed on their frail frames through the police and other mass incarceration agencies, their numbers continue to grow. The continual human drift from impoverished rural areas into the urban slums of big cities ensures the movement of more children in search of basic survival. Yet, as children, the law enshrines the right of the child to basic health, well-being, and education. As we shall see below, the UBEC Act 2004 of Nigeria follows the Dakar Declaration in asserting children's right to free and compulsory primary education. Hence the conflicting signals that seem to permeate many policies toward children's welfare in the urban jungle that is the city. However, the current coronavirus pandemic has exacerbated the crisis of this generation. In poorer countries, the crisis of an already neglected generation becomes more evident as the bite of closures, curfews, and clampdowns deepens the anguish of this post-COVID generation. Yet, the life chances of *almajirai* are further diminished by the perceived hopelessness and irrelevance of their "vocation" as beggars of food and purveyors of dangerous crimes. The *almajiri* has always been viewed with suspicion in the urban landscape of many West African cities. A combination of attitudes toward Muslim itinerary scholarship and regional disparities forms part of the narrative of alienation that the *almajiri* experiences in daily encounters with fellow citizens. The coronavirus pandemic has worsened the onslaught of this negative perception to the point where a direct connection between the virus and the *almajiri* is imputed. Witness the massive operation in Nigerian cities of forcibly removing and transporting children to their presumed localities in the midst of the pandemic in Nigerian cities! This massive exodus of children is discussed in greater detail below in the section dealing with *almajirai* as vectors and super-spreaders.

It is against this background that this chapter seeks to explore how representation can work to demonize and dehumanize the victim further by defining a whole epistemology in terms of a virus without cure. In the rest of the chapter, we will explore the nature of itinerant scholarship within Muslim theology and examine how it fits with the pursuit of the good life in a post-modern, coronavirus-afflicted Nigeria. In this respect, the *almajiri* is situated in the historical context of his vocation. Within that context, we explain the rationale and rationality of the quest for knowledge even in the face of urban adversity that daily impacts upon *almajiri*'s determination to survive. In both the real world of Nigeria's sprawling urban landscape and the fictional world of African literature, we point out the changing fortunes of the *almajiri*, whose journey from a mystical character of wisdom, knowledge, and humanity to a child made monstrous by the new economy of inequality remains a recurring decimal in transhuman movement. The coronavirus pandemic, we argue, is a juncture in the continuing saga of children without hope or help. All of these issues of representation and perception will be critically addressed using sources as diverse as novels, newspapers, institutional reports, edicts, personal histories, and encounters. In theoretical terms, we look at representation as a conceptual paradigm through which meaning is created and circulated (Hall 1997) and situate the current disavowal of *almajiri* practices as an aspect of this representational narrative in fiction and in everyday description. In our concern to fully specify how representation works at both of these levels, we have attempted to link them to the contrasting and, at times, complementary concepts of semiotics (Barthes 2012 [1972]) and discourse (Foucault 1980), respectively. We also explore the trajectory of the language and practice of disavowal, which resulted in mass deportation of *almajirai* at the peak of the COVID-19 pandemic in Nigeria. We will examine the consequence of such translocation both to the children and the national landscape which permits such movement in the midst of a health emergency without the supporting infrastructure. We will also endeavor to situate the conditions under which the almajirai find themselves within the wider global context of child poverty, deprivation, and health inequality. Finally, we suggest how best to accommodate the practice of Muslim discipleship without demonizing children and denying them the right to a future of opportunities from which Nigeria can benefit and prosper. Our claim is that the representation of almajirci as a product of a patently discredited system of Muslim acculturation highlights the representational gap between reality and perception.

Itinerant Scholarship in Local Muslim Theology

One of the most oft-cited prophetic traditions in Islam related learning to journeys beyond one's locality and imagination. It spoke of the importance of seeking further knowledge wherever it may reside. Thus, the life of learning for those Muslims wishing to "drink deep" had involved the metaphor of learning as a (difficult, but rewarding) journey in Hausa:

tafiya mabuɗin ilmi ("travelling is a source of knowledge"); *karatu, farkonka maɗaci, ƙarshenka zuma* ("learning is bitter in the beginning, and sweet in the end"). The journey could be as short as a walk to the local school in the neighborhood or the early morning walk of the *Malam* in search of further knowledge. At times, however, the journey could involve thousands of kilometers as was the case of famous itinerant West African Sufi scholars travelling to Sokoto, Nigeria, in search of further knowledge (Bâ 2008).

This journey of learning and devotion was often undertaken on foot, and on a shoestring, on the belief that *Allah Ka Bai, Allah Ka Hanawa* ("God gives and God deprives"). Small acts of labor would be undertaken as well, in exchange for food and shelter. At other times, the seeker of knowledge would have to rely on the kindness of strangers along the route of learning. Many a *Zango* quarter in West Africa started as a listening and resting post for itinerant *malam* and other transhuman travelers searching in the borderless world of Islamic epistemology, *duniya ta Allah ce* ("the world belongs to God") (Adamu 1978). Alhassan Dantata (1877-1955), one of the wealthiest merchants of West Africa, was said to have begun his incredible journey into international trade through itinerant *almajiri* discipleship and in the process left a legacy of business acumen that has been passed down to the current billionaire Dantata extended family, including Aliko Dangote, a grandson, and the wealthiest man in Africa today. The classic quest journey of *Shaihu Umar* (1966) exemplifies both of these trajectories.

In effect, the discourses of the wandering *almajiri* represent a great tradition of learning as a universal quest, and it is important to keep this assumption in mind, as we move into the examination of the life and tribulations of the *almajiri* as a representation of a (post-) COVID generation. We begin however with a description of the lived experience of an *almajiri* in fiction.

Ambiguous Adventure and the Fictional World of *Almajirai*

Cheikh Hamidou Kane's *Ambiguous Adventure* opens with a glimpse of the life of an *almajiri*, who, in this context, is no "ordinary" beggar-disciple. Samba Diallo is a noble prince of the Diallobe country, and his sojourn at the hearth of the revered teacher, Thierno, is part of the long tradition of his people to send crown princes to learn to lead by following in the footsteps of their ancestors. This tradition entails a period of dislocation from the sheltered confines of the local palace to a different environment in which the prince becomes one of the many disciples that are voluntarily sent to the master Sufi to learn to recite and memorize the Qur'an. Away from home, with only learning on their minds, the young disciples must also fend for themselves as part of the knowledge architecture of Islamic sufism that promotes self-denial, ascetism, and other deprivatory practices, including begging. Begging was an essential component of the learning process, for it instils in the disciple, according to this school of thought, an awareness of the irrelevance of material prosperity. Mastering the Qur'an is viewed as the first step toward enlightenment and proximity to the very essence of godliness.

The process of mastering the word for *almajiri* Samba Diallo necessarily involves "the strength to master his suffering" (Kane 1972: 1). Such suffering comes from beatings, but also from the very act of dislocation from one's immediate family at a very young age. In this period of extreme deprivation, all disciples must beg to feed and feel the essence of subsistence through leftovers from families for whom the prayers of the beggars at the beginning of the working day serve as a form of cleansing and absolution:

> Under the morning wind, Samba Diallo improvised edifying litanies, with interpolations by his comrades, at the closed door of his cousin, the chief of the Diallobe. The disciples would go about so, from door to door, until they had collected victuals enough for their day's nourishment ... [The disciples squatted in the dust and set to on their first meal of the day. When they had eaten enough to satisfy their hunger, they put the rest in their wooden bowls, against possible future need. With his bent index finger

> Samba Diallo thoroughly cleaned the plate, and put the little ball of food, thus recovered into his mouth ...] Tomorrow the same quest would begin again. While seeking God, the disciples would know no other way of supporting life than by begging, whatever their parents' wealth might be. (Kane 1972: 14)

In this vivid description, we have a glimpse of the life of the wandering *almajiri* disciple. Beyond assuaging the hunger of the moment, nothing else takes precedence over learning to recite the Qur'an—a book whose mystery becomes open to them in a long time to come. This particular form of spiritual resilience is considered the antidote to the ravaging march of modernity.

In the contrasting world of the Diallobe and that of the French colonizer, Cheikh Hamidou Kane is conflicted. The issue for him was how to achieve harmony between the new school's "ways of joining wood to wood" and the old school's learning, in which "what we teach the children is God [so that] they forget ... themselves, their bodies, and the futile dream which hardens with age and stifles the spirit' (Kane 1972: 34). There was always the fear that these two ways of seeing and being to which the Diallobe were bound would lead to the impasse, eloquently put forward by Hamidou Kane through Thierno, the teacher: "can one learn *this* without forgetting *that*, and is what one learns worth what one forgets?" (Kane 1972: 34). As the Diallobe would find out, there is no easy solution to an existential problem for all colonized societies. On the one hand, the march of modernity, globalization, and more recently economic nationalism forces poor and impoverished ex-colonies to swallow the pills of consumption capitalism with the active collusion of rigged multilateral systems. On the other hand, their knowledge production capacities have been maligned, decimated, and broken by the permanent allure of urban economy and culture.

Yet the narrative of *almajiri* practice is filled with stories of redemption, (re-)discovery, and emancipation. Nigeria's late prime minister Tafawa Balewa's *Shaihu Umar* (1966) exemplifies the transformative effect of knowledge acquired through the path of itineracy. In this quest novella, the protagonist, Shaihu Umar, recalled his journeys of (mis) adventure through time and space to the gathering of his own *almajirai* disciples. He recounted his capture, enslavement, and trafficking into the hands of the Arabs before finally becoming the most learned scholar throughout sub-Saharan Africa. He was later to find his way back to his homeland and settle in the northeastern city of Bauchi, the location of his recollection. And in the course of this grand narrative, we were invited to participate in the unmasking of a borderless Africa of immense diversity, complexity, and transformations, where slaves became masters and descendants of masters knelt before slaves to receive learning, wisdom, and healing. The unbounded nature of *Shaihu Umar*'s journey was not only linked to slavery but also to the cosmopolitan and migratory interactions of the various Muslim peoples of Africa (Kane 2016). In that process, circulation and exchange of knowledge is also engendered, in addition to commerce and cultural brokerage (Brenner 2000). Let us bear this in mind as we ponder about the role of the humanities in contextualizing the *almajirai* and the local knowledge production system they are deploying to challenge their own "ambiguous adventure" through a dominant ideology of Islamic education.

Interestingly, the knowledge architecture of *almajiri* education displays a definitive pattern of knowledge transmission within the Muslim Sufi brotherhood throughout West Africa. In a non-fictional scholarly context, Ousmane Kane, the Harvard historian and a member of a prominent Sufi Tijjaniya lineage in Senegal, presented his diary of knowledge navigation at age six and over, as he moved between secular French lycée and the Islamic madrasa in 1960s Senegal (Kane 2016: 3). The present authors are also products of this parallel co-mingling of the "old" school of spirituality, *makarantar Allah* ("faith school"), and the "new" school of modernity, *makarantar boko* ("secular school").

COVID-19 Pandemic and the Wandering *Almajiri* Child

Almajiri, as a term of religious and social acculturation, has expanded to cover all manner of migratory practices, including those that sit firmly within the realm of child trafficking, child labor, and exploitation. In this respect, the *almajiri* shares many of the terrible conditions in which girl-child house help, child traders, and other minors find themselves in Nigerian cities (Khalid 2020). In its classical form, a Malam and his *almajirai* pupils embark on a scholarly journey, locally called *yawon bundi* (literally "wandering-of-tail"). It requires the *Malam* to take over the responsibility not only of the Qur'anic education of the children under his care but also their general health, well-being, and safety. Parents will ordinarily send some food and clothing items and, at times, cash for the basic upkeep of the child. However, this is neither regular nor compulsory, as part of the character strengthening of the *almajiri* disciple will depend on his forbearance and the kindness of strangers. It is also important to note that the Malam may be on his own quest for greater knowledge and enlightenment, as he seeks residency with his potential teacher. Needless to say, there is no exchange of money at any stage in the learning process for both the *almajiri* and his *Malam*. (The emphasis of male membership of the *almajiri* group underscores the virtual absence of girls as *almajirai*.)

Thus, the daily life of the *almajiri* before the pandemic was characterized by uncertainty in essentials as basic as food and clothing. A typical *Almajiri* wakes up to roam around begging for daily meals in tattered clothes. Some of them identify with the homes of families helping with house chores in exchange for a meal and a little allowance. Other than these chores, they stay around their school with the Malam to learn the recitation of the Qur'an. Their accommodation with the Malam is mostly congested and lacks basic sanitation facilities like toilets and water. Hoechner's (2018) extremely valuable insights into the lives of *almajirai* make a compelling case for understanding and recognition of the underlying poverty and alienation dictating their changing fortunes. She situated her extensive study within a broader conceptual context "bringing insights from education studies, poverty research, and childhood and youth studies" (Hoechner 2018: 7). And, perhaps, for the first time, we heard from the *almajirai* themselves, who pointed out that the practice provides a platform for learning how to cope with their inescapable and impoverished condition through "patience and humility." As Hoechner (2018: 5) noted, "patience and humility ... are central elements of faith." These attributes are also part of the characteristics of the "perfect-person" in Hausa society (see Buba 2020). Instructively, the local personality with the perceived highest perfection was Shehu Usmanu Danfodiyo, the revered itinerant Malam who founded the Sokoto Caliphate in the nineteenth century. Yet, the *almajirai* continue to experience extreme prejudice and stigmatization, as their dehumanization during the current COVID-19 pandemic shows. For Hoechner (2018: 225), it is the society that needs reform, in order "to fight the stigma attached to poverty, and to promote respect on the basis of one's worth as a human being rather than as a function of one's position within social hierarchies."

While this is the reality of their daily experience, an interview conducted by the second author with some of the families patronizing the *almajiri* services in Sokoto revealed that the *almajiri* phenomenon also represents an adaptive strategy for the economic necessity of rural-urban migration and search for better life opportunities. One of the interviewees revealed that there were many economic benefits to the *almajiri* children in the kind of domestic work they provide. She explained that immediately the help begins, the *almajirai* get smarter with improved cleanliness, concentrate more on their learning, and aspire to join public school. She recalled her *almajiri* domestic help buying a bicycle for his younger brother from the stipend he received. Another *almajiri* house help bought livestock from the money he sent home. He would also use the money to buy brocades and related fabrics as he sets out to visit his family in the village. However, even where they find solace in the above patron-client relationship, Hoechner (2018) argued that the transaction was largely one of unequal exchange, and the "good boss" is a rare occurrence in the lived experience of the *almajirai* in her research study. Clearly, then, modernity in the form of urbanization and extreme inequality has eroded many of these lofty ideals.

Almajirai as Vectors and Super-spreaders

In common with the rest of the world, the COVID-19 pandemic in Nigeria exposes the extreme inequality which exists in the new knowledge economy. Poor and "unlettered" citizens were left to fend for themselves, although their daily paid manual jobs have virtually disappeared due to restrictions in human and vehicular movements. In addition to these two devastating factors, there is the persistent insecurity that has engulfed most part of the non-industrialized northern Nigeria. This part of Nigeria relies heavily on agriculture both for internal consumption and for export to other parts of Nigeria. In exchange for food, particularly cattle, manufactured goods are bought and brought to the north. This trade has been going on for many centuries, but it came almost to a halt as a result of the twin tragedies of COVID-19 and insecurity in the north.

In this atmosphere of restriction and deprivation, the *almajiri* suddenly became the focus of anger, where newspaper headlines began to exploit the vulnerability of this "minor" and indefensible group. There was a strident attempt to merge the images of scavenging little boys in tattered clothes and a well-worn bowl in hand with the discourses of demonization. Labels of "terrorists," "criminals," "menace," "plague," "virus," and "threat" feature prominently in these discourses of demonization. There was, for example, the story carried in *The Sun* Nigeria (October 22, 2020) of the concern expressed by the Christian Association of Nigeria (CAN) in Anambra State over the "distribution of almajiris from Kano to other parts of the country." In the report, spokesman of CAN in the state quoted a news report in *Vanguard* Nigeria (May 15, 2020), in which "fear gripped A[kwa]-Ibom residents as Taskforce intercepts another trailer conveying 32 Northerners." The concern, according to the *Vanguard*, was related to "alleged transportation of Almajiris suspected to be COVID-19 positive from some states in the north to the southern states," as well as "the invasion of some states in the region by suspected terrorist groups from the north." In the same vein, the Igbo pro-Biafra group, IPOB, warned, in a *Daily Post* (May 4, 2020) news report, about "the ploy … to export coronavirus from its epicenter to other parts of Nigeria", noting also that "Everybody knows that almajiris are wanderers causing uprising, mayhem and crises in the whole of North." In Rivers State, Nigeria, the Governor, in a state broadcast, reported in *PM News*, Nigeria (April 29, 2020), "directed the Commissioner of Social Welfare to round up and deport all vagrants, including the almajiris, to their States of origin to protect our people from the threat they present to the transmission of this pandemic."

An extensive review of the demonization of *almajirai* by all sections of the Nigerian society has been undertaken in Hoechner (2018). In that study, she quoted scholarly studies and influential public intellectuals, such as Wole Soyinka, who described *almajirai* as Boko Haram "foot soldiers … bred in madrassas." (See Hoechner [2018:4ff] for a fuller critical overview of these negative portrayals.) Yet, Hoechner (2011) reported the tendency of the *almajirai* to "occupy moral high ground" and restrain themselves from retaliating "bad treatment," which is in contrast with the common perceptions earlier quoted that make them the pool for Boko Haram recruitment.

Managing the *almajiri* situation, however, was also one of the major issues of the COVID-19 pandemic period in most northern Nigerian states, where the number of *almajirai* includes the "expelled" and "deported." This did not come as a surprise considering that the life of the *almajiri* children—roaming about the street begging for their daily meal—is irreconcilable with the lockdown that authorities imposed to curve the spread of the pandemic. Thus, the *almajirai* were caught in the crossfire of the demands of the pandemic for restricted movement and a political leadership that was ill-prepared for the emergency. What followed was a statement from the Northern Governors Forum on April 21, 2020, banning the *almajiri* and the resolve to return them to their states of origin. Some northern State Governors started enforcing the decision of their regional forum leading to what a feature on May 12, 2020, by the BBC considered "the biggest ever state organized mass movement of minors" in the country, with evident contradiction of repatriating thousands of children in crammed vans across state borders in the midst of a travel ban to control the spread of the virus. In May 12, 2020, *The Guardian* Nigeria reported that "not fewer than 435 of such vulnerable children were returned by Kano to Katsina." Governor Abdullahi Umar Ganduje of Kano Sate also announced a plan to immediately return 524 to neighboring Jigawa state. Kaduna State's response was more prominent with the *Premium Times* (May 20, 2020) quoting about 30,000 as the number of *almajirai* "who have been sent back to their home states so far."

Sentiments brewed in divergent ways from the decision and action of the states to repatriate the *almajirai*. The revered head of the Muslim population in Nigeria, Sultan of Sokoto, was reported by *Premium Times* (May 20, 2020) to have distanced Islam from "laziness, ignorance and idleness as exemplified by itinerant *almajiri*," confirming the main opinion of the report, which celebrated the pandemic as "a golden opportunity to change the [almajiri] narrative and put the plague behind us once and for all." And, in a statement during the pandemic, Secretary to the Government of the Federation, who doubles as the Chair of the Presidential Task Force on COVID-19, described the *almajirai* as "instruments for faster transmission of COVID-19 virus in the society" in addition to their pre-existing threat of "grooming future members of Boko Haram." The discourse of apprehension here, as elsewhere, was one of deportation and expulsion in addition to banishment and evacuation. As the *almajiri* children were rounded up, arrested, detained, and then deported, COVID-19-positive cases within their confined spaces increased. On what to do with them when they arrived at their intended destination, no statement was forthcoming. There was a muted indication of coordinated effort among the governors of northern Nigeria, for example, but little came of it in the form of policies and provisions for the dispersed *almajirai*.

While the state actors are being ambivalent about the responsibility for taking care of the *almajirai*, and proceeding with the action of repatriating them, civil society groups were unequivocal in challenging the deportation. Human Rights Agenda Network (HRAN) condemned the deportation as "illegal and unconstitutional," supporting the position with Section 41 of the 1999 Constitution that guarantees the rights of citizens to stay in places of their choice within the federation. The Coalition of Kano Civic Groups made a related statement and considered the action of the Governors as "fundamentally wrong."

Supporting *Almajirai* in the Pandemic Expulsion Aftermath

Since the announcement and implementation of the *almajiri* expulsion, several initiatives emerged to provide alternative views and actions on managing the situation. The moment also bolstered other already existing initiatives to renew their commitment on the issue. Prominent among such initiative is the proposed National Almajirci Summit which, according to a report in the *Tribune* Nigeria (October 18, 2020), was "borne out of the recent move by states governors to stop *almajiri* in their respective domains." The National Coordinator of the Summit described any attempt to stop the practice of *almajirci* as "a shame" for Muslims. Instead, the Summit proposed reforms and plans to mobilize all stakeholders for technical sessions on critical issues around sustaining the *almajiri* system ahead of the national summit. Coordinators of this initiative worked to mobilize the identified stakeholders, led technical cohorts, and developed draft documents on the history of *almajiri* system in Nigeria with its models and challenges. They also understudied related models in other Islamic countries, as well as proposed mechanism for funding and logistics and identified strategies for outreach and enlightenment.

Although an affiliate of the planned summit, the independent effort of the Almajiri Child Right Initiative (ACRI) in mobilizing support for the *almajiri* toward reform deserves a special mention. ACRI led and participated in a series of webinars and advocacy with the support of United Nations platforms, particularly UNICEF, with a view to providing alternatives to deportation. One of those webinars was on the occasion of World Children's Day on November 20, 2020, with a multi-stakeholder's perspective to address "the rights of *Almajiri* children." Speakers included the UN Deputy Secretary General, the Ambassador of the European Union to Nigeria, and ECOWAS President.

Another dimension of the deportation debate was the awareness of practical interventions that impact the life of *almajiri* and are worth emulating. Prominent among these was the intervention of the Emir of Gombe who was known to cater for the basic needs of hundreds of *almajirai* in his emirate. He spoke in a webinar organized by *Noor Takaful* in June 2020 and called for an integrated National Policy on *Almajiri*. Another effort that started a few months before the COVID-19 repatriation fiasco and continued throughout the period was the intervention of a National Assembly member from Sokoto State, Nigeria, Dr. Balarabe Shehu Kakale. The intervention targeted 1000 *almajirai* with skills and decent learning environment during 2021. *Daily Trust* Nigeria (January 11, 2021) reported that the legislator distributed 9 vehicles, 33 motorcycles, 60 sewing machines, and 40 grinding machines, among others, to the first set of *almajirai* beneficiaries. The national legislator was also one of the main sponsors of the bill seeking to repeal and enact UBEC Act 2004, so that vulnerable groups such as *almajirai* are captured in its provisions. He was reported to have called for "a total overhaul of the *almajiri* education system ... [through] Recognition, Reform and Mainstreaming (RRM)."

Critical Considerations

It is important, however, that we do not take this narrative of the *almajiri* as a health hazard and an economic embarrassment at face value. It has a broader context in representation theory, where culture, in this case Muslim Hausa (Sufi) religious culture and its representation in the everyday lived experience, is widely condemned as "other." In his many engagements with culture as an overarching principle of understanding society, Stuart Hall warned us that everyday life is, in fact, an essential component of the economic and political life of the people. He noted that how "ordinary" people speak, what they watch, what they eat, as well as the company they keep, all feed into their perception and how they are perceived in the society. He went on to advocate for acute awareness of how these cultural artifacts of a society could inform its political and economic behavior. In short, Stuart Hall had always sought to put the humanities at the center of his studies of representation. According to Hall (1997:15):

> Representation connects meaning and language to culture ... [and] is an essential part of the process by which meaning is produced and exchanged between members of a culture. It does involve the use of language, of signs and images which stand for or represent things — semiotic and discursive.

In focusing attention on the semiotic and discursive roles of representation, Hall (1997) was appealing to the wider concerns of Roland Barthes and Michel Foucault. He argued, following Barthes (2012 / 1972), that representation can proceed from consensus-building denotation features of signs, be they individuals, objects, or events, to their indeterminate connotative attributes for which interpretation becomes the source of meaning. Furthermore, connotative interpretation is rooted in a "social ideology," which serves to represent "the general beliefs, conceptual framework and value system of society" (Hall 1997:39). Hence the creation of a "myth" around which members of a society construct their own sense of belonging and membership. In explaining how interpretation proceeds in this context, Hall (1997: 39) summarized Barthes' (2012 / 1972) exemplification of the mythology of French greatness through the image of a black soldier "giving the French flag a salute." At the level of connotative interpretation, it symbolized both a progressive nation and its "imperiality," now celebrated at the level of a myth.

With respect to Foucault's (1980) notion of discourse, Hall pursued it as a function of "the production of knowledge through language." In this context, language has been supplanted by discourse, which now describes the relation between power and knowledge production. Discourse, according to this representation paradigm, is where meaning resides, and it is through such discursive practices that we uncover both the specificity of the representation and the historical context of its interpretation. In addition, the meaning of a discursive practice is subject to continuous change and interpretation with the passage of time.

In this connection, it is interesting to note how the *almajiri* represents a particular form of learning culture and is, in turn, represented and defined by a different form of learning culture. As we noted elsewhere, the *almajiri* represents a great Sufi tradition of learning whose ultimate aim is communion with God and the radiation of such communion as ethics to the wider community. The transitional vagrancy and victual satiation of hunger that are associated with his vocation are components of the disciple's "regime of truth" test along the path of freedom from wants and needs (see Foucault 1980). This path is, of course, not the same for everyone, but no one is spared from experiencing part of the journey, precisely because it is the only path to salvation for (Hausa) Muslims. The obligatory Muslim daily prayers, for example, require individuals to memorize portions of the Qur'an through practice and perseverance. This is the same for the Ramadan fasting during which all Muslims must eschew food, leisure, and pleasure from dusk to dawn for the full lunar month in a year's cycle. And here lies an aspect of the powerful discourse of power and knowledge production behind the resilient and resistant posture of *almajiri* as a cultural practice (See Hall 2016).

Viewed in this way, *almajiri* practices and ethos have resonance in the wider Muslim practices in the society. In fact, it was the dominant discourse of power, knowledge, and religious conduct for more than three centuries of Islamic propagation in Nigeria and beyond. The current appearance of *almajirai* as pitiful and their subsequent dehumanization as the "virus" itself, then, arose from a "new" interpretation of their relevance and the sufficiency of the "message" they project in the society. For local Muslims, whose new religious culture directly connects to Wahhabi Sunni traditions of Mecca and Medina, *almajiri* practice is a peculiar Sufi practice that privileged a clerical lineage with tight control over knowledge production and dissemination. That hierarchical ordering of society has since been replaced officially by the colonial "meritocratic" education system and unofficially by the leveling effect of Madrasa-to-Medina Salafism of urban Muslim Hausa (Thurston 2018). The efficacy of their prayers, amulets, and *rubutu* written potions has been publicly destabilized by the overwhelming presence of *Izala* ritual practices beginning with the declaration of *Where I Stand* by Sheikh Abubakar Gumi since the 1970s (see Gumi and Tsiga 1992; Kane 2012). Having noted this, the services of the Malam and his *almajirai* to the sprawling urban poor for health and healing continue with an unbroken regularity.

For the wider Nigerian population, the continued presence of the *almajiri* as a permanent feature of the urban landscape in Nigerian cities is a confirmation of a historic tradition of conservatism, illiteracy, religious fanaticism, and endemic poverty. In particular, the conflation of the itineracy of the *almajiri* with Islamic radicalization and subsequent recruitment into the Boko Haram terror group represents a potential danger to the society. The evidence for this apprehension is not supported even by one of the most detailed studies of Boko Haram in Nigeria (Walker 2016). In addition, many parts of Nigeria are already experiencing the unwelcome encroachment of Fulani herdsmen, whose cattle rearing has come under severe scrutiny as a kidnapping and murderous ring. Here too, the "northern" dimension of this transhuman movement is stressed, as is its "recolonization" and "Islamization" agenda. Yet, for hundreds of years, movement, settlement, and exchange had taken place among peoples and cultures currently within the borders of Nigeria. Resident Muslim Hausa communities, particularly in the southwest of Nigeria, have found *Sabo* "new" settlements and inter-married with the local Yoruba communities in these areas. Trade between the north and south has continued to flourish even in the face of rampant violence and kidnappings along the bad roads of Nigeria. Islam is also a constant reminder of the intersectional nature of the relationship between the dominant ethnic groups in Nigeria. Crucially, Lagos remains the pre-eminent commercial nerve center of Nigeria, necessitating the massive influx of fortune seekers from all parts of the country. One of the "night jobs" of *almajiri* in these areas, as well, have always included participating in the burgeoning "prayer economy" of a citizenry living with uncertainty (Adamu 1978; Falola 2016; Walker 2016).

Almajiri and the "National Question" in Focus

It seems, then, that the anxiety about a super-spreader marauder in the form of *almajiri* was much more than a concern with health. After all, the *almajirai* were herded together and transported to other epicenters of the disease without any protocols in place on how to handle their cases when they arrived at their destination beyond the optics of media coverage. Worse, there was no indication that there was any data source against which their actual state of origin could be confirmed. Presumably, these states relied on the information supplied by the children themselves, which will serve to explain the harried manner of their evacuation.

Fundamentally, the circumstances of the *almajirai* evacuation to a putative state of origin were an indication of state's failure. Quite apart from the constitutional rights of all citizens to roam and remain in any part of the country, as noted earlier, children have specific rights under the Child Rights Act 2003. In the act, children's safety from harm and education are to be guaranteed by the state, agencies, and the individuals caring for them. However, most northern states have not incorporated the act into their laws, meaning that effective enforcement of the rights of children under the act is in abeyance. How then could they be evacuated and handed over to states where their rights as children are unenforceable? One of such rights is a constitutional requirement of the right to education, which has also been enshrined in the Universal Basic Education Commission (UBEC) Act 2004. The UBEC Act 2004 was fashioned to align with the goals of Dakar Declaration on Education for All (EFA) which Nigeria ratifies. The declaration sets out to ensure, for example, that "all children, with special emphasis on girls, children in difficult circumstances and from ethnic minorities, have access to complete, free and compulsory primary education of good quality." Hence, the agitation of National Education Summit on *Almajiri* for UBEC to use its funds to support the *almajiri* schools. Unfortunately, here, too, aspect of these rights has been ceded to states with respect to primary education. In other words, local provision regarding children education will apply to evacuated *almajirai* in many of these impoverished states. At any rate, the current school infrastructure is totally inadequate even for the children enrolled in mainstream state schools. Even with the expanding role of Arabic Boards, which now cater for a bigger school intake than mainstream schools, places for the "newcomers" will be non-existent in these states. The Arabic boards, ordinarily established by states at their discretion, cater mainly for Integrated Qur'anic Schools (IQS), which promote the integration of national curriculum subjects such as English, Science, and Arithmetic into their religious education curriculum of memorization and exegesis.

Related to this incapacity to address the needs of *almajirai* is the underlying current of national "conflicts" of resource control, resource allocation, and resource mismanagement. As one of the most intractable national malaises, these "conflicts" are at the heart of the use of indigeneship to determine the statehood of citizens whose right to residency anywhere in Nigeria is guaranteed by the constitution. However, given the current revenue allocation formula, states, usually high-income generating ones, have been placing the hurdles of the formula in the path of "non-indigenes." This hurdle, often determined through language and ethnicity, is in addition to considerations of biosecurity and criminal conduct that were used to exclude *almajirai* from affluent states' "imaginary borders." Currents of political polarization and re-alignment, as the wind of change blows in the direction of the 2023 presidential election, should also not be discounted in the hawkish posture of regions jostling for power.

Way Forward

What existed prior to COVID-19 on policy that relates to the specific situation of the *almajiri* was the sponsorship of the Child Destitution Bill by the senator representing Sokoto Central Senatorial district in 2017. The bill sought to establish a National Commission on Child Destitution to meet the basic livelihood needs of children without caregivers. The debate on *almajiri* deportation during the COVID-19 pandemic re-enacted the importance of the bill with *Almajiri* Child Right Initiative (ACRI) calling for its passage into law.

Another aspirational move also emanating from Sokoto was the proposal to adopt the Indonesian Pondok model "as an alternative to the existing *almajiri* system in the state" as reported by the *Vanguard* Nigeria (March 1, 2020). This intent was expressed when the State Governor received the Indonesian Ambassador to Nigeria in the state According to the report, Pondok utilizes mosques and other traditional centers to provide integrated learning for Islamic and formal education. The Governor assured that Sokoto State was not in a hurry to ban the *almajiri* system like other states until an alternative system was provided.[1]

In the global arena, UNICEF has been providing interventions to the Integrated Qur'anic Schools (IQS) for more than a decade. One of the

[1] For a detailed study of the Pondok system in Malaysia, see Omar (1993).

most recent of such interventions was through the Girls Education Project (GEP3) with funding from the Foreign, Commonwealth & Development Office (FCDO). Some of the interventions include grants for building learning centers, as well as provision of materials and training to support the integration of literacy and numeracy in the schools. HASKE and RANA programs are part of GEP3 and have reached over 2500 Qur'anic schools in five states in northern Nigeria with foundational learning materials, training, and support.

A related initiative from the World Bank, managed by Better Education Service Delivery for All (BESDA), also targets the Qur'anic Schools with a view to the integration of Basic Education curriculum in their routine learning. These trends point to the initiatives of taking responsibility on the life of the *almajiri* as a child with rights enshrined by global and local statuses through a combination of literacy, numeracy, and vocational skills with their spiritual learning of the Qur'an as the best and humane way forward to the situation during and beyond COVID-19.

Concluding Remarks

Thus, the specific phenomenon of *almajiri* discipleship in Nigeria has continued to be addressed in relation to (a) the Arabian model (Islamiyya), (b) the Western (faith schools) model, and lately (c) a proposed Indonesian model, but the underlying issues of poverty, social exclusion, and misallocation of resources as elements of the narrative of representation must first be addressed. Already, there is a deafening silence regarding the allocation of N400 billion for vaccine importation, while young people of all ages are facing uncertain futures as a result of COVID-19 school closures and the loss of economic livelihood by millions of caregivers on whom they depend. A World Bank report on the negative impact of COVID-19 indicated that the pandemic has the potential for increasing the number of children in learning poverty by 72 million over the 382 million count before the shock. The future for *almajirai* in this uncertain time is even more dire as the contest between the epistemologies of "useful knowledge" and "deep learning" continues to arrest their development into active and confident members of the wider community. The humanities must endeavor to push for a parallel system of access to educational opportunities that produced much of the creative talents in northern Nigeria well into the 1980s. There is space and scope for both "useful knowledge" and "deep learning" to flourish in the same environment, as it did in the past with positive outcome for the *almajirai* then broadly defined to include all Hausa children undergoing their rites of passage in Muslim Hausa households.

References

Adamu, M. 1978. *The Hausa Factor in West African History*. Zaria: Ahmadu Bello University Press.

Balewa, A.T. 1966. *Shaihu Umar*. Zaria: The Northern Nigerian Publishing Company.

Barthes, R. 2012 [1972]. *Mythologies*. Trans. Richard Howard. New York: Hill and Wang.

Bâ, A.H. 2008. In *A Spirit of Tolerance: The Life of Tierno Bokar*, ed. Roger Gaetani. Bloomington, Indiana: World Wisdom Inc.

Brenner, L. 2000. *Histories of Religion in Africa*. London: School of Oriental and African Studies, University of London.

Buba, M. 2020. Mutuntaka 'Personhood' as a Paradigm of African Epistemology and its Implication for Governance in Africa. *Asian Journal of African Studies 47*: 145–170.

Falola, T. 2016. *The Humanities in Africa*. Austin, TX: Pan-African University Press.

Foucault, M. 1980. In *Power/Knowledge: Selected Interviews & Other Writings 1972-1977*, ed. Colin Gordon. New York: Pantheon Books.

Gumi, A., and I. Tsiga. 1992. *Where I Stand*. Ibadan: Spectrum Books.

Hall, S., ed. 1997. *Representation: Cultural Representations and Signifying Practices*. Milton Keynes: The Open University.

———. 2016. Cultural Studies 1983. In *Slack and Lawrence Grossberg*, ed. Jennifer Daryl. Durham and London: Duke University Press.

Hoechner, H. 2011. Striving for Knowledge and Dignity: How Qur'anic Students in Kano, Nigeria, Learn to Live with Rejection and Educational Disadvantage. *European Journal of Development Research* 2011 (23): 712–728. https://doi.org/10.1057/ejdr.2011.39.

———. 2018. *Quranic Schools in Northern Nigeria: Everyday Experiences of Youth, Faith, and Poverty*. Cambridge: Cambridge University Press.
Kane, C.H. 1972. *Ambiguous Adventure*. Nairobi: Heinemann.
Kane, O. 2012. *Muslim Modernity in Post-colonial Nigeria*. Leiden; Boston: Brill.
———. 2016. *Beyond Timbuktu: An Intellectual History of Muslim West Africa*. Cambridge, MA: Harvard University Press.
Khalid, S., 2020. Almajiranci Phenomenon and Child Abuse in Northern Nigeria: The Urgency for Massive Advocacy and Sensitization on Muslim Crises in Nigeria. Unpublished paper.
Omar, A. B., 1993. In Quest of Islamic Ideal of Education: a Study of the Traditional Pondok Institution in Malaysia. Ph.D. Dissertation, Temple University.
Thurston, A. 2018. *Salafism in Nigeria: Islam, Preaching, and Politics*. Cambridge: Cambridge University Press.
Walker, A. 2016. *"Eat the Heart of the Infidel": The Harrowing of Nigeria and the Rise of Boko Haram*. London: Hurst & Company.

12

Quarantining the Holy Spirit: Africa and the Pentecostal Economy of COVID-19 Pandemic

Asonzeh Ukah

When a planet wants you dead, you die. (Gaal Dornick (Foundations, 2021))

Introduction

In the early months of 2020, the world was hit by a ravenous coronavirus (COVID-19) pandemic, the like of which had not known for over a hundred years.[1] In epidemiological jargon, the causative virus of

[1] Research for this chapter was partly supported by the National Research Foundation of South Africa (Reference number [uid] 85,397). The opinions, findings and conclusions or recommendations expressed are those of the author; the NRF accepts no liability whatsoever in this regard. I am grateful to Banchiliyew Getahun Silewondim for assistance during the revision and editing of this chapter. The usual caveats hold.

A. Ukah (✉)
University of Cape Town, Cape Town, South Africa

University of Leipzig, Leipzig, Germany

F. Egbokhare, A. Afolayan (eds.), *Global Health, Humanity and the COVID-19 Pandemic*, https://doi.org/10.1007/978-3-031-17429-2_12

COVID-19 is SARS-Cov-2, a severe type of pneumonia. The initial outbreak was reported around the city of Wuhan in China, specifically, among dealers and vendors at the Wuhan Huanan Seafood Wholesale Market. However, the origin of the virus has been shrouded in controversies, unproven theories, allegations and accusations.[2] The "mysterious" and uncertain origins of the virus have lent some credence to its increasing spiritualisation by some believers, especially Christian evangelicals around the world. Historically, however, what is known and beyond controversy is that every known pandemic leaves an indelible mark on society, especially in its religious epistemology and relationships to both the material and the metasocial worlds (Ranger and Slack 1992). Such an indelible mark could be a loss of "cultural self-confidence" or permanent destruction of culture by disease (Ranger 1992: 241). As Pierluigi Consorti (2020: 17) pointedly asserts, "The COVID-19 epidemic is … unavoidably destined to produce effects … on religious cultures, on the way of being of religions and on their laws". It could also be how the epidemic elicits religious reasons and specifically the types of responses and reactions that are produced as modes of understanding, interpreting and explaining it. Making sense of adversities such as pain and suffering or death and sickness is a hallmark of religious epistemologies, myths and rituals.

The COVID-19 pandemic, like all epidemics, is primarily a public health problem that impacts all aspects of society and in significant ways revises a people's understanding of death and its aftermath. Because it is transmitted by touch or contaminated surfaces, it calls for the institutionalisation of particular social and cultural infrastructure and regimes of bodily and public hygiene to contain and control its transmission. Such new structures and reorganisation of social connectivity call into

[2] In a detailed 120-page WHO-China joint report, "WHO-Convened Study of Origins of SARS-CoV-2", the World Health Organisation and association with Chinese scientists ranked four possible theories about the origins of virus from "very likely to extremely unlikely", namely, i) an intermediate host, ii) direct zoonotic introduction, iii) introduction through cold/food chain and iv) introduction resulting from a laboratory incident. Yet, some claim it was an accident from some bioweapons' experimentations which occurred elsewhere in Europe or the United States. The report concluded with a call "for a continued scientific and collaborative approach to be taken towards tracing the origins of COVID-19" (p. 120). (See: https://www.who.int/publications/i/item/who-convened-global-study-of-origins-of-sars-cov-2-china-part).

question already established conviviality which religious communities are known for and which they attribute to their connection to a metasocial realm. Moreover, these regimes materialise what it means to live in an age of anxiety and a permanent condition of personal and social risk. With more than 6.5 million confirmed deaths from the epidemic, according the the World Health Organisation, the COVID-19 pandemic has produced an excess of deaths and suffering, anxiety, worry and fear (Ranger and Slack 1992; Fleisher and Norman 2016).[3] This is essentially because there are no known and generally available and accessible cures or remedy for it. COVID-19 is a pandemic of excesses. In this sense, it resembles Pentecostalism as preached and practised in Africa: it is a religion that erases moderation and preached the excess of wealth as a sign of God's blessing and health and human flourishing as ends in themselves in this world. Religion has also played an important role in the meaning and purpose of death and its aftermath. Some scholars have argued that religion emerged from humanity's attempt to make sense of death and what happens after death (Chidester 2002; Harari 2014: 303–306).

The present pandemic, therefore, has particularly produced marked responses and challenges to the Pentecostal communities of Africa where the Pentecostal spirituality has blossomed and attracted intense public fervour because of its theology of prosperity and healing claims. As a religion of power (and also a "public religion"[4]), the pandemic provides not just theological, socioeconomic and practical challenges but opportunities for Pentecostalism to demonstrate its community-making resources and the resilience of theological creativity in dealing with human suffering. The Pentecostal theology and rhetoric of power, miracle, healing and prophecy are all, it seems, put to the test by the COVID-19 pandemic. The too-muchness of Pentecostal promises, especially from the activities of the megachurches (Ukah 2020d), appears to have been modelled for a

[3] The global death toll from COVID-19 as at 28 October 2022 stands at 6,566,610; there has been a total of 626,337,158 reported and confirmed cases of COVID-19 infection. (see WHO Coronavirus (COVID-19) Dashboard, https://covid19.who.int/).

[4] I characterise "public religions", as active social movements intent on transforming members, renovating social structures and reconfiguring society according to the priorities and inspirations from metasocial considerations or other-worldly sources or text such as scriptures (see Marty 1998: 393–4; Casanova 1994; Ukah 2020c)

human catastrophe such as a pandemic. Moreover, in the history of Christianity, there is much that apparently would, it is supposed, prepare Pentecostal leaders and communities for epidemics of global proportions such as the COVID-19 pandemic. The early church was characterised as a community of mercy, love, kindness and empathy. These factors would predispose the Pentecostal communities of Africa to respond in specific, theologically consistent ways to a pandemic. It is, therefore, important to understand how in reality these flourishing Christian communities in Africa responded and continued to respond to the emergence of the COVID-19 disease to put into context the place of religion and religious organisations in post-colonial Africa, where states are known to be under-performing and unable to meet their obligations to their citizens. This chapter critically examines how the Pentecostal communities in Africa responded to doing church from a distance and making sense of a human tragedy of unimaginable proportion, now called the COVID-19 pandemic.

Lockdown and the Quarantining of the Holy Spirit

The fear, dread of death and sickness occasioned by the outbreak of the COVID-19 pandemic caused state governments and public health officials across the world to institute strict and hitherto unprecedented measures and regulations such as lockdown of society, social or physical distancing between people, restrictions of the sales of certain goods and the unavailability of some social services. The closedown of schools and public gatherings such as sporting events and the insistence on the wearing of facial coverings and use of hand sanitisers were sufficient sources of panic and distress to many people. For many individuals, because these new public regulations restricted personal freedoms such as public gathering, in some cases gathering in private homes too, and movement, the pandemic also impacted the relationship between faith communities and public laws. As religious communities of all stripes could not come together to worship or exercise their liberties of worship, panic set in and resistances to the new rules emerged. It was not just a test of the power of the state to make new laws and implement them but also the test of the nature and extent of public trust in government or public officials and the state infrastructures that they oversee. For many African Christians, however, it was a test of their faith in God and a search for a new meaning or explanation for evil and suffering, death and human frailty in the face of a supposedly just, all-powerful, loving, caring and righteous God. Like all problems of evil, COVID-19 is a challenge to believers' understanding and conception of a benevolent deity in the face of human finitude which pain and death evoke and which the global death toll of the disease presents to believers.

The initial panic and draconian nature of the rollback of societal connectivity and common life elicited sharp, sometimes negative, reactions from some sectors of societies. Among those with sustained and uncooperative reactions, at least at the onset of the pandemic, have been faith-based organisations and leaders. Among these, evangelical Christians of which the Pentecostals are a subset, predominate. The Pentecostal segment, because of their mastery and penetration of modern social media, has acquired a larger-than-life influence among their followers and a sizeable section of African communities. For these communities, the COVID-19 pandemic represents a direct attack on protected rights and freedoms such as those pertaining to movement and gathering or association. More importantly, some of the public measures directly interfered with their understanding of their religion and of God, as the maker, master and controller of the universe. Furthermore, the (sometimes confusing, even contradictory) public health messaging by governments and state agencies created a cloak of secrecy and misinterpretation which some believers took to be directed at the very foundation of their faith in a higher power. Thus, the distrust of the state and its officials started a sustained and confusing circulation of alternate explanations and interpretations based on faith and religious convictions. Pentecostal leaders have been very vocal about their views partly because of their access to modern social media and partly because of their belief in an all-knowing deity who is also a source of accurate information about the world and its organisaton. Pentecostal sermons and other forms of communication have frequently been posted on Twitter, Facebook, YouTube and Instagram giving Pentecsotal leaders' views a large footprint and uptake.

Understanding the reactions and responses of some religious leaders to the Covid pandemic would help in better situating African conceptions of evil and healing amid global flows of information and technologies of mass communication. For example, was it the need for community or healing or income that informed the challenges to social distancing and lockdown mounted by Pentecostal leaders? Because the coronavirus pandemic and the attendant restrictive legal regime hurriedly instituted to contain its effects impinged on economic and legal rights and liberties, some of the implications directly and adversely affected the economic rights of religious clergy to earn a living. The primary income of Pentecostal clergy derives from the financial collections (offertory, donations, tithes, etc.) they take during religious events. These events include the Sunday worship event but also other ritual activities such as bible study, healing services, and prayer meetings among others. Lockdown regulations largely compromised incomes and revenues from these sources. Pentecostal leaders' near-collective opposition to the new legal and social regimes dealing with the pandemic might have arisen from a diversity of sources: theological, social, legal and economic. For these groups of clergy who are functionally religious entrepreneurs, religious freedoms are economic freedoms. These freedoms are discursively and conceptually separate but practically and realistically the same. The coronavirus pandemic, therefore, has presented a constitutional conundrum for many African countries (such as Nigeria, South Africa, Uganda and Malawi) regarding the complex and complicated (incomplete or is it impossible?) relationship between religion and the state and the limits of each sphere's authority (Asamoah-Gyadu 2020, 2021; Ukah 2020a; Tengatenga et al. 2021). Religious leaders claim authorities beyond the realm of the state, but the state exercises the regulatory authority on religious association and public conduct. Across Africa, religion provided a canopy for interrogating state laws and regulations of the public sphere; religious leaders articulated alternatives to both official [state, see Fig. 12.1 below, for example] or scientific interpretations and explanations of the disease as well as possible solutions to it. The effective exercise and implementation of state authority and regulations required the co-operation

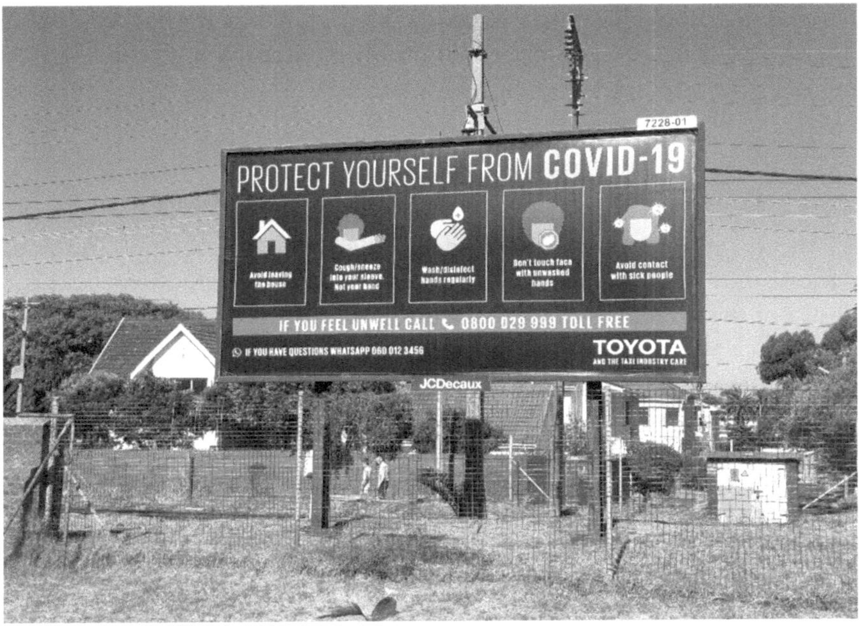
7228-01
PROTECT YOURSELF FROM COVID-19
Avoid leaving the house
Cough/sneeze into your sleeve. Not your hand
Wash/disinfect hands regularly
Don't touch face with unwashed hands
Avoid contact with sick people
IF YOU FEEL UNWELL CALL 0800 029 999 TOLL FREE
IF YOU HAVE QUESTIONS WHATSAPP 060 012 3456
TOYOTA
AND THE TAXI INDUSTRY CARE
JCDecaux

Fig. 12.1 A public message about COVID-19 (Photo: author 2021)

and co-optation of religious leaders. Religion provides anchor and direction to many but also, during the COVID-19 era, religion demonstrated its overaching influence as a destabilising rhetoric for many others in the face of fear, panic and the unknown (Prempeh 2021). Pentecostal communities and their leaders were in the forefront of making their views public in response to government actions and regulations vis-à-vis the pandemic. Their initial reactions were that of confusion and powerlessness; leaders revolted but soon retraced their steps, retracted some of their initial opinions and revised their actions. The confusion that ensued could be attributed to the direct and immediate impact of the lockdown which also foreclosed pastors' exercise of "Holy Ghost Power", the rhetoric of invincibility which the pulpit affords them when they preached. When Pentecostal healers failed to perform their rituals of healing and miracles, they resorted to cursing and binding the coronavirus. Perceived as evil, cursing and binding the pandemic became a strategy of performing ritual power by Pentecostal leaders. Not being able to do this in physical religious assemblies was a severe setback and challenge to many Pentecostal leaders (Asamoah-Gyadu 2021).

COVID-19 and Spiritual Inoculation

As the ongoing coronavirus pandemic has exposed the limitations of African state powers and authority—in the area of public trust and the power of the state to respond to the needs of their citizens—so also it has shown the weakness of African religious systems and their leadership capabilities. The reactions and responses of both African state governments and religious organisations to the pandemic and attempts at containing the spread of the virus or managing the disease illustrate "a web of religious prevarication and state fragility" which partly inform "the prevailing perception of the virus as eschatological and nihilistic among citizens" (Chidume et al. 2021: 1). In a pandemic, trust in the powers and reliance on the resources of groups and entities above the individual is critical. This is where trust in the powers of the state comes in. But for so many people, more trust is invested in the powers of religion or the entities around which religious rituals revolve than in the structures of the state; for some Christians, their trust is in God. For Pentecostal Christians especially, more trust is reposed in the power of the Holy Spirit—to bring healing and sustenance, for example—than in human structures and knowledge such as the state or science.

By far the most far-reaching shock for many Africans and their physical and economic well-being and livelihoods in the twenty-first century is the coronavirus outbreak and the COVID-19—the disease caused by the virus—pandemic that has since January 2020 ensued. African countries, with weak institutional structures—such as healthcare facilities, technological production, political institutions and economic bases—are affected by the pandemic in different and perhaps more adverse ways than many non-African countries and societies. Statistically, while Africa has not experienced high rates of infection and deaths from COVID-19 disease, the socio-economic consequences of the outbreak seem far-reaching than in more developed societies with robust medical and politico-economic institutions and networks.[5] In the weak and under-performing post-colonial African states, religion and religious organisations have become crucial actors in the public management of disaster and vulnerability. Religious actors—Christian, Islamic and indigenous—have historically exercised significant influences in bringing members of societies together and reassuring them through various methods and means of the powers of the unseen world and entities in restoring wholeness and broken harmony. Harmony, which is the primary religious quest in the African worldview and order of things, is only meaningful in the context of discordant desires and forces or sources of disharmony such as illness and disease, poverty and lack, suffering and pain, confusion, disorder and dislocation. All this has characterised contemporary African societies in the wake of the COVID-19 pandemic. The COVID-19 era has, therefore, heightened the quest to re-establish harmony as a first step towards achieving human and societal flourishing.

Pentecostalism promises its adherents life lived in abundance (Jn 10:10) which is made manifest in health, wealth, success and prosperity in life. Pentecostal promise of salvation in terms that strongly resonate with the cultural worldview of Africans accounts for its wildfire-like popularity, especially in urban centres and cities. In the past fifty years, scholars of African Pentecostalism have described the explosion and spread of this new form of pneumatic spirituality and Christianity as a "revolution" (Gaiya 2002; Ojo 2004; Marshall 2008; Burgess 2008). However, none of those who so generously and eloquantly described Pentecostalism as a revolution supports such a description with an in-depth, empirically driven analysis of what a "revolutionary religion" means or the many-layered features of a revolution (e.g. see Cherstich et al. 2020).[6] Based on the capacity of Pentecostal leaders to mobilise and seize the public and keep throngs of people spell-bound over hours and days—ostansibly for

[5] Alex Eze, Michael Silverman, Saverio Stranges & Janica Adams, "The impact of COVID-19 has been lower in Africa. We explore the reasons", Conversations, 17 August 2021, https://theconversation.com/the-impact-of-covid-19-has-been-lower-in-africawe-explore-the-reasons-164955.

[6] What may be apparent is that "revolution" and "revolutionary" are used relative to the influence or impact of African Pentecostalism and its leadership on the African landscape in a metaphorical rather than analytical sense. However, concepts such as revolution or decolonisation do not have synonyms and so need a great deal of care and analytical clarity in their application (see Tuck and Wayne Yang 2012).

revivals and retreats—some scholars have concluded that Pentecostalism is the fastest-growing religion in Africa with a capacity to transform urban ecology and structure, among other aspects of social life. In the sphere of urban regeneration and reconstruction, Pentecostal leaders have built massive prayer camps that have slowly enlarged into ritual cities, sometimes with self-sustaining facilities. They have also actively engaged in the real estate industry developing in some peri-urban areas of Africa large swaths of prime real estate, primarily for their wealthy members. Pentecostal Christians have also made their imprint on the political life of many African countries where their participation in multi-party democracy and partisan politics have been very visible. In Nigeria, Pentecostals have swayed voting outcomes and as a result have been intensely courted by politicians aspiring for elective public positions. This leads to such claims, like that of Ebenezer Obadare (2018), albeit prematurely, it seems, that there is a "Pentecostal Republic" within the Republic of Nigeria. In Zambia, the popularity of Pentecostalism nudged Frederick Chiluba, the country's erstwhile president (from 1991–2002), to declare it a "Christian republic". In the past sixty years or more, Pentecostal theological schools have also emerged across many African cities where local clergy are trained in culturally relevant methods of theological education. Further, in East, West and southern Africa, Pentecostals have also engaged with public education, particularly at the tertiary education market, where they own and manage universities and vocation centres, thus, influencing the training of Africa's future elite. In all these areas, it is apparent that the new Pentecostal paradigm of power is obvious, palpable, even visible. The varied and diverse African publics can see, touch, feel, and smell the material manifestation of African Pentecostal social and ritual life and spirituality. This was so until the emergence of the COVID-19 pandemic.

In the course of the unfolding COVID-19 pandemic, this characterisation of Pentecostal public face and force has come under severe scrutiny. African Pentecostalism as a people-centred revolutionary impulse has come under intense re-examination and recharacterisation. There are many reasons for this. Broadly, Pentecostalism is recognised as a religion of the "Spirit and Power" (Miller et al. 2013). The "spirit" is usually but not exclusively understood as the Holy Spirit that believers recognise as the engine and energy that drive and propel the believing community but that empowers in the sense of 'bringing to be' new forms of life and socialites in the community. The spirit is associated both in the African worldview and in Pentecostal theology with life and vitality (on African concept of vitality, see Magesa 1997; Molefe and Maraganedzha 2022). As Matthew Engelke (2018: 288) rightly points out, in many African languages the word for *spirit* is synonymous with breath, air, wind and life. Pentecostalism claims to be internally animated by the breath of life that indicates the central role of the Holy Spirit in its scheme of things. The claim is that It is the Holy Spirit that informs its rituals, teachings, leadership style and structure, and work. Above all, the claim continues, the Holy Spirit is the power that believers and leaders exercise in speaking in tongues and performing miracles. Many of these assumptions and claims of power and its practices have been challenged by the emergence and impact of the COVID-19 pandemic.

For Africans, life is a force, a power, and energy for action, a capability to perform (Sogolo 1993: 91–118; Kamalu 1998: 51–75); hence, human life is often characterised as participation in a "life-force", "a divine power manifesting itself in everyone and everything in the universe … a world of faith which is the crown of culture" (Ruch and Anyanwu 1981: 163). Pentecostal claims to, and of, power and its performance are totalising, encompassing all aspects of life and society (Lindhardt 2012; Endong and Essoh 2019; Premack 2019; Soothill 2019), which would mean that under the vitiating influence and impact of the COVID-19 pandemic, the Pentecostal spirit and practice should constitute a mitigating impulse in believers' experience. As Wynand J. de Kock (2000) observes, Pentecostal theology of power is a "doing" rather than a "thinking" activity; it is action-oriented and driven. As such, it privileges action and praxis over reflection and reflexivity. This aspect of the religion is easily evident in the way its leaders advertise their activities as sights and scenes of change and transformation, of healing, repair, regeneration, restoration and miracles as radical and positive realignment and self- and social-repositioning. The Pentecostal concept of power often revolves around the role of charismatic leaders as spiritual mediators of the capability to bring about human wellness and the "wellbeing of [hu]mankind" (Endong and Essoh 2019: 371). Thus, well-being is comprehensive and all-encompassing in the diverse ways in which power is advertised in Pentecostal discourse and praxis.

Pentecostal practices of the Holy Spirit and performances of power are intimately linked to health and all the diverse ways in which this key cultural religious and spiritual quest is threatened and compromised. Because the natural and the supernatural interlock and intertwine, the quest for health and healing are spiritual exercises. What threatens, hinders and compromises physiological or biological well-being and wellness is connected to and believed to be of spiritual consequence. African understanding of health—and by extension the Pentecostal conception of health and wellness as a comprehensive physical, mental, physiological, social and spiritual well-being—is consistent with the World Health Organisation's definition of health.[7] Such conception recognises the complexities of the human person, condition and aspiration. The appreciation of both the comprehensiveness and the complexities of health indicates that it is more of an ideal, an approximation and an unrelenting quest than a practice, achievement or goal. The search for well-being and the desire to explain the presence and cause of misfortune (in order to prevent it) in human experience have animated the Pentecostal imagination and praxis, and remains an enduring attraction for many Africans. This is all the more so under the conditions of a public health epidemic such as COVID-19. More importantly, the claim by prominent Pentecostal figures across Africa to have the power to heal, restore, cure, or provide remedy remains a strong selling point for Pentecostal entrepreneurs. The COVID-19 pandemic, it would seem, presented a near-perfect condition for Pentecostal entrepreneurs to market their healing wares and exercise their gifts of realigning the social distortions and dislocations many people experienced and still experiencing. Presented as a healing strategy, Pentecostalism may, therefore, be construed as a public welfare and health facility, a mechanism that enables and restores broken harmony and empowers believers with optimal capability to discharge their responsibilities, personal and social. Conceived in this manner, the Holy Spirit in the life of the believer can be likened to a spiritual inocula-

[7] WHO's Constitution, signed on 22 July 1946 by representatives of 22 states, is available at https://www.who.int/about/governance/constitution.

tion, a vaccine against lack, illness and malevolent forces. Again, this is until the onset of the COVID-19 pandemic when the global social order was so abruptly disrupted and disorganised, and, as it turned out, the Holy Spirit and its powers of healing—as claimed by many Pentecostal entrepreneurs—were challenged and quarantined by state public health regulations enforced and backed up by state power and bureaucracy.

COVID-19 Pandemic and the Power of the Holy Spirit

Understanding the generalised and nuanced reactions of believers to adverse events, especially sudden and unexpected adverse events, is important in understanding religious behaviours and the implications for religiously induced social change. As Diego Meza (2020: 218) states, fear of the unknown "motivates religious faith" and religious faith "mitigates fear". From the experience of past pandemics in history, religion has been prominent in both supplying explanations and interpretations as well as responses to human adversity (Stark 1997; Ellwood 2009; Ukah 2020b: 446–457). In the economies of evil, human suffering and death, religion thrives (Lopez and Gillespie 2015). For example, Omololu Fagunwa (2020: 52) claims that the 1918–1919 influenza pandemic in West Africa "overlapped with the move of the Holy Spirit in the life of indigenous African Christians". The "move of the Holy Spirit" referred to is the emergence of the Aladura (*adura*, Yoruba for prayer; Aladura, people of prayer) Church movement in southern Nigeria during this time (Peel 1968: Mitchell 1970) as well as the first group of Pentecostal churches in Nigeria. According to dam Mohr (2020: 220), "the 1918–1919 influenza pandemic, a destructive disease … led to a religious revolution" in West Africa. That "revolution" was the emergence of 250 faith-healing churches in West Africa all of which traced their roots to the Faith Tabernacle Congregation in Philadelphia.

In the face of a health crisis, spiritual resources such as divine healing assume new and reinforced resonance. Both religious beliefs in higher powers and ritual practices provide certain degrees of assurances and regularities during crises moments that mitigate the unpredictability of unfolding health emergencies such as an epidemic of massive proportion. While the problem and presence of death have remained a key issue in religious doctrines and the search for life's purpose, the sheer volume of deaths during a pandemic comes with a heightened awareness of human vulnerability and mortality (Chidester 2002). Across Africa, many new religious movements sprang up as a direct response to the flu pandemic of 1918–1919. According to J.D.Y Peel (2016: 79), the Aladura movement in West Africa, which was established during this time, sought to make the power of prayers more available than in the older Protestant churches "for such this-worldly objectives as health, fertility, protection against witchcraft and danger, guidance, prosperity, and success—in sum, that state of all-round well-being …". Sickness and large numbers of deaths occurring in very short intervals cause panic and a feeling of helplessness and distrust in existing structures of interpretation and mitigation. For some Africans, COVID-19 has turned their previously flourishing family trees into wasteland twigs due to the high fatality rate of the virus. The shredding and jarring experience nudges them to re-evaluate their religious spiritual beliefs and standpoint. Religion supplies beliefs in higher powers and supernatural capabilities in dealing with the anxiety caused by the imminence of death and human frailty. This may explain the manifest spiritualisation of the meaning and interpretation of the COVID-19 pandemic among African Pentecostals.

The outbreak of the coronavirus pandemic from the beginning of 2020 onward is a case in point in assessing and understanding the impact of Pentecostal beliefs and practices in many parts of the world. This is more so in Africa where the religion of the Holy Spirit has many adherents and where high-profile Pentecostal leaders have emerged over the decades claiming unusual powers to heal and restore people to health and to empower and promote believers to function optimally in all aspects of life. Prophecy, as one of the highly sought-after gifts of the Holy Spirit, has played a visible role in the making and marketing of Pentecostal innovators and entrepreneurs. The most prominent African Pentecostal innovators have been those who claim to have the power of prognostication. Those religious leaders who promise to provide insights into their clients' private lives and hidden explanations regarding the outcome of future events have attracted large patronage. Often during religious events, these leaders have in various ways tried to meet the expectations of their clients by supplying what many of their followers claim to be predictions of future events or a demonstration of the foreknowledge of hidden events or experiences attributed to the power of the Holy Spirit. In this respect, two important and pre-eminent Pentecostal prophets in Africa will illustrate the place and role of prophecy in times of existential uncertainty. From the 1990s through to his sudden and shocking demise on 05 June 2021, Temitope Balogun Joshua, founder-owner of the Synagogue of All Nations Church (SCOAN) and Immanuel satellite television station, was the most important religious entrepreneur and innovator in Africa. His rise to prominence was partly on account of his claims to accurately predict high profile deaths of politicians or voting outcomes in many countries across the world or football matches (Ukah 2016; McNaught 2021). The dramatic ritual services and the power of satellite television drew a global audience and followership to Joshua's Lagos headquarters of SCOAN. Joshua's popularity came with great wealth and his wealth reinforced and expanded his spiritual empire and disciples who come from all walks of life and socioeconomic classes (McNaught 2022). Similarly, Emmanuel Makandiwa of United Family International Church is a famous Pentecostal prophet from Zimbabwe whose claim to fame revolves around his prophetic goods and services (Biri 2021). By prying into the future and gaining insights about what is to happen before they happen, these pastors and many others like them claim to guide and inform believers' decisions through the inspiration of the spirit of God. Such insights, they claim, come from their intimate relationship with a metasocial or divine source, usually the Holy spirit such that the words they speak are not theirs but those of the mind of deity. This explanation notwithstanding, the practice of foretelling the future or prognostication (which is different from prophecy as "the mediation and interpretation of the divine mind and will" [Vawter 1990:187]) is something that ties these Pentecostal actors to the African religious and cultural worldview and praxis. In both African religions and Pentecostal practices, prophetism could rightly be regarded as a kindred institution or practice; Pentecostal prophets are diviners by a different name. These two pillars of Pentecostal innovators have featured prominently in the attempts to make sense of and contend with the COVID-19 pandemic. While the latter claimed to have foretold the coming of the coronavirus in a series of pronouncements in 2015, 2016 and 2017, the former made no such claims. However, Makandiwa's claims only became known after the virus had gained ground around the world. It is puzzling, therefore, to consider the worth and purpose for such prophecy when it did not lead to any redemptive, amiliorative or mitigating action.

At the end of 2020, T.B. Joshua, who called COVID-19 "the affliction" and a "monster", prophesied that the pandemic has three stages, the first of which was nearing its end, while the remaining two parts would be more devastating and "tougher" than the first stage but only for a few unnamed countries rather than involving all the world.[8] For the African Pentecostal community, the emergence of the pandemic was a rude shock to the claimed ability of its principal prophets to speak, mediate and interpret the mind of God to their followers and the larger society. Pentecostal prophecy, which in the past is credited with predicting the demise of politicians and other socially significant people, failed to predict the death of a large number of the human population which includes politically exposed and significant personalities such as John Jerry Rawlings of Ghana (22 June 1947 – 12 Nov. 2020), (former)President John Magufuli of Tanzania (29 Oct. 1959 – 17 March 2021), Abba Kyari (23 Sept. 1952 – 17 April 2020) and Obediah Mailafia (24 Dec. 1956 – 19 Sept. 2021) both of Nigeria. The singular consistent interpretation of the coronavirus that emerged from the Pentecostal community is that it is a plague, a "demonic spirit" sent by God to punish humanity for their failings. Some church leaders, such as Helen Ukpabio, founder-owner of Liberty Gospel Church, Nigeria, further asserted that what she called the "plague" was designed and devised by humans who mistakenly allowed it to get out of hand and control (more on COVID-19 as a

[8] Muhaimin Olowoporoku, "COVID-19: What God told me would happen in 2021, says TB Joshua", 1 January 2021, https://pmnewsnigeria.com/2021/01/01/covid-19-what-god-told-me-would-happen-in-2021-says-tb-joshua/ (accessed 01.10.2021).

plague shortly). In that accident, she sees the hand of God in penalising humanity for its intransigence.[9]

The effervescence of Pentecostalism in Africa as well as on many Global South centres has been widely documented and different explanations and interpretations offered about its appeal. Central to these explanations and interpretations is the place and role of the Holy Spirit in the life of believers and communities, the organisation of ritual practices and activities. Pentecostal theologians of repute have come to describe Pentecostalism as a pneumatological religion. The Holy Spirit, according to these scholars, is believed to be active and operational in the lives of individual believers, empowering them to speak in the language of the spirit, understood only by the Spirit and characterising its power to overcome barriers and produce manifold embodied experiences and expressions. Such characterisation is often linked historically to the events described in the second chapter of the New Testament book of Acts of the Apostles where a handful of fearful followers of Jesus Christ hid in the Upper Room on the Day of Pentecost—while their neighbours celebrated the Jewish feast—experienced an unusual occurrence. The occurrence was the coming of the Holy Ghost which was described as "a sound of violent wind … [which] appeared to them tongue as of fire [that] came to rest on the head of each of them".[10] What is significant for this chapter is that the followers of Jesus self-quarantined in fear of the larger Jewish community. The coming of the Holy Spirit under the conditions of self- or group-isolation also (effectively) quarantined the Holy Spirit. In like manner, under the conditions of the coronavirus pandemic, one of the first non-pharmacological interventions to mitigate the spread of the virus was social distancing, isolation and quarantining of exposed persons or groups and the prohibition of mass gathering. Even when reinterpreted as an apocalyptic instrument of divine anger, the coronavirus epidemic was a re-enactment of Christian origin stories of fear, isolation and quarantining. Further, such reinterpretation that the Pentecostal community

[9] Helen Ukpabio, "Corona Virus Plague Reveals God's Anger", https://www.facebook.com/ ladyapostlehelenukpabio/videos/533021300734044/ (the sermon was preached on Sunday, February 23, 2020).

[10] Acts of the Apostles 2: 1–3 (*The New Jerusalem Bible*, Standard version translation (London: Darton, Longman & Todd Ltd., 1985).

favours connects contemporary experience with the history and rereading of the ten plagues of Exodus (Ex.7:8-13:16) and the seven plagues of Revelation (16:2-21).

Salvation, Starvation and Suffering

As sickness caused by COVID-19 infections caused many deaths, physical and social distancing devastated economic livelihoods. Across African cities, usually characterised by endless cycles of Pentecostal gatherings such as revivals, night vigils and other mass events, city life went dormant and silent. According to a United Nations' projection of the socio-economic impact of the COVID-19 pandemic in Africa, "more than $200 billion" would be needed and mobilised to stabilise African economies which would "include direct support that will help keep households afloat and businesses solvent" (2020: 3).[11] Ordinarily, the need to safeguard communities from the risk of food shortages, especially for the most vulnerable such as young children, women and older people and

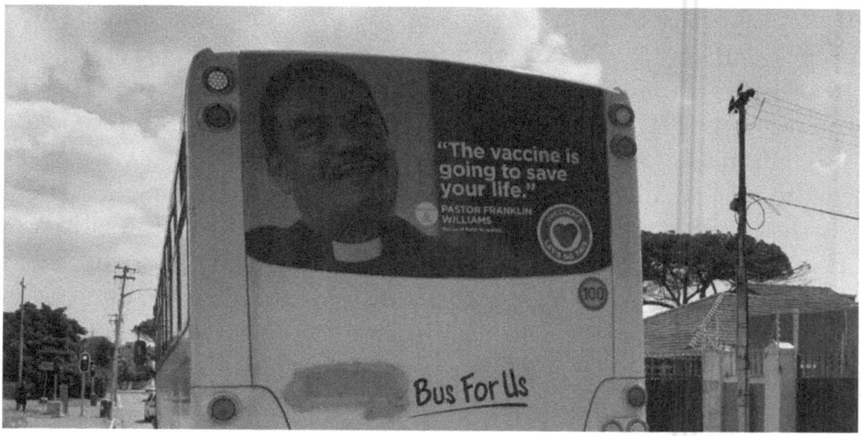
"The vaccine is going to save your life."
PASTOR FRANKLIN WILLIAMS
100
Bus For Us

Fig. 12.2 A Public Service advertisement to curb religion-induced vaccine hesitancy in South Africa (Photo: author)

[11] United Nations, "Policy Brief: Impact of COVID-19 in Africa", 20 May 2020, https://unsdg.un.org/resources/policy-brief-impact-covid-19-africa.

other at-risk groups, evokes a powerful response from religious communities. It was the case for the early church during the epidemics of the second and third centuries of the Common Era when the early church members mobilised resources in support of its diverse communities. The trust deficiency which many Africans have with their government officials and the formal state makes it possible for them to believe and trust what their religious officials and leaders tell them. African states are fragile in the sense of not adequately meeting the citizenship and governance needs of their people, not providing adequate security of lives and property and not being responsive to the yearnings and aspirations of the populations. Under such fraught social conditions, religious organisations and their leaders often step in the gap to fulfil some of those important needs which these populations cannot often meet on their own (Prempeh 2021; Chidume et al. 2021). In the immediate aftermath of COVID-19 in Africa, however, Pentecostal organisations which prioritised health and wealth doctrines in their self-marketing and public representation, responded differently.

Pentecostal leaders called for more prayers and prayer gatherings, in some instances explicitly against public health regulations and state directives of social and physical distancing and lockdown. In Kenya, for example, some clergy argued that the limited number of persons permitted in indoor services during the early relaxation of the lockdown was unfair, and that the one-hour stipulated by the government for church service was not enough. In some cities, security officials had to use brute force such as whipping and tear gassing to disperse congregations who, encouraged by their leaders, had gathered in churches for prayers.[12] It must be added, however, that the forcible dispersal of worshippers happened across the religious spectrum and not just restricted to the Pentecostal churches.[13] It does, then, seem that in the context of the unfolding disas-

[12] Sotho Molosankwe, "Soweto Pastor and His congregations arrested after Worshippers Attack Cops, Damage Patrol Cars", 1 May 2021, https://www.iol.co.za/news/soweto-pastor-and-his-congregants-arrested-after-worshippers-attack-cops-damage-patrol-cars-7d34a193-bd69-4e07-ad81-c465871e3dea; Dickens Olewe, "Coronavirus in Africa: Whipping, shooting and snooping", https://www.bbc.com/news/world-africa-52214740.

[13] "Worshippers flee as police flog them out of Catholic Church", https://naijabanging.com.ng/worshippers-flee-as-police-flog-them-out-of-catholic-church-photos/.

ter, Africans sought religious answers more than scientific, legal or bureaucratic responses. More importantly for both congregants and the leadership, many ignored the obvious capacity and potential of religious community-making tendencies to accelerate and escalate the spread of COVID-19 and the social transmission of the disease. As a result, in many parts of Africa, such as South Africa, Pentecostal groups became super-spreaders of the coronavirus because they wilfully and deliberately ignored government regulations and the new regime of social infrastructure put in place for controlling the spread of the virus. One reason why these Pentecostal leaders ignored these new public health rules could be traced to the belief in the power of prayer, especially the power of the Holy Spirit as healer and saver of believers from diseases and dangers. Another reason is that Pentecostal pastors largely depended on their congregations for their livelihoods, which come from donations, collections and tithes. Not being able to gather, then, deprived the leaders of a sure means of income and thereby threatened their means of livelihood. It is also important to consider another reason: the exercise of religious freedom as well as the assumption that "religious freedom" is an unlimited or unrestricted human right. Many religious leaders argued that the exercise of religion was a form of human right was also an "essential service" requiring exemption from the general COVID-19 restrictive regimes (Tengatenga et al. 2021). Worship as essential service is more about salvation of the soul than serving people from starvation and meaningfully responding to human suffering. In many different ways, Pentecostal actors assuming a superior source of knowledge and social power constituted formidable hindrances to government regulations and management of the COVID-19 pandemic. Hence, some states made deliberate efforts to court the support of some clergy in the implementation of state policies on COVID-19 (Fig. 12.2).

COVID-19 Pandemic and Pentecostal Prophetic Chaos

> Money comes to money, and poverty to poverty. Education comes to education, and ignorance to ignorance (Yuval Noah Harari, 2014: 161).

COVID-19 pandemic created, among other wide-ranging consequences, global instability, uncertainty and chaos. The largest numbers of people falling sick from infection with the virus, the unsightly scenes of crowded hospitals and the elevated numbers of fatalities destabilised social routines and processes forcing government and states to roll back social connectivity by enforcing lockdowns and physical distancing, among other precautionary measures. These two measures (physical distancing and lockdown) directly and viciously stabbed at the heart of religious communities which are sustained by conviviality and connectedness. Indeed, it seemed that when believers needed divine intervention, the measures against the virus deliberately undermined such intervention. This is especially so among the poor who live in crowded homes who derive their livelihoods from petty businesses and with little reserved resources to fall back on under lockdown conditions. The disorienting condition likely nudged many to seek spiritual help or lean on the resources that religion and religious belonging offer. One important function of religion has been to make sense of chaos, to generate certainty in times of confusion and crisis through myth and rituals, and also to provide interpretations of human experiences of unknowing. Consistent with totalising Pentecostal beliefs and practices, leaders were quick to offer a spiritual interpretation for the COVID-19 pandemic. Religious interpretation and explanation of the pandemic became a viable and meaningful resource in the face of the often confusing government policy and communication or the frequently inaccessible scientific jargons about the disease provided in the media. Even those Pentecostal leaders who failed to predict and foresee the coronavirus outbreak were quick to claim that the affliction was a form of communication of divine displeasure from a metaphysical realm. Helen Upkabio, the Nigerian religious entrepreneur and moviemaker, claimed that the pandemic was a plague sent by God to demonstrate divine displeasure at how humans, especially westerners, have sought to dethrone God from his majesty and enthrone the idol of science, technology and human knowledge cum ignorance. This type of understanding of the pandemic as plague or a divine visitor, gained traction among many Pentecostal Christians in Africa. The reinterpretation of the pandemic as a plague is in line with the story of the destruction of Sodom and Gomorrah in the Bible as well as the Ten Plagues (מכות מצרים) that afflicted the Egyptians (Ex. 7: 14–12: 30). The plague interpretation of COVID-19 pandemic is also consistent with "evidentialist religious epistemology" of the Old Testament whereby believers consistently sought to discern or decipher "the finger of God" in human history (Gerike 2012: 376). Identifying the finger of God in human affairs is a claim to revelation as well as an argument for and an appeal to a divinely sanctioned cosmic and moral order. As Jaco Gericke (2012: 376) argues, the attractiveness of evidentialist religious epistemology is its "foundationalist assumptions" about 'knowledge of Yhwh". Those religious leaders who claim that the sudden eruption of the COVID-19 pandemic was a sacred visitation assume that they know and understand the mind of God and divine intentions for the cosmos, not just for the human world. As a pneumatological religion, Pentecostalism prides itself as a veritable means and source of understanding and knowing the mind of God; Pentecostal leaders have always claimed they could speak authoritatively about this to the believer. The claim to the inscrutable knowledge of God is the foundation and basis upon which other beliefs and practices (e.g. prophecy, miracle, speaking in tongue, healing) are erected. According to the Pentecostal train of thought, knowing the mind of God does not countenance the probabilities of chance since God "does not play dice with the universe", as Albert Einstein would say (Born 1971: 91). Undergirding this Pentecostal epistemology which presupposes that the COVID-19 is an act willed by divine intention is the freedom of God to act decisively towards his creation. God's freedom cannot be discounted or contended with by the power of human knowledge, science or technology. For those who believe that the COVID-19 was an unleashing of divine displeasure, they implicitly acknowledge and recognise the power of the Christian God as creator-owner of the universe and the ethical imperative to govern the affairs of the world according to certain discernible rules. As a plague, COVID-19 is both a punishment for human sins and misbehaviour and a demonstration of God's power, ownership and dominion over the earth and all creations; using the coronavirus as instrument of war against humankind, the COVID-19 pandemic is construed according to this narrative as a holy war in which God manipulates natural elements in inflicting harm on humans and in manifesting his sole divinity. The virus, thus, serves as an instrument of divine anger and majesty at the same time. The coronavirus, for those who conceive it as a plague, signifies an eschatological judgement of cosmic proportion since the pandemic affected more than human beings: water, air, animals and the general environment. In this judgement, there is salvation, and Pentecostal leaders and actors are purveyors and key to unlocking this new salvific dispensation.

There are, however, some problems with interpretations of social calamities along this line. It is difficult to read COVID-19 as being about human arrogance and disobedience. This is because the pandemic equally affected the non-human populations; animals such as pets and zoo-kept animals were also known to have contracted the disease and some of them had died or suffered immensely as a result. It is, therefore, difficult to understand why these co-habitants of the world with humans should suffer for the misdeeds of a section of the human population against God. Further, westerners who are, according to the interpretation of COVID-19 as divine wrath, responsible for the plague, constitute a small minority of the human species. COVID-19 and its devastation savaged non-Western societies which cannot, arguably according to proponents of the divine wrath argument, be accused of usurping the throne of God through their arrogance, science and technology and economic dominance of world affairs. As it turns out, the suffering and pain wrought by the COVID-19 pandemic brought more wealth to the Western societies, economic institutions and scientific establishments. The invention and selling of COVID vaccines and other related health-care products made Western pharmaceutical companies wealthier than they were during the pre-COVID era. COVID-19 vaccines were invented and manufactured in all continents by their respective scientists except in Africa, where a vaccine production facility was open in South Africa by Aspen and another in Algeria by Saidal—both non-African pharmaceutical companies. Pentecostal leaders who claim COVID-19 is a punishment from loving God fail to explain those who are supposed to be punished are made wealthier at the same time while the apparently righteous and religious Africans depend on donations of vaccines and food and equiptment to survive the pandemic.

The unfolding pandemic illustrates the chaos and confusion, inconsistencies and contradictions of Pentecostal interpretation of the problem of evil. What amounts to a theory of Pentecostal Chaos needs a bit of explanation. Many events happened in quick succession or simultaneously precipitated the COVID-19 panic and pandemic, creating a sense of end-time anxiety that appealed to a religious mindset which needed to reorder the events to make sense of it. Prediction is governed by regularities and patterns, but the outbreak of the pandemic followed no discernible pattern as randomness and irregularities seemed to be at the heart of the responses by states and corporations. For example, the shutting down of international travels and boundaries and the enforcement of stay-at-home orders disrupted livelihoods and neighbourhoods. Furthermore, the sheer complexities of global events and the many different moving parts in the COVID-19 scenario created a degree of chaos that baffled and confounded Pentecostal prophets who were used to working with smaller groups of believers or discerning patterns in routinised global affairs and contexts. The suddenness of the ensuing events caused more irregularities than disorder and within the apparent chaos, lurked a degree of religious orderliness: the need for an omnipotent power to reveal a pattern, a purpose and possible outcomes.

What some scholars have called the "distanced church" was one outcome out of apparent COVID-19 disorder (Campbell 2020). The distanced church, made possible by Internet connectivity and media technologies, illustrates the uncoupling of society under the pandemic. This period marked the increased intensification of how offline and online religious spaces and practices merged, entangled, intersected and blurred (Campbell and Evolvi 2020). The blurring of virtual and physical religious spaces restructured the meaning of religious community, liturgy as a public religious service, religious authority and identity and the place of technology in accessing divine grace and salvation. Furthermore, in an important sense, it also changed the religious economy of many societies, especially how religious entrepreneurs recruited pecuniary resources from their clients. Under the COVID-19 era, the assumptions on which Pentecostal churches were built and gained popularity in Africa—mass energy, the ready availability of miraculous cure, or the promises of these, the promise of the presence and power of the Holy Spirit—were challenged and undermined because they no longer fit present realities. Every aspect of the pandemic such as mass deaths and sickness, hunger under lockdown, and the disruption of economic and livelihood activities seemed to be directed to the Pentecostal promise of power and prosperity, healing and wholeness but these practices failed to adequately respond to these present realities. Before the pandemic, Pentecostalism flourished in Africa on the assumptions of what its clients and consumers wanted and what was considered meaningful in their lifeworlds. COVID-19 scuttled these assumptions and undermined and reorganised the religious market in significant ways. The state asserted its powers to regulate society by making new rules and enforcing these in a draconian manner in some cases. The state became a supplier of material salvation goods such as sanitisers and personal protective equipment, food rations, etc. In the context of mass deprivation following the aggressive implementation of pandemic regulations, the Pentecostal crisis of imagination became evident as religious leaders were unable to adequately respond to the needs of their members, followers and the larger society. The usual Pentecostal rhetoric of power, of healing miracles and power to make people prosperous, or even the explanation and answers to the problem of evil fell short of reality. This is what I call the prophetic chaos.

By discounting the validity of scientific explanations and interpretations of COVID-19 and attributing the cause of the crisis to a spiritual realm, Pentecostal leaders proffered a spiritual solution to the unfolding crisis. According to many of them, only prayer was needed to resolve and dissolve the problem. When their members starved as a result of the lockdown and shutdown of economic activities, many megachurches failed to respond with the provision of charity to their flocks. It is perhaps instructive to quote at length the views of one of the staunchest and persistent disseminators of the African Pentecostal views on the pandemic, Helen Ukpabio,

> Christians generally believe that it is the devil's instigated agenda for this last day in conformity with satanic schemes for one-world government. If their agenda works then it is time for Satan to take over the world [...] As you can see, homosexuality, lesbianism, the Church of Satan, non-acceptance of one's gender, wickedness and hatred towards Christianity and their tenet of faith, persecution of the church and believers and openly discrediting the Bible and inciting people to hate it and many such things simply shows [*sic*] that the pandemic is part of their bid to force Christians to receive satanic marks via the vaccine and tampering with certain human genes to corrupt it especially people of the third world countries. The entire covid [sic] is manmade. [...]. All the controversies surrounding the pandemic notwithstanding, government is interested in using it to advance their [sic] selfish interest instead of embarking on [a] rescue mission.[14]

In the above quote, which resonated among many conservative religious groups, western governments and their African allies are those being riled against as trying to foist and instigate a Satanic world government. Views such as these are shared by a large section of African Pentecostal Christians, both lay members and leaders, as other studies have also found (Ossai 2021; Wild-Wood et al. 2021). Bishop David Oyedepo, founder-owner of Living Faith Church, Worldwide (A.K.A. Winners Chapel), for example, claims there is no longer coronavirus but "antichurch virus" and a "satanic plot against the church",[15] a position that aptly summerises Ukpabio's opinion that the coronavirus has produced a "hatred towards Christianity". Chris Oyakhilome of Christ Embassy Church, with branches across Africa, Europe and North America, adds a specific element to the mix of causes: human technology; specifically, the 5G mobile telephony. The pastor claimed 5G, rather than coronavirus infections, was responsible for the deaths in Wuhan and the motivation for the stay-at-home orders issued by different governments around the world. Similar to the views of Helen Ukpabio, Oyakhilome claimed that some unnamed but powerful forces were ushering in a "new world order"

[14] Helen Ukpabio, personal communication, 11 September 2021.

[15] Xavier Moyet, "Appraisal of the discourses of two Nigerian Megachurch leaders about vaccination against Covid-19", https://religiousmatters.nl/appraisal-of-the-discoursesof-two-nigerian-megachurch-leaders-about-vaccination-against-covid-19/.

through 5G technology. The global COVID-19 lockdowns were a pretext to stealthily build and instal 5G structures without public notice or disruption. For Oyakhilome, the *real* objective of the new lockdowns and social distancing regimes were not containing and controlling a viral epidemic, but to "create the antichrist and go after the church of Jesus Christ".[16] As the COVID-19 pandemic protracts, Oyakhilome has also developed his 5G theory and connected it to nanotechnologies and the development of vaccines. According to this evolved version of his claim, the COVID-19 vaccines are embedded with nanoparticles actionable through the 5G network. In May 2020 and again in January 2021, Oyakhilome was found guilty of disseminating disinformation through his televised sermons which was potentially harmful to his mostly Christian audience about COVID-19.[17] Ukpabio, Oyakhilome and Oyedepo all dissuade their audiences from getting the COVID-19 vaccines. In his opposition to vaccination, Oyedepo says mandatory vaccination is immoral, inhuman and very likely illegal. He claims taking the vaccine makes a person "a guinea pig": "The world is confused but the church is lighted. They are confused. But the church has the answer. Did you see any outbreak of virus here? How will it enter the gate?". It was as if the Pentecostal assembly was supernaturally or mystically immune from coronavirus infection.[18]

Another prominent Pentecostal leader in Africa who has weighed in on the issue of vaccination is Pastor Enoch Adeboye of the Redeemed Christian Church of God. Addressing his congregation during the monthly Holy Ghost Service on 02 October, 2021, he said:

[16] Aanu Adeoye, "Misinformation at the pulpit" (12 May 2020), https://restofworld.org/2020/nigeria-covid-5g-misinformation/.

[17] For disseminating "inaccurate and potentially harmful claims about coronavirus", Oyakhilome's LoveWorld television broadcasting station, the United Kingdom broadcast regulators, Office of Communications, fined the television station £125,000 in January 2021. See: "Christian Broadcaster Fined £125,000 for Covid-19 conspiracies", (31 March 2021) https://www.independent.co.uk/news/media/christian-tv-channel-ofcom-covid-conspiracy-b1825259.html, Jibril Ibrahim, "Covid-19 in Nigeria: Once Again, Religion Stands in the Way" (29.06.2020), https://www.fes.de/referat-afrika/neuigkeiten/covid-19-in-nigeria-once-again-religion-stands-in-the-way.

[18] Kayode Oyero, "I won't take COVID-19 vaccine, I'm not a guinea pig –Oyedepo", *Punch* (Lagos), 17 April 2021, https://punchng.com/i-wont-take-covid-19-vaccine-im-not-a-guinea-pig-oyedepo/.

> I never said to you don't be vaccinated, you have never heard that from me. Rather than living in fear or doubt, get vaccinated. If you believe that getting vaccinated would put your mind at rest, then go ahead If there are nations in the world that say I cannot come to preach the gospel there because of vaccination, I will do anything for Jesus Christ. If vaccination is going to hinder me from doing the work that God has called me to do, if they asked me to get vaccinated 10 times, I would be vaccinated.[19]

The equivocation or prevarication in Adeboye's speech cannot be missed. It is disingenuous, even dubious, to link vaccination with evangelism rather than the social good of public health. The love of neighbour (Matthew 22:35–40, Mark 12:28–34, Luke 10:27) and hospitality towards the other Christian principles and premise for private and public action are clearly lacking in the self-serving rhetorics of many African Pentecostal leaders on COVID-19 and the need for vaccination. A religion that emphasises salvation as a private and personal pursuit rather than a collective endeavour would also miss the notion in the teaching of Jesus Christ and in the early church that the religious and non-religious "other" is not simply an object for missionary fervour or conversion but a neighbour to love and keep safe (Yong 2008). Still, understanding that Pentecostalism does not articulate a principle of the public or common good as social virtue,[20] one may begin to explain, that is, theorise the emergent Pentecostal chaos in the face of public health emergencies.

What comes out in these views of popular African Pentecostal leaders is the tension in the interplay between certain kind of religions or faith, the complex and complicated nature of contemporary public health issues and scientific inquiries as well as the interpretation of illness and disease in the age of global science and technology. In the Pentecostal views discussed above, one sees an attempt to mobilise the claims about the power of the Holy Spirit to provide answers and explanations to contemporary suffering and illness as well as for the clergy to

[19] Sam Eyoboka, "Why I will Take the COVID Vaccine—Pastor Adeboye", *Vanguard* (Lagos), 03 October 2021, https://www.vanguardngr.com/2021/10/why-i-will-take-covid-vaccine-pastor-adeboye/.

[20] (See Cartledge 2016 on how *charismata* in Pentecostal-Charismatic churches could be used for the benefit of the wider society).

play prominent roles as responsible and dedicated public health providers. In the attempt to reposition religion, or rather, the brand which they produce and market, as perennially relevant in the face of the ongoing pandemic, these Pentecostal leaders grapple with the relationship between science and technology and divine revelation or the interpretation of sacred texts. In the unfolding scenario of COVID-19 pandemic, a section of African Pentecostal community transmuted into what might be called "ConPentecostalism": the emergence of conspiracy Pentecostalism as a public force or public religion in relation to attempts to explain and interpret the COVID-19 pandemic and its toll on human sociabilities and sensibilities (on how conspiracy beliefs are created and sustained, see Albarracín et al. 2022).

Conclusion

In the Pentecostal economy, sickness and diseases are not aspects of human experience that is at variance with a theology of abundance and flourishing; they are to be commodified in framing a religious entrepreneur's miracle-working capabilities. Pentecostalism claims to be a religion of social, spiritual and economic power; a religion infused and driven by the power of the Holy Ghost which produces radical change and cures for human ailments. In many parts of Africa, it also claims to be both a social force and political powerhouse for determining how society is to be structured and governed in line with the will of God. African Pentecostal leaders have developed intricate theologies of health and wellness, wealth and prosperity, and have built immense and expansive entrepreneurial empires on these claims. The COVID-19 health emergency has put these claims to the test. Prophets failed to predict or anticipate the emergence of the pandemic; they spiritualised its origins and cause and actively resisted government and scientific interpretation of the virus. When their initial efforts failed, or when the force of public opinion or state implementation of a new social and cultural infrastructure became overwhelming, many of them revised their actions and opinions and reluctantly encouraged their followers to adhere to state regulations. Furthermore, Pentecostal leaders have been at the forefront of disseminating COVID-19 and vaccine disinformation; hence, creating and reinforcing vaccine hesitancy among their followers. The ongoing pandemic graphically illustrates how religion, specifically Pentecostalism and its entrepreneurial leaders, stands in the way of development and the production of social good. The alternative to the vaccine recommended by these leaders is prayers to "the true God"—as Ukpabio frames it —and Oyedepo says, the "church is light" that the darkness of a pandemic is unable to extinguish or dim. If the church in Africa is light, it is difficult to understand why and how Africa and Africans still dwell in the crushing darkness of poverty, vaccine scarcity, political failure and unending conflict. In their public pronouncements and preaching about COVID-19, African Pentecostal leaders provide a moral critique of the west; however, they fail to apply their own standards to why and how Africa is the way it is: the least developed continent in the world (Okeja 2017).

The pandemic has thrown a serious challenge to Pentecostal spirituality, theology and practices. The rituals of casting and binding evil or illness have not worked with COVID-19; the rituals of performing miraculous healings have spectacularly failed too. More importantly, as a religion that claims the power of the Holy Spirit to foretell the future and to guide humankind in understanding the mind of deity, Pentecostal leaders and prophets did not notice the approaching tsunami of COVID-19. When the pandemic unfolded, what ensued was a scrambling for responses in the face of chaos. Pentecostal chaos, the apparent confusion that follows the simultaneous occurrences of many different events, generated dissonance and confusing responses from different leaders. Also, the complex networking and the rapidity of the scientific invention that went into the production of a range of vaccines caught African Pentecostal leaders unprepared but also challenged their claims to healing ability. Almost all continents except Africa produced their vaccines. Africa, with fragile states and weak structures, demanded and relied on vaccine donations from mainly Europe and North America. The dependency reinforced the perception of the west foisting a New World Order as claimed by some of these Pentecostal leaders.

However, the presence of Pentecostal chaos does not imply the complete absence of order and pattern within the African Pentecostal field. It shows that the field is composed of a wild array of actors whose actions collectively cannot be predicted or predetermined because there is a clear absence of a single organising principle. For example, African Pentecostal actors lack a nuanced understanding of the principle of social good or the common good: goods, services, values, resources, basic/collective rights and freedoms that benefit *all* members of society. Hence, a concept such as "public health" is alien to their practice, which explains why Adeboye would link his taking the COVID-19 vaccine to the need for evangelism rather than helping to secure and promote the good of himself and others around him. He would not take the vaccine voluntarily unless it is mandated by governments as a condition to achieve other ends. Such instrumentalist thinking is embedded in the Pentecostal principle; the need to achieve personal rather than collective objectives such as personal prosperity and salvation. Making sense of the apparent Pentecostal chaos means figuring out and making sense of the undergirding and underlying principles governing the field of practice and the real interests that drive Pentecostal actors. The discussions in this chapter demonstrates how African Pentecostalism is driven by a set of religious entrepreneurs acting in a competitive religious economy which compels each actor to show relevance and visibility or be relegated to the sidewalks of the Pentecostal market and field. It is reasonable to assume that African Pentecostalism is an integral aspect of the social economy needed to redress a post-crisis society. It is, however, in crisis and would be unable to assert its influence appropriately. For the Pentecostal church in Africa to regain its vigour and play a similar role that the early church played during the epidemics of the second and third centuries, the Holy Spirit needs to be freed from the quarantine which African Pentecostal leaders have imposed on it. For the church to make the needed impact that serves the needs of the people of God, African Pentecostalism needs to be born again, reimagined and recaliberated in the COVID-19 era to usher in a post-Covid world relevant to the suffering people of God in Africa.

References

Albarracín, Dolores, Julia Albarracín, Man-Pui Sally Chan, Kathleen Hall Jamieson (eds). 2022. *Creating Conspiracy Beliefs: How Our Thoughts are Shaped*. London: Cambridge University Press.

Asamoah-Gyadu, Kwabena J. 2020. *Christianity and Faith in the COVID-19 Era: Lockdown Period from Hosanna to Pentecost*. Accra: Step Publishers.

Asamoah-Gyadu, Kwabena J. 2021. Pentecostalism and Coronavirus: Reframing the Message of Health-and-Wealth in a Pandemic Era. *Spiritus: ORU Journal of Theology* 6 (1): article 12. http://digitalshowcase.oru.edu/spiritus/vol6/iss1/12.

Biri, Kudzai. 2021. Pentecostalism in Zimbabwe and the Revitalization of African Traditional Religions: A Comparative Analysis of the Newer Religious Movements. In: Ezra Chitando (ed.), *Innovation and Competition in Zimbabwean Pentecostalism: Megachurches and the Marketization of Religion*, (pp. 21–32). London: Bloomsbury Academic.

Born, Irene. 1971. *The Born-Einstein Letters*. Trans. I. Newton-John. London: Macmillan Press Ltd.

Burgess, Richard. 2008. *Nigeria's Christian Revolution: The Civil War Revival and Its Pentecostal Progeny (1967–2006)*. Cumbria: Paternoster.

Campbell, Heidi A., ed. 2020. *The Distanced Church: Reflection on Doing Church Online*. Texas: TAMU NNMR&DCS.

Campbell, Heidi A., and Giulia Evolvi. 2020. Contextualizing Current Digital Religion Research on Emerging Technologies. *Hum Behav & Emerg Tech* 2: 5–17.

Cartledge, M.J. 2016. Renewal Theology and the 'Common Good'. *Journal of Pentecostal Theology* 25 (1): 90–106. https://doi.org/10.1163/17455251-02501011.

Casanova, José. 1994. *Public Religions in the Modern World*. Chicago: University of Chicago Press.

Cherstich, Igor, Martin Holbraad, and Nico Tassi. 2020. *Anthropologies of Revolution: Forging Time, People, and Worlds*. California: University of California Press.

Chidester, David. 2002. *Patterns of Transcendence: Religion, Death and Dying*. 2nd ed. California: Wadsworth Press.

Chidester, David. 2002. *Patterns of Transcendence: Religion, Death and Dying*. 2nd ed. MIchigan: Wadsworth Publishing.

Chidume, C.G., C.N. Oko-Out, and G.C. Aro. 2021. State Fragility and COVID-19 Pandemic: Implications on the Political Economy of Nigeria. *Social Science & Humanities Open* 3 (1): article 100127: 1–7. https://doi.org/10.1016/j.ssaho.2021.100127.

Consorti, Pierluigi. 2020. Religion and Virus. In *Law, Religion and COVID-19 Emergency*, ed. P. Consorti, 15–18. Pisa: DiReSom.

De Kock, Wynand J. 2000. Pentecostal Power for a Pentecostal Task: Empowerment through Engagement in South African context. *Journal of Pentecostal Theology* 8 (16): 102–116.

Ellwood, Robert. 2009. *Tales of Darkness: The Mythology of Evil*. London: Continuum Books.

Endong, Floribert Patrick, and Eugenie Grace Essoh. 2019. The Concept of Power in the Nigerian Religious Discourse: A Study of Advertising Copies by Pentecostal and Charismatic Churches. In *Handbook of Research on Consumption, Media, Popular Culture in the Global Age*, ed. Ozlen Ozgen, 371–396. Hershey, PA: IGI Global.

Engelke, Matthew. 2018. Spirit. In *Critical Terms for the Study of Africa*, ed. Gaurav Desai and Adeline Masquelier, 288–301. Chicago: Chicago University Press.

Fagunwa, Omololu Ebenezer. 2020. African Pentecostalism and the 1918 Influenza Pandemic: The Supernatural amid the fearful and Implications for the COVID-19 Pandemic. *Christian Journal for Global Health* 7 (5): 52–64.

Fleisher, Jeffrey, and Neil Norman, eds. 2016. *The Archaeology of Anxiety: The Materiality of Anxiousness, Worry, and Fear*. London: Springer.

Gaiya, Musa. 2002. *The Pentecostal Revolution in Nigeria*. Occasional Papers, Centre of African Studies, University of Copenhagen.

Gerike, Jaco. 2012. *The Hebrew Bible and Philosophy of Religion*. Atlanta: Society of Biblical Literature.

Harari, Yuval Noah. 2014 [2011]. *Sapiens: A Brief History of Humankind*. Trans. Y.N. Harari, J. Purcell, and H. Watzman. London: Penguin Books.

Kamalu, Chukwunyere. 1998. *Person, Divinity & Nature: A Modern View of the Person and the Cosmos in African Thought*. London: Karnak House.

Lindhardt, Martin. 2012. *Power in powerlessness: A Study of Pentecostal Life Worlds in Urban Chile*. Leiden: Brill.

Lopez, Patricia J. and Kathryn A. Gillespie. 2015. *Economies of Death: Economi Logic of Killable Life and Grievable Death*. New York: Routledge.

Magesa, Laurenti. 1997. *African Religion: The Moral Traditions of Abundant Life*. New York: Orbis Books.

Marshall, Ruth. 2008. *Political Spiritualities: The Pentecostal Revolution in Nigeria*. Chicago: The University of Chicago Press.

Marty, Martin. 1998. Public Religion. In *Encyclopedia of Religion and Society*, ed. William H. Swatos and Peter Kivisto, 393–394. Walnut Creek: Altamira Press.

McNaught, Matthew. 2021. From Lagos to Winchester: How a Divisive Nigerian Pastor Built a Global Following. *The Guardian*. London, September 9. https://www.theguardian.com/news/2021/sep/09/tb-joshua-scoan-church-divisive-nigerian-pastor-global-following.

McNaught, Matthew. 2022. *Immanuel*. London: Fitzcarraldo Editions.

Meza, Diego. 2020. In a Pandemic are we more Religious? Traditional Practices of Catholics and the COVID-19 in Southwestern Colombia. *International Journal of Latin American Religions* 4 (4): 218–234.

Miller, Donald E., Kimon H. Sargent, and Richard Flory, eds. 2013. *Spirit and Power: The Growth and Global Impact of Pentecostalism*. Oxford: Oxford University Press.

Mitchell, Robert Cameron. 1970. "Religious Protest and Social Change: The Origins of the Aladura Movement in Western Nigeria". In: Robert I. Rotberg and Ali Mazrui (eds), Protest and Power in Black Africa, New York: Oxford university press: 458-496.

Mohr, Adam. 2020. Faith Tabernacle Congregation, the 1918–19 Influenza Pandemic and Classical Pentecostalism in colonial West Africa. *Studies in World Christianity* 26 (3): 219–238.

Molefe, Motsamai and Mutshidzi Maraganedzha. 2022. African Traditional Religion and Moral Philosophy. *Religious Studies*, 1–16. https://doi.org/10.1017/S0034412522000543.

Obadare, Ebenezer. 2018. *Pentecostal Republic: Religion and the Struggle for State Power in Nigeria*. London: Zed Books.

Ojo, Matthews A. 2004. *The End-time Army: Charismatic Movements in Modern Nigeria*. Trenton, NJ: Africa World Press.

Okeja, Uchenna. 2017. Evaluating Societies Morally: The Case of Development and 'Developing' Societies. *Analysis & Kritik, 39*(2), 241–263.

Ossai, Emmanuel Chiwetalu. 2021. 'It is the anti-christi. Can't you see?' Perceptions of COVID-19 among Nigeria's Christians and the Religion—Health Debate. *Studies in World Christianity* 27 (1): 48–64.

Peel, J.D.Y. 1968. *Aladura: A Religious Movement among the Yoruba*. Oxford: Oxford University Press.

———. 2016. *Christianity, Islam, and Orịṣa Religion Three Traditions in Comparison and Interaction*. California: University of California Press.

Premack, Laura. 2019. Bless US With Children: Pregnancy, Prosperity, and Pragmatism in Nigeria's Christ Apostolic Church. In *Spirit on the Move: Black Women and Pentecostalism in Africa and the Diaspora*, ed. Judith Casselberry and Elizabeth A. Pritchard, 181–195. Durham: Duke University Press.

Prempeh, Charles. 2021. *"Religion and the State in an Episodic Moment of COVID-19 in Ghana", Social Sciences & Humanities Open* 4 (1): art. 100141. https://doi.org/10.1016/j.ssaho.2021.100141.

Ranger, Terence. 1992. Plagues of Beasts and Men: Prophetic Responses to Epidemic in Eastern and Southern Africa. In *Epidemics and Ideas: Essays on the Historical Perception of Pestilence*, ed. Terence Ranger and Paul Slack, 214–268. Cambridge: Cambridge University Press.

Ranger, Terence, and Paul Slack, eds. 1992. *Epidemics and Ideas: Essays on the Historical Perception of Pestilence*. Cambridge: Cambridge University Press.

Ruch, E.A., and K.C. Anyanwu. 1981. *African Philosophy: An Introduction to the Main Philosophical Trends in Contemporary Africa*. Rome: Catholic Book Agency.

Sogolo, Godwin. 1993. *Foundations of African Philosophy: A Definitive analysis of Conceptual Issues in African Thought*. Ibadan: Ibadan University Press.

Soothill, Jane. 2019. A Critical Approach to the Concepts of 'Power' and 'Agency' in Ghana's Charismatic (or Neo-Pentecostal) Churches. In *Spirit on the Move: Black Women and Pentecostalism in Africa and the Diaspora*, ed. Judith Casselberry and Elizabeth A. Pritchard, 151–179. Durham: Duke University Press.

Stark, Rodney. 1997. *The Rise of Christianity: How the Obscure, Marginal Jesus Movement became the Dominant Religious Force in the Western World in a few Centuries*. New York: Harper-SanFrancisco.

Tengatenga, James, Susan M. Tengatenga, and Duley and Cecil J. Tengatenga. 2021. *Zimitsani Moto*: Understanding the Malawi COVID-19 Response. *Laws* 10: 20. https://doi.org/10.3390/laws10020020.

Tuck, Eve, and K. Wayne Yang. 2012. Decolonization Is Not a Metaphor. *Decolonization: Indigeneity, Education & Society* 1 (1): 1–40.

Ukah, Asonzeh. 2016. Prophecy, Miracle and Tragedy: The Afterlife of T. B. Joshua and the Nigerian State. In *Religious Freedom and Religious Pluralism in Africa: Prospects and Limitations*, ed. M. Pieter Coertzen, Christian Green, and Len Hansen, 209–232. Stellenbosch: SUN PReSS.

United Nations. 2020. *Policy Brief: Impact of COVID-19 in Africa*, https://unsdg.un.org/resources/policy-brief-impactcovid-19-africa.

———. 2020a. 'God Reload': The Pentecostal Political Transgression and Africa's Non-Secularity. In *Religion in the Era of Postsecularism*, ed. Uchenna Okeja, 148–170. New York: Routledge.

———. 2020b. Prosperity, Prophecy and the COVID-19 Pandemic: The Healing Economy of African Pentecostalism. *Pneuma* 42 (3–4): 430–459. https://doi.org/10.1163/15700747-bja10010.

———. 2020c. *From Excess to the Apocalyptic: Media and the Production of Religious Surplus in Africa*. Keynote presented at a workshop on Media and 'Public' Islam in Africa & Elsewhere, January 23–24, The Centre for Global Islamic Studies, 404 Grinter Hall, University of Florida.

———. 2020d. Sacred Surplus and Pentecostal Too-Muchness: The Salvation Economy of African Mega-Churches. In *Handbook of Megachurches*, ed. Stephen Hunt, 323–344. Leiden: Brill.

Vawter, Bruce. 1990. "Introduction to Prophetic Literature". In R. E. Brown, S.S, J. A. Fitzmyer, S.J. and R. E. Murphy, O. Carm. (eds), *The New Jerome Biblical Commentary*, (pp. 186–200). New Jersey: Prentice-Hall.

Wild-Wood, Emma, et al. 2021. The Public Role of Churches in Early Responses to COVID-19 in Africa: Snapshots from Nigeria, Congo, Kenya and South Africa. *Studies in World Christianity* 27 (1): 65–84.

Yong, Amos. 2008. *Hospitality and the Other: Pentecostal, Christian Practices, and the Neighbor*. New York: Orbis Books.

13

On Pandemic Planning and the Frontline Workers in Nigeria

Damilola Victoria Oduola

Introduction

In December 2019, a novel disease identified as SARS-CoV-2/COVID-19 broke out in Wuhan, China. This novel virus has resulted in a pandemic with over 190 million infected cases and over 4 million deaths across 188 countries and territories (WHO 2021a). However, although in July 2020, COVID-19 vaccines such as the Pfizer/BioNtech, the AstraZeneca and the Moderna were developed and over 3.4 billion doses have been administered globally, yet, in late 2020, new variants such as the COVID-19 Alpha, Beta, Gamma and Delta variants were identified and they have continued to pose increased risk to global health (WHO 2021b, c). The emergence of the COVID-19 virus and its variants has continued to raise a number of medical, scientific and ethical questions about the plans and strategies put in place to identify its cause, facilitate proper diagnosis and treatment, and develop effective methods to limit the spread and to deal with future occurrences. It is common knowledge

D. V. Oduola (✉)
Department of Philosophy, University of Ibadan, Ibadan, Nigeria

F. Egbokhare, A. Afolayan (eds.), *Global Health, Humanity and the COVID-19 Pandemic*, https://doi.org/10.1007/978-3-031-17429-2_13

that pandemics, whether mild, moderate or severe, often affect a large proportion of the population and that it could result to a large number of casualties if mismanaged. For this reason, most countries develop response plans that incorporate operational procedures and strategies for managing possible pandemic outbreaks. In preparation for such pandemic occurrences like the COVID-19 pandemic, Nigeria, in 2011, established the Nigeria Centre for Disease Control (NCDC) and in 2013, the National Pandemic Influenza Preparedness and Response Plan (NPIPRP) with the mandate to lead the preparedness, detection and response to infectious disease outbreaks and public health emergencies.

This chapter, however, contends that the NCDC and the NPIPRP have not properly conceptualized and attended to the rights and responsibilities of the Nigeria health workers (NHWs) within the context of pandemic planning. We argue that the Nigerian pandemic response plan has not addressed this significantly important age-long question: do healthcare workers have the duty to treat patients during pandemics, especially when doing so exposes the workers themselves to significant risks of harm and even death? This chapter, divided into four sections, will examine this question within the scope of ethical and medical considerations. The first section will examine pandemics and pandemic planning from a historical perspective. The second will discuss the Nigerian pandemic influenza preparedness and response plan within the context of pandemic planning. The third will critically engage a critical omission in the Nigerian pandemic response plan, that is, the neglected discourse on the rights and responsibilities of the NHWs. The last section will interrogate the significances or implications of the NHWs rights and responsibilities for pandemic planning in Nigeria.

On Pandemics and Pandemic Planning: A Historical Overview

Throughout the history of humankind, one of the greatest catastrophes ever, if not the greatest is the outbreak of a pandemic. As a matter of fact, very few phenomena throughout human history have shaped human societies and cultures the way outbreaks of infectious diseases and pandemics have. As Ashoka (2021) comments, pandemic outbreaks have had terrible consequences on the human society throughout history, but also, paradoxically, it has cleared the way for innovations and advances in sciences, economy, and political systems. Etymologically, the word "pandemic" is derived from two Greek words *pan*, "all" and *demos*, "people" which therefore suggests "an outbreak of a disease that occurs over a wide geographic area and typically affects a significant proportion of the population" (Merriam-Webster 2021).

Human population, throughout history, has experienced several outbreaks of pandemics ranging from the plagues, the earlier form of smallpox and tuberculosis and HIV/AIDS to the influenza virus pandemics of the twentieth and twenty-first centuries. However, the first global pandemic that brought devastating consequences on human societies across the globe was the 1918/1919 Spanish flu. The Spanish flu, an H1N1 influenza virus strain, referred to as the "greatest medical holocaust in history" is believed to have infected over half of the world's population at the time and caused about 50–100 million deaths (Saunders-Hastings and Krewski 2016: 4). As Saunders-Hastings and Krewski (2016: 4–5) opine, during the Spanish flu outbreak, effective vaccines and antibiotics to prevent and treat influenza were unavailable, public health systems were grossly unprepared, and there was little or no meaningful international coordination and cooperation among jurisdictions as regards the prevention and control of infectious diseases. At this time, doctors were clueless about the novel disease and the weak health system that was in place was overwhelmed in no time. These factors therefore contributed to the high mortality rate and the severe economic meltdown that accompanied the Spanish flu pandemic.

Subsequent years after the Spanish flu outbreak, the international community established the World Health Organization (WHO) and the International Health Regulations (IHR) in recognition of the view that since the human community is constantly faced with the threat of pandemics that could have devastating effects on the whole human population, there is the need for effective approaches and models that would be geared towards the development and improvement of pandemic preparedness and response capabilities. Apropos of this, the WHO, in 1999, established the influenza pandemic plan which outlined the roles of the WHO and public health leaders in responding to future threats of pandemic outbreaks. The roles of the WHO would be to "collect and analyse data on the occurrence of influenza viruses around the world; provide information to health authorities, the media and the general public about current influenza vaccine recommendations; and develop proposals to help guide national policy makers or those implementing national policies" (WHO 1999: 8). On the other hand, the roles of public health leaders would be to establish National Pandemic Planning Committees in their various countries, and these committees would be responsible for drafting the overall contingency plans for responses to a pandemic (WHO 1999: 21–22).

In 2005, however, the 1999 WHO influenza pandemic plan was revised and replaced with the WHO global influenza preparedness plan aimed at assisting member countries and those responsible for public health, medical and emergency preparedness to respond to threats and occurrences of pandemic outbreaks (WHO 2005: 1). The 2005 preparedness plan redefined the phases of public health risk associated with influenza virus, recommended actions for national authorities and outlined the responsibilities of the WHO in the event of a pandemic (WHO 2005: 1). Since 2005, however, the WHO preparedness and response plan has continued to witness several reviews and updates such as the WHO strategic action plan for pandemic influenza (2006/2007), the WHO pandemic influenza preparedness and response (2009), the WHO guide to revision of national pandemic influenza preparedness plans (2017) and the recent 2019 novel coronavirus (2019-ncov) strategic preparedness and response plan. Following the publication of the WHO pandemic preparedness plan and the growing concerns about the threats posed by influenza viruses, however, many countries of the world began to invest in developing, publishing and improving their preparedness plan. Between 2005 and 2009, about 43 countries in the European Union (EU) published their pandemic preparedness plan (Nicoll et al. 2012). Before 2007, fifteen Latin American countries published their preparedness plan (Mensua et al. 2009), between 2002 and 2006, about six Asian-pacific countries published their response plans (Coker and Mounier-Jack 2006) and between 2005 and 2017, about 35 African countries also published their national pandemic plan (Sambala et al. 2018). In spite of this, the COVID-19 pandemic has revealed that even with the advancement in medicine and pandemic planning, global preparedness for pandemics is still very weak as most countries have one or more important gaps to address. Hence, as LePan (2020) notes, there is an urgent need for countries to review, improve and update their preparedness plans in order to address important shortcomings as well as combat future challenges of disease outbreaks.

Pandemic Planning and the Nigeria Pandemic Response Plan

The prevalence of contagious diseases and the increasing possibility of new disease outbreaks in modern times have become an issue of concern not only to the international community but also to nation states. In recognition of this and the directives of the WHO, the Nigerian government established the Nigeria Centre for Disease Control (NCDC) as a regulatory institution with the mandate to lead the preparedness, detection and response to infectious diseases outbreaks and public health emergencies in Nigeria (NCDC 2020). Upon its formation in 2011, the NCDC became responsible for preventing and responding to disease outbreaks; stockpiling and prepositioning of supplies for outbreak response in the states; developing guidelines and checklists for emergency preparedness; supporting states in responding to small outbreaks and leading the response to large disease outbreaks in Nigeria (Njidda et al. 2018: 2). However, as part of its institutional function to coordinate preparedness and response to diseases outbreak in Nigeria, the NCDC, in 2013, established the Nigerian National Pandemic Influenza Preparedness and Response Plan (NPIPRP) to serve as a blueprint for a coordinated strategy to prepare for and respond to pandemics.

The NPIPRP, modelled after the WHO pandemic preparedness plan, identified six alert phases of pandemic outbreaks and the expected responses of the NCDC and other health agencies to each of the phases. As outlined in the document, the first phase of the pandemic response plan starts when the WHO announces that there are no viruses circulating among animals which is known to cause infections in humans (NNPIPRP 2013: 8). In the second phase, the WHO identifies an animal influenza virus which is known to have caused infection in humans, and is therefore considered a potential pandemic threat (NNPIPRP 2013: 8). The third phase is signalled when the WHO announces an animal or human-animal influenza virus, which has caused sporadic cases or small clusters of disease in people, but has not resulted in human-to-human transmission sufficient to sustain community-level outbreaks (NNPIPRP 2013: 8). At the fourth phase, the WHO announces verified human-to-human transmission of an animal or human-animal influenza virus that is able to cause "community-level outbreaks" (NNPIPRP 2013: 8). It is at this fourth phase that the NPIPRP would identify the following:

Phase 4a: No confirmed or suspected cases within Africa, Nigeria or neighbouring countries (Benin, Niger, Chad, and Cameroon).

Phase 4b: Confirmed or suspected cases in Africa, but no cases within Nigeria or any of the countries immediately bordering Nigeria (Benin, Niger, Chad, and Cameroon).

Phase 4c: Local Outbreak: First confirmed or suspected case in Nigeria or one of the countries immediately bordering Nigeria (Benin, Niger, Chad, and Cameroon).

Phase 4d: Regional Outbreak: Confirmed or suspected cases in Nigeria and at least one country bordering Nigeria (Benin, Niger, Chad, and Cameroon).

Phase 4e: Widespread Regional Outbreak: Confirmed or suspected cases in Nigeria and at least three countries immediately bordering Nigeria (Benin, Niger, Chad, Cameroon).

Phase 4f: High-Risk Regional Outbreak: Confirmed or suspected cases in Nigeria and at least three countries immediately bordering Nigeria (Benin, Niger, Chad, Cameroon) and widespread confirmed cases in schools.

Phase 4 g: Deceleration/Resolution: Weekly incidence rates of pandemic influenza decline by at least 10% per week for at least two weeks (NNPIPRP 2013: 8).

The fifth phase commences immediately when the WHO confirms human-to-human spread of the virus into at least two countries in one WHO region (NNPIPRP 2013: 9). This also prompts the NPIPRP into a series of processes:

Phase 5a: No confirmed or suspected cases within Africa, Nigeria or neighbouring countries (Benin, Niger, Chad, and Cameroon).
Phase 5b: Confirmed or suspected cases in Africa, but no cases within Nigeria or any of the countries immediately bordering Nigeria (Benin, Niger, Chad, and Cameroon).
Phase 5c: Local Outbreak: First confirmed or suspected case in Nigeria or one of the countries immediately bordering Nigeria (Benin, Niger, Chad, and Cameroon).
Phase 5d: Regional Outbreak: Confirmed or suspected cases in Nigeria and at least one country bordering Nigeria (Benin, Niger, Chad, and Cameroon).
Phase 5e: Widespread Regional Outbreak: Confirmed or suspected cases in Nigeria and at least three countries immediately bordering Nigeria (Benin, Niger, Chad, and Cameroon).
Phase 5f: High-Risk Regional Outbreak: Confirmed or suspected cases in Nigeria and at least three countries immediately bordering Nigeria (Benin, Niger, Chad, and Cameroon) and widespread confirmed cases in schools.
Phase 5 g: Deceleration/Resolution: Weekly incidence rates of pandemic influenza decline by at least 10% per week for at least two weeks (NNPIPRP 2013: 9).

The sixth phase of the process demands that the WHO makes the announcement of a global pandemic outbreak (NNPIPRP 2013: 9). Consequently, the NNPIPRP would also activate the following:

Phase 6a: No confirmed or suspected cases within Africa, Nigeria or neighbouring countries (Benin, Niger, Chad, and Cameroon).
Phase 6b: Confirmed or suspected cases in Africa, but no cases within Nigeria or any of the countries immediately bordering Nigeria (Benin, Niger, Chad, and Cameroon).

Phase 6c: Local Outbreak: First confirmed or suspected case in Nigeria or one of the countries immediately bordering Nigeria (Benin, Niger, Chad, and Cameroon).

Phase 6d: Regional Outbreak: Confirmed or suspected cases in Nigeria and at least one country bordering Nigeria (Benin, Niger, Chad, and Cameroon).

Phase 6e: Widespread Regional Outbreak: Confirmed or suspected cases in Nigeria and at least three countries immediately bordering Nigeria (Benin, Niger, Chad, and Cameroon).

Phase 6f: High-Risk Regional Outbreak: Confirmed or suspected cases in Nigeria and at least three countries immediately bordering Nigeria (Benin, Niger, Chad, and Cameroon) and widespread confirmed cases in schools.

Phase 6 g: Deceleration/Resolution: Weekly incidence rates of pandemic influenza decline by at least 10% per week for at least two weeks (NNPIPRP 2013: 9–10).

In response to the pandemic alert phases 4a, 5a, and 6a, the NCDC and other health agencies (e.g. NEMA, Federal Ministry of Health and other cognate ministries) are to focus on monitoring the global situation and increasing surveillance and pandemic preparedness efforts (NNPIPRP 2013: 18). The alert phases 4b, 5b, and 6b demand monitoring the global situation, with special emphasis on the situation in Nigeria and West Africa (NNPIPRP 2013: 21). With the phases 4c, 4d, 5c, 5d, 6c and 6d, the NCDC and national, state and local health agencies are to step into heightened surveillance and the activation of protocols to reduce viral spread and actions to address existing and anticipated medical caseload (NNPIPRP 2013: 24). Alert phases 4e, 5e and 6e compel the NCDC and national, state and local health agencies to focus on community mitigation measures to minimize spread of the virus and its economic and societal impact (NNPIPRP 2013: 28). In the alert phases 4f, 5f and 6f, the risks associated with the pandemic outbreaks are at their highest, and thus, the NCDC and other health agencies are to ensure continued community mitigation measures to minimize the spread of the virus and its economic and societal impacts, and to also ensure the maintenance of critical government services, as well as those provided by private sector businesses upon which the government and general public are dependent (NNPIPRP 2013: 32). In the alert phases 4 g, 5 g and 6 g, the health risks associated with pandemic outbreaks begin to diminish. Hence, the NCDC and all national, state and local health agencies are to ensure continued mitigation measures to minimize any additional pandemic-related economic and societal impacts; conduct assessments of the pandemic's impact on the society; and work with international and regional organizations to ensure societal stability and to assist in post-pandemic recovery (NNPIPRP 2013: 37).

The NPIPRP and the Nigeria Health Workers

A pandemic outbreak often puts a great strain on the healthcare system. During pandemics, the entire health community is expected to exhibit day-to-day resilience and commitment towards mitigating morbidity and mortality that the pandemic instigates. This suggests that effective pandemic preparedness also requires the total and active engagement of healthcare workers—the "frontline soldiers" in the war against infectious diseases. As Adindu and Asuquo (2013: 2) comment, the Nigeria health workers (NHWs) which comprise of doctors, nurses, midwives, pharmacists and other health-related personnel are the diverse highly trained health professionals who provide direct health services and support delivery of such services to the Nigerian population. Ojo and Akinkunmi also comment that the Nigerian health professionals, who are involved in activities primarily devoted to enhancing health in the absence of which clinical and public health services cannot be delivered to the population, constitute a significant component of the healthcare system and are important in the delivery of smooth efficient, effective and quality healthcare services (2015: 377). However, in the event of a pandemic outbreak, the responsibilities of the NHWs—indeed of the entire health community—become heightened. During this period, patients and the public expect healthcare workers to employ their knowledge and skills to manage the situation effectively. They will be generally required to go beyond their routine roles to take on tasks with which they are less familiar and which they will, most likely, have to carry out under stressful conditions and environments (Asghari and Tehrani 2020: 4). During outbreaks, some of the tasks that would be required of health workers as illustrated in the recent WHO COVID-19 Rights, Roles and Responsibilities of Health Workers (RRRHW) document include: following established occupational safety and health procedures; using provided protocols to assess, triage, and treat patients; treating patients with respect, compassion, and dignity; and reporting suspected and confirmed cases of infected persons (WHO 2020a: 1).

In the discharge of these duties, however, there is the need to situate the WHO pandemic preparedness plan within the context of a postcolonial healthcare system like Nigeria's. The Nigerian health workers, in dealing with epidemics and pandemics, are often exposed to significant risks and hazards such as pathogen exposure and infection, long working hours, psychological distress, fatigue, stigma and in most cases, unpaid salaries and allowances. This is apart from the deep institutional and systemic dysfunction within which they are expected to operate efficiently. During the recent coronavirus outbreak, for instance, many NHWs were exposed to high risk of COVID-19 infection as a result of their close contact with infected patients and the unavailability of the needed personal protective equipment (PPEs) (Adejumo et al. 2020: 42). As reported by the WHO external situation report 11, between 25 February and 12 May 2020, 401 Nigeria health workers were already infected with coronavirus (WHO 2020b: 2), and by 27 May 2020, an updated WHO external report 13 showed that the number of the infected health workers had increased from 401 to 606 (WHO 2020c: 3). Apart from the risk of infection, NHWs also suffer other challenges such as increased workload, traumatic stress, discrimination, unpaid allowances, and at the worst, death. An instance of this is the indefinite strike embarked upon by the National Association of Resident Doctors in Nigeria (NARD) on 15 June 2020, due to the failure of the government to provide adequate personal protective equipment for health workers and to pay hazard allowances to doctors working on COVID-19 patients (Adejumo et al. 2020: 42). Also, in an interview with *PUNCH HealthWise*, the National president of The Nigerian Union of Allied Health Professionals (NUAHP) commented that the association had recorded about 150 infection cases among its members and 25 fatalities arising from complications of the coronavirus due to the lack of PPEs (Folorunsho-Francis 2020).

These challenges encountered by the NHWs especially during pandemic outbreaks raises the question as to whether health workers have a duty to treat or care for patients especially when doing so exposes them to significant risks of harm and even death. That is, can a physician legitimately refuse to treat a patient who, for instance, is suspected of having COVID-19 because the doctor is not adequately protected and such a patient would put the physician at risk of contracting the virus and possibly dying? In response to this, Heidi Malm et al. argue that "common morality holds that we all, in virtue of our shared humanity, have a moral duty to aid others in great need when we can do so at minimal risk to ourselves" (2008: 6). This means that individuals have some general duties to others, and these duties do not rest on any kind of special relationship between the individual and the others except that of common humanity. In contrast, however, as Malm et al. further argues, the duty to treat is a special duty because there is the existence of a special "role-related relationship" between the health worker and the patient which grounds the duty (2008: 6). According to them, this special relationship can obligate health workers to incur greater risks than would be required of persons in general because first, the health worker had expressed or implied his/her consent to treat when signing up for the job; second, the health worker had received some special training to aid others at minimal risk; third, the health worker has the duty to reciprocate or give back to the society, and lastly, the health workers had submitted him/herself to the oaths and codes of conduct guiding the profession (2008: 7–15).

In the same vein, Chalmers Clark (2003: 1) argues that there are motivating and practical reasons for health workers to care for patients in the face of personal danger because health workers are in a form of binding social agreement with their patients and the public. Clark (2003: 1) argues further that not only is it the physician's duty to provide treatment at some personal risk, but also public expectations for hazardous duty are justified as a result of the physician's choice of joining a profession aimed at combating disease and the physician's implicit promise of readiness in perilous times. Consequently, doctors and other health workers have the duty to treat simply because they have given their consent to join the medical profession. Now, if it is the case that health workers indeed have a role-defined duty to treat even when doing so poses significant risk, then we may want to ask if there is a limit to what this duty demands of them. In other words, do health workers have the obligation to tolerate every form of risk especially during pandemic outbreaks? In response to this, Clark contends that "doctors need not become abjectly self-sacrificing in medical emergencies .... doctors and other health workers should have first access to inoculations and other protections required by those who toil on the front lines of illness" (2003: 1). Samuel Huber and Matthew Wynia (2004: 9) argue similarly that the physician's duty to treat should be mediated with the doctor's responsibility not to become a patient herself, and so, risks must be balanced against one's capacity to do good in the future. They argue further that the physician-patient relationship is a kind of reciprocal social relationship and since physicians have the obligation to treat even at personal risks, then it suggests that communities in turn have obligations towards physicians and the entire health community (Huber and Wynia 2004: 9). More importantly, clarification on how to handle predictably very high-risk situations and the level of expertise that is required for caring during such high-risk situations should be subjected to open dialogues within and between the profession and the society (Huber and Wynia 2004, 9).

The above discussion therefore suggests that the responsibilities of health workers are very germane or significant during pandemics because they are the frontline workers who, in the face of significant harm or risks, are expected to provide essential health services to the general public and ensure minimal spread of the virus. In the same vein, there should be corresponding expectation of some reciprocal social obligations that should be geared towards the rights (welfare and protection) of health workers, especially during pandemics. This means that although the NHWs' duty to treat especially during pandemics is sacrosanct, their rights are equally important. As Onigbinde et al. remarks, during outbreaks, "if a catastrophe will be averted, the healthcare delivery system must be safeguarded. The health and safety of healthcare workers must also be well-taken care of to sustain public health and recoveries" (2020: 1). Bringing this discourse into the context of pandemic planning, Draper et al. argue that "healthcare workers are essential personnel in any response to emergencies and will be in the frontline of exposure to infection during pandemic outbreaks. Hence, effective pandemic planning would need to rely on the majority of health services staff in responding to outbreaks" (2008: 2).

This simply suggests that heath workers are central figures not only during pandemic outbreaks but also in pandemic planning because effective pandemic preparedness would have to rely on their professional services. Thus, if health workers are central to pandemic planning, then, it simply follows that their rights and responsibilities are also very important and must be considered when preparing for a pandemic. According to the Center for Disease Control and Prevention, "to ensure optimal workforce performance during a severe pandemic, an organization's pandemic plan, pre-pandemic work culture, and safety procedures must reflect the importance of health protection and, where feasible, provide services that enhance personal and professional resiliency of health worker" (CDC 2020: 3). This therefore reveals that effective pandemic preparedness requires not only taking into consideration the rights and responsibilities of health workers but also outlining them in the pandemic response plans.

The submission gleaned from the CDC and the WHO with regard to the rights and responsibilities of health workers instigates a re-examination of the NPIPRP document and how it affects the rights and responsibilities of the Nigeria health workers. The NPIPRP was designed to achieve five major objectives, namely: contribute to an effective national and local level response to influenza pandemic; reduce influenza-related morbidity and mortality; minimize disruption of critical social, economic and medical services during pandemics; mitigate pandemic-related impacts on critical infrastructure; and facilitate post-pandemic recovery operations (NPIPRP 2013: 3). These objectives are to be carried out through ten functional operational areas: surveillance and laboratory; triage and patient care; infection control measures; antivirals acquisition, storage, distribution and use; vaccine acquisition, storage, distribution and use; mass fatalities management; mental health; mass care and logistics; communications and public education; and command and control and continuity of operations (NPIPRP 2013: 11). Unfortunately, out of these ten operational areas outlined in the NPIPRP, the only operational area that made reference to the NHWs is the mental health operational area which states that

> The primary recommendations for workforce support focus is the establishment of psychosocial support services that will assist workers in managing emotional stress during response efforts to an influenza pandemic, and resolving related personal, professional, and family issues .... Hospitals in Nigeria are encouraged to develop a mental health component to their influenza pandemic plans to ensure that healthcare staff and their families receive adequate mental health support during any pandemic disaster. Staff members in hospitals and other healthcare facilities should be trained in behavioural techniques to help employees cope with grief, stress, exhaustion, anger and fear during an emergency. (NPIPRP 2013: 56)

Sadly, the NPIPRP only mentioned issues pertaining to the mental health of NHWs and paid less attention to other fundamental rights such as adequate protection against risk of infection, payment of allowances and provision of reliable compensations for the families of those who die while fulfilling their duties. Also, the NPIPRP failed to spell out the specific responsibilities of the NHWs as well as the extent or limit of these responsibilities during pandemic outbreaks. This critical omission therefore reveals a shortcoming in the NPIPRP that should be addressed.

Lessons to Learn: Pandemic Planning and the Nigeria Health Workers

A pandemic outbreak is largely an unpleasant event but its severity depends on the preparedness of a community in its response to it. Pandemic planning is expected to be all-encompassing as it requires the ability of public health officials, healthcare professionals, researchers and scientists to work together to devise a plan and to strengthen their capabilities to prepare and respond to outbreaks. Pandemic planning, therefore, becomes very vital in developing preventive and cost-effective mitigating measures against pandemic threats (Bollyky and Patrick 2020). As Oppenheim et al. (2019: 2) note, epidemic preparedness reflects the capacity of institutions such as public health authorities, health systems and emergency response bodies to detect, report and respond to outbreaks; and in the event of a pandemic, health institutions, healthcare workers and public health systems are required to identify, investigate, monitor and manage infected persons through the mobilisation of personnel and resources.

As mentioned earlier, the duties of health workers during pandemics would often go beyond the conventional roles as they would be required to receive additional knowledge, skills and trainings to protect themselves, protect others and as well work safely and effectively. However, if it is the case that health workers would be required to go beyond their conventional duties to take on additional responsibilities during pandemics, then it becomes necessary to spell out these roles accordingly. In pandemic outbreaks, health workers are often saddled with overwhelming responsibilities, and if these responsibilities are not clearly stated and understood, health workers may not be able to carry out their duties or respond effectively. A vivid example can be drawn from the 1918 Spanish flu pandemic which had an estimated case mortality rate of 2.5% and caused more than 40 million deaths worldwide (Schoch-Spana 2001: 32). According to Schoch-Spana, "during the 1918 influenza pandemic, health care workers were just as vulnerable to influenza as their patients. In some instances, fear of contagion kept caregivers from performing their duties. Practitioners and public health nurses faced overwhelming caseloads and frequently fielded demands for care among crowds in the street" (2001: 33). At this time, pandemic planning was nonexistent and health workers were mostly clueless about what to do or how to respond to the ravaging disease, and this, in a way, contributed to the high mortality rate that accompanied the pandemic. This implies that the absence of a pandemic preparedness plan that recognises and outlines the responsibilities of health workers during pandemics may lead to confusion, poor response and management of the disease which could ultimately lead to a surge in the mortality rate and a collapse of the overall health system.

In the same vein, the increased vulnerability of healthcare workers during pandemics clearly justifies the need to highlight and recognise the rights of health workers in pandemic planning. During pandemics, healthcare workers often face significant exposure to infectious materials, and if there is no corresponding provision and/or clear indication of their welfare and protection in the form of adequate provision of PPE supplies, occupational health and safety training, compensation, rehabilitation, mental health and counselling, conducive working conditions and practices among others, then health workers may end up becoming patients themselves. To illustrate this, Madhav et al. (2018: 324) note that during the first Ebola outbreak in the Democratic Republic of Congo (DRC) in 1976, the Yambuku Mission Hospital at the epicentre of the outbreak was closed because 11 out of the 17 staff members had died of the disease. During the Kikwit Ebola outbreak in 1995 in the same DRC, 24% of cases occurred among known or possible healthcare workers. Similarly, during the Ebola disease outbreak in Guinea, Liberia and Sierra Leone, health workers accounted for 3.9% (815/20,955) of all confirmed and probable cases reported (WHO 2015: 4). This reveals that without adequate welfare and protection, health workers may end up being causalities of "pandemic war" and if this happens, health systems may become overwhelmed as a result of scarce health workforce. Invariably, overwhelmed health systems among other indirect effects may contribute to a 2.3-fold increase in all-cause mortality during pandemics (Madhav et al. 2018: 323).

So what lessons does this hold for pandemic planning in Nigeria? Our discussion so far has revealed some critical omissions in the NPIPRP. It has also shown the need for a review of the NPIPRP. While it is quite essential that pandemic planning develops strategies for reducing influenza-related morbidity and mortality and mitigating pandemic-related impacts on critical infrastructure, however, it is also expedient that it recognises and highlights the rights and responsibilities of NHWs as they are critical personnel in the fight against "pandemic wars". Hence, substantive recognition of the rights and responsibilities of NHWs as well as the political will to implement this recognition must be at the core of any emergency response plan for there cannot be an effective healthcare system without a health workforce that is protected and capable of meeting the needs of the population (WHO 2015: 2).

Conclusion

Much has been written about pandemic planning, and the recent coronavirus outbreak has shown that much is still needed to be done. There is the need for the Nigerian government to welcome new perspectives, adjustments and revisions as regards pandemic planning and preparedness. As much as there is a need to pay attention to the operations of healthcare delivery systems, the socio-economic systems and the political systems in pandemic planning, it is equally crucial that the rights of Nigeria healthcare workers at the forefront of managing the pandemic are adequately protected. The recent WHO *Coronavirus disease (COVID-19) outbreak: rights, roles and responsibilities of health workers, including key considerations for occupational safety and health* (RRRHW) document, which outlines the rights and responsibilities of health workers as well as employers and managers in health facilities, is a step in the right direction. It is, therefore, advisable that the Nigerian government, in partnership with the Nigeria Centre for Disease Control, come up with such a document and also, take necessary practical steps to give it legal validity in order to provide a firm legal basis for its implementation and enforcement. Also, efforts should swiftly commence on the review of the Nigerian national pandemic influenza preparedness and response plan to accommodate the rights and responsibilities of the Nigeria health workers.

References

Adejumo, O.A., A.O. Adejumo, and F.E. Okonofua. 2020. Rights Versus Responsibilities of Health Care Workers in Nigeria: Changing the Narrative in the COVID-19 Era. *African Journal of Reproductive Health* 24 (2): 41–45. https://doi.org/10.29063/ajrh2020/v24i2s.6.

Adindu, A., and A. Asuquo. 2013. Training Human Resource for 21st Century Nigerian Health Sector. *Global Journal of Human Resource Management* 1 (3): 1–11.

Asghari, F., and S.S. Tehrani. 2020. Ethical Issues in Responding to the COVID-19 Pandemic: A Narrative Review. *Advanced Journal of Emergency Medicine* 4 (2): 1–8.

Ashoka, J.P. 2021. Human Response to Pandemics in History and Medico-anthropological Correlates. *Royal Society of Chemistry*. July 21. https://www.chemistryworld.com/the-coronavirus-pandemic-and-the-future/human-response-to-pandemics-in-history-and-medico-anthropological-correlates/4013237.article.

Bollyky, T.J., and S.M. Patrick 2020. Improving Pandemic Preparedness: Lessons from COVID-19. *Council on Foreign Relations*, October. https://www.cfr.org/report/pandemic-preparedness-lessons-COVID-19/findings

Centre for Disease Control and Prevention. 2020. *Psychological and Social Support for Essential Service Workers During an Influenza Pandemic*. United States: Centre for Disease Control and Prevention. https://stacks.cdc.gov/view/cdc/5356.

Clark, C.C. 2003. In Harm's Way: Service in the Face of SARS. *The Hastings Center Report* 33 (4): 1. http://www.jstor.com/stable/3528383.

Coker, R. and Mounier-Jack, S. 2006. "Pandemic Influenza Preparedness in the Asia–Pacific Region." The Lancet, 368, Issue 9538: 886-889. Doi: https://doi.org/10.1016/S0140-6736(06)69209-X

Draper H., S. Wilson, J. Ives, C. Gratus, S. Greenfield, J. Parry, J. Petts, and T. Sorell 2008. Healthcare Workers' Attitude towards Working during Pandemic Influenza: A Multi Method Study. *BMC Public Health* 8 (192): 1–7. http://www.biomedcentral.com/471-2458-8-192.

Folorunsho-Francis, A. 2020. COVID-19: 150 Health Workers Infected, 25 Dead, Says NUAHP. *Punch Healthwise*, July 24. https://healthwise.punchng.com/covid-19-150-health-workers-infected-25-dead-says-nauhp/.

Huber, S.J., and M.K. Wynia. 2004. When Pestilence Prevails: Physician Responsibilities in Epidemics. *American Journal of Bioethics* 4 (1): 5–11. https://doi.org/10.1162/152651604773067497.

LePan, N. 2020. *Ranked: Global Pandemic Preparedness by Country*. Published 20th March, 2020. https://www.visualcapitalist.com/global-pandemic-preparedness-ranked/. Accessed 14 Oct.

Madhav, N., B. Oppenheim, M. Gallivan, P. Mulembakani, E. Rubin, and N. Wolfe. 2018. Pandemics: Risks, Impacts and Mitigations. In *Disease Control Priorities: Improving Health and Reducing Poverty*, ed. D.T. Jamison, H. Gelband, S. Horton, P. Jha, R. Laxminarayan, C.N. Mock, and R. Nugent, 315–345. Washington, DC: International Bank for Reconstruction and Development / the World Bank.

Malm, H., T. May, L.P. Francis, S.B. Omer, and D. Salmon. 2008. Ethics, Pandemics, and the Duty to Treat. *The American Journal of Bioethics* 8 (8): 4–19.

Mensua, A., S. Mounier-Jack, and R. Coker. 2009. Pandemic Influenza Preparedness in Latin America: Analysis of National Strategic Plans. *Health Policy and Planning* 24 (4): 253–260. https://doi.org/10.1093/heapol/czp019.

Merriam-Webster Dictionary. Pandemic. https://www.merriam-webster.com/dictionary/pandemic. Accessed 20 July 2021.

Nicoll, A., C. Brown, F. Karcher, P. Penttinen, M. Hegermann-Lindencrone, S. Villanueva, M. Ciotti, L. Jean-Gilles, S. Rehmet, and J. Nguyen-Van-Tam. 2012. Developing Pandemic Preparedness in Europe in the 21st century: Experience, Evolution and Next Steps. *Bulletin of the World Health Organization* 90 (4): 311–317. https://doi.org/10.2471/BLT.11.097972.

Njidda, A.M., O. Oyebanji, J. Obasanya, O. Ojo, A. Adedeji, N. Mba, J. Oladejo, and C. Ihekweazu. 2018. The Nigeria Centre for Disease Control. *BMJ Global Health* 3: 1–3. https://doi.org/10.1136/bmjgh-2018-000712.

Ojo, T.O., and A.F. Akinwunmi. 2015. Doctors as Managers of Healthcare Resources in Nigeria: Evolving Roles and Current Challenges. *Nigerian Medical Journal* 56 (6): 375–380.

Onigbinde, O.A., A.O. Ajagbe, and O. Babatunde. 2020. The Welfare of Healthcare Workers Amidst COVID-19 Pandemic in Sub-Sahara Africa: A Call for Concern. *Ethics, Medicine and Public Health* 15: 1–4. https://doi.org/10.1016/j.jemep.2020.100555.

Oppenheim, B., M. Gallivan, N.K. Madhav, N. Brown, V. Serhiyenko, N.D. Wolfe, and P. Ayscue. 2019. Assessing Global Preparedness for the Next Pandemic: Development and Application of an Epidemic Preparedness Index. *BMJ Global Health* 4 (1): 1–9. https://doi.org/10.1136/bmjgh-2018-001157.

Sambala, E.Z., T. Kanyenda, C.J. Iwu, C.D. Iwu, A. Jaca, and C.S. Wiysonge. 2018. Pandemic Influenza Preparedness in the WHO African Region: Are We Ready Yet? *BMC Infectious Diseases* 18 (567): 1–13. https://doi.org/10.1186/s12879-018-3466-1.

Saunders-Hastings, P.R., and D. Krewski. 2016. Reviewing the History of Pandemic Influenza: Understanding Patterns of Emergence and Transmission. *Pathogens* 5 (66): 1–19.

Schoch-Spana, M. 2001. Hospital's Full-Up: The 1918 Influenza Pandemic. *Public Health Reports* 116 (supplement 2): 32–33.

The Nigeria Centre for Disease Control. 2013. *The Nigeria National Pandemic Influenza Preparedness and Response Plan (NPIPRP)*. Abuja: The Nigeria Centre for Disease Control. https://ncdc.gov.ng/diseases/guidelines.

———. 2020. *About the NCDC*. https://ncdc.gov.ng/ncdc. Accessed 21 Oct.

World Health Organization. 1999. *Influenza Pandemic Preparedness Plan: The Role of WHO and Guidelines for National and Regional Planning*. Geneva: World Health Organization. https://apps.who.int/iris/handle/10665/66155.

———. 2005. *WHO Global Influenza Preparedness Plan: The Role of WHO and Recommendations for National Measures before and During Pandemics*. Geneva: World Health Organization. https://apps.who.int/iris/handle/10665/68998.

———. 2015. *Health worker Ebola Infections in Guinea, Liberia and Sierra Leone: A Preliminary Report.* Geneva: World Health Organization. https://www.who.int/csr/resources/publications/ebola/health-worker-infections/en/.

———. 2020a. *Coronavirus Disease (COVID-19) Outbreak: Rights, Roles and Responsibilities of Health Workers, Including Key Considerations for Occupational Safety and Health*. Geneva: World Health Organization. https://www.who.int/publications/i/item/coronavirus-disease-(covid-19)-outbreak-rights-roles-and-responsibilities-of-health-workers-including-key-considerations-for-occupational-safety-and-health.

———. 2020b. *COVID-19 WHO African Region: External Situation Report 11/2020*. WHO Regional Office for Africa. https://apps.who.int/iris/handle/10665/332078.

———. 2020c. *COVID-19 WHO African Region: External Situation report 13/2020*. WHO Regional Office for Africa. https://apps.who.int/iris/handle/10665/332199

———. 2021a. *Weekly Operational Update on COVID-19—20 July 2021*. Geneva: World Health Organization. https://who.int/publications/m/item/weekly-operational-update-on-covid-19–20-july-2021.

———. 2021b. *WHO Coronavirus (COVID-19) Dashboard*. https://covid19.who.int/. Accessed 20 July.

———. 2021c. *Tracking SARS-CoV-2 Variants*. https://www.who.int/en/activities/tracking-SARS-CoV-2-variants/. Accessed 20 July 2021.

14

Dialogism and Polyphony in the Interpretations of COVID-19 Discourse in Zimbabwe

Tobias Marevesa and Esther Mavengano

Introduction

The genesis of the COVID-19 pandemic brought untold suffering to humankind the world over. The problematic nature of the virus is evident in the emergence of multiple narratives and perspectives which define the pandemic discourse. The main contention in this study is that the

T. Marevesa (✉)
Department of English and Media Studies, Great Zimbabwe University, Masvingo, Zimbabwe

Research Institute for Theology and Religion, College of Human Sciences UNISA, Pretoria, South Africa

E. Mavengano
English and Media Studies Department, Faculty of Arts, Great Zimbabwe University, Masvingo, Zimbabwe

Georg Forster Postdoc Research Fellow at Alexander von Humboldt, TU (Techische Universistat Dresden) Institut of English and American Studies Department of English, Dresden, Germany

F. Egbokhare, A. Afolayan (eds.), *Global Health, Humanity and the COVID-19 Pandemic*, https://doi.org/10.1007/978-3-031-17429-2_14

COVID-19 pandemic narrative, just like any other human discourses, is complex and multifaceted, and this calls for a multidisciplinary approach adopted in this chapter through the interface of linguistics and religious studies. Chugh and Sharma (2012) posit that language is the most salient gift to humankind utilised to present worldviews. This observation is pertinent because even religious perspectives are constructed and presented in language. Olimat (2020) also contends that words are powerful weapons to shape the public views and perceptions about the coronavirus. It is imperative to examine the linguistic framing of COVID-19 and religious perspectives that shape the interpretations of the pandemic discourse. The following research questions guide the claims, discussion and submissions in this study:

- How does the language in COVID-19 discourse shape the perceptions and interpretations of the pandemic?
- What is the interpretation of the COVID-19 pandemic from three religions in Zimbabwe?
- How is the pandemic conceptualised from Bakhtin's notions of the dialogic and polyphonic?

Dialogic Theory and the Monologic Sense of Truth in COVID-19 Pandemic Discourse

Mikhail Bakhtin is a Russian philosopher whose ideas on language have been used in linguistics, religious studies, philosophy, education, literary criticism, among other disciplines (Mavengano et al. 2020). Bakhtin (1981) introduces the term metalinguistics which is a philosophy of language that celebrates multiplicity of worldviews and recognises the sociopolitical and ideological dimensions of discourse (Mavengano 2020). In other words, Bakhtinian metalinguistics framework focuses on languaging in a particular discourse and heuristic problem due to polysemantic, dialogic and polyphonic nature of language. Although Bakhtin made his primary reference to poetics, particularly the novel genre, his ideas have been extended to the understanding of human language in different disciplines such as linguistics and religious studies in numerous contexts. Dialogism underscores contradictions or conflicting perspectives and the unfinalisability of sense-making in discourses. This is a departure from mainstream linguistics and its monolingual closure of the text (Bakhtin 1981; Mavengano 2020). The interpretations of COVID-19 are moulded in dialogic and polyphonic spaces of the pandemic discourse. Bakhtin (1981) contends that language is dialogic by nature and using it is participating in dialogue in which divergent views compete with each other. He affirms that the multiplicity of conflicting worldviews is realised in the realm of language. Dialogism acknowledges the multiplicity of voices and dynamics of the relations between individuals and society. Bakhtin (1984) contends therefore that the meaning of an utterance or word (*slovo*) is always half someone else's. His observations have significant implications about the nature of human language and discourses such as COVID-19.

What Bakhtin underscores here is that meanings are not individually constructed by the author /participant in discourse but rather emerge from interactional relationships. This is a remarkable shift from traditional linguistics and religious studies because from a Bakhtinian sense, the text is no longer the source of meaning production as established in the structuralist perspective. Similarly, Mavengano (2020) comments that Bakhtin's concept of dialogism regards language as a porous, hybrid and open-ended phenomenon. Interestingly, Bakhtin (1981/1984) argues that languaging in discourse is a site for dialogic interaction and contestation of multiple perspectives which thereby creates semantic dissonance. This means that reality in a discourse is provisional, ever-evolving and always contested through re-interpretation. Dialogic interpretation of COVID-19 discourse is attentive to the interplay of a cacophony of voices or plurality of unmerged autonomous consciousnesses or perspectives. The most fascinating aspect is the emphasis on the coexistence of different worldviews (polyvocal nature of texts or discourses), active interaction involved in sense-making (addressivity and responsivity), and an acknowledgement of the presence of other.

Polyphonic Theory and the Plurality of Consciousnesses

Polyphony, from Bakhtin's (1981/1984) theorisation of language and discourse, refers to the existence and manifestation of several conflicting but valid opinions. Bakhtinian thinking refutes the idea of a single reality or monolithic truth. This then raises the issue of multiperspectivality in the understanding of reality, as well as the problematisation of the idea of a single truth (Mavengano 2020). Bakhtin (1981) argues that human discourse is an interactive space in which diverse voices or worldviews "speak back" to one another. Discourse captures and represents the human world defined by difference in interacting perspectives or worldviews (Bakhtin 1981/1986). His dialogic and polyphonic concepts refute any notion of a fixed truth. Explaining his metalinguistics theory, Bakhtin (1981/1984) further postulates that meaning does not exist in isolation but rather springs from historical, religious and social milieu in which language is utilised. This argument significantly points at the contextual or situational dimension of language in discourse which further provides several avenues for sense-making.

What this suggests is that perceptions about COVID-19 pandemic are not formed in a vacuum but rather influenced by contextual factors, what Bakhtin (1981) calls the outsideness of language. Such arguments make a compelling case against Saussurean and Chomsky and linguistics in which contextual factors are not accorded much attention in the study of language. The significance of context is emphasised in Bakhtinian framework since a verbal utterance (*slovo*) is not merely lexical but also contextualised (Mavengano 2020). For instance, John Mangwiro, the Zimbabwe's Deputy Minister of Health, cited what WHO stated at the beginning of 2021, "the entire Zimbabwe has been declared a coronavirus hotspot for a new variant of COVID-19 in the second wave" (Moche 2021: 2). The Deputy Minister also argued that World Health Organisation claimed that the infection rates rose drastically in all the provinces of Zimbabwe. If one compares the statistics of new cases and deaths in South Africa and Zimbabwe, not to mention the Western world, the truth value of this statement from WHO is challenged and refuted. Yet, WHO's claim has some sociopolitical, health and economic connotations. WHO's utterance can only be relevant and meaningful when the Zimbabwean's prevailing sociopolitical, health and economic conditions are taken into consideration. Thus, the meaning of this statement is derived from factors beyond verbal (lexical) content. In other words, mere linguistic and religious descriptions in interpreting the COVID-19 discourse are insufficient. The concept of polyphony is relevant when examining the linguistic framing of COVID-19 and religious perspectives present in the pandemic discourse. Polyphonic discourse accommodates the plurality of independent perspectives and unfinalisability or open-endedness of meaning-making. In other words, the examination of COVID-19 discourse in this study is done in pursuit of various perspectives.

Linguistic Landscape, Languaging and Semantics of Metaphorising in COVID-19 Discourse

The outbreak of the coronavirus pandemic brought some very interesting linguistic items to describe the pandemic. Language plays an essential role in communicating information and realities about COVID-19 pandemic. Language is employed by political figures as an instrument with the intention to shape the public perceptions about the lethal coronavirus disease. The political function of language when used by politicians is described by Crespo-Fernandez (2007/2013). Former president of the United States, Donald Trump, described the coronavirus as "foreign virus and invisible enemy" that demands "aggressive and comprehensive" effort coordinated by him as "wartime president." By employing the adjectival terms "foreign" and "invisible" the former president brings to fore the controversial subject about the genesis of coronavirus and also stresses the strangeness of the disease (Olimat 2020). Another critical possible reading of Trump's perception of COVID-19 speaks to the politics of representation. The politics of representation is embedded in Trump's linguistic framing of coronavirus as a "China virus," "Chinese virus" and Wuhan virus (Su et al. 2020: 2; Aljazeera News, 17 March 2020) Marcus (2020) observes that the battle between the US and China over the genesis of the coronavirus is conveyed in Trump's selection of linguistic items, revealing his perception of the virus as a Chinese invention. In self-defence, The New York Times on 19 March 2020 reported that China Spins a tale that the "U.S Army started the coronavirus epidemic." The Chinese government dialogically refutes the allegation by the American president and labelled COVID-19 as an "American virus" (The New York Times 2020; Shanapinda 2020).

The foreignness of the virus, aggravated by the lack of epidemiological information, magnifies its threat and arouses public fear (Olimat 2020). Cognisance of the fact that Trump is a prominent politician, his utterances can be interpreted as circumlocutory language that is ambiguous but politically charged. For politicians, language is a powerful instrument to shape public perception (Olimat 2020). He implicitly but deliberately influences public worldview about the origin of COVID-19 by framing the virus as a strange phenomenon in America (Shanapinda 2020). The dysphemistic metaphor of war in the adjectival/noun phrase employed by Trump foregrounds urgency and justifies political actions taken by his administration. Both *The Guardian*, *The BBC* and *The New York Times* reported that Trump views himself as a "wartime president" and puts the US on war footing to combat the outbreak (Smith 2020: n.p.). He declares, "I am a wartime president. This is a war. A different kind of war than we've ever heard" (Remarks 2020g cited in Smith 2020: 3). Bates (2020) condemns Trump's use of metaphors as a means to shape public's understanding of the coronavirus. Bates (2020) posits that war metaphor is a strong frame employed to compel the public to support radical political decisions from his government because, according to Trump, the COVID-19 environment demands immediate political actions. In war situations, presidents have obligation to defend their territories, and radical actions can be taken against the invading enemy. For Trump, the coronavirus disease threatens lives the same way as wars.

It is imperative to note that Trump's claim about the genesis of the coronavirus is contested by the Chinese government in a dialogic space of COVID-19 discourse. The public perceptions of the virus are shaped by the two conflicting truths because, according to Bakhtin (1981), truth is located at the point of converge of multiple and divergent consciousnesses. Yet, this study problematises Bakhtinian argument because it is also possible that what the American and the Chinese government's claim to be true could be false. This is so because the law of logic states that if one of them is true, then the other must be false. So, the question is, contrary to Bakhtin, is truth always what is involved in discursive disagreements? In other words, the question of truth remains problematic and contested. Significantly, the political and socio-economic background provides shades of meanings to these perspectives from the US and Chinese governments which have been in political and economic conflict for some time (Shanapinda 2020). This implies that the interpretive process is informed by both the verbal content from the two governments as well as contextual dimension of languaging in discourse.

COVID-19 has created "a state of exception," to borrow Agamben's (1998) term which justifies the use of authoritarian mechanisms as demonstrated through Trump's COVID-19 policy when he blocked the disbursement of fiscal aid to cash-starved states and cities. In the state of exception, "the sovereign has legal power to suspend the validity of the law, [and] legally places himself outside the law" (Agamben 1998: 15). Interestingly, Trump did not initially believe the coronavirus was a grave danger to Americans, only to take a turn around and declare himself a "wartime president" (BBC News 2020; The New York Times 2020; Shanapinda 2020), ready to fight the "invisible enemy" from China. It is thus appropriate to argue that Trump politicised COVID-19 pandemic discourse after he realised that he was becoming unpopular due to his laissez-faire leadership style. In a different context but relevant to the present discussion, Flusberg et al. (2018) argue that from a cognitive linguistics perspective, the prototype of war as source domain of the target domain (COVID-19 in this case) triggers emotional response such as anxiety and fear. Such metaphoric framing of COVID-19 heightens anxiety in American citizens. For a more robust linguistic understanding of the COVID-19 discourse, it is imperative to examine counter statements about the pandemic from different presidents from Africa. For instance, the Zimbabwean President Mnangagwa claims that the solution of COVID-19 should come from the appeasement and veneration of ancestors who are perceived by the Zimbabwean President to be angry. The appeasement according to Mnangagwa can only be done by traditional leaders at *Ematonjeni* which is a traditional sacred place. Mnangagwa's remarks suggest that COVID-19 is a punishment from the ancestors. Ironically, President Mnangagwa's perception of the pandemic differs greatly from that of Zimbabwe's Minister of Defence, Oppah Muchinguri, who claims that, "the coronavirus pandemic is the work of god punishing countries that imposed sanctions on us [Zimbabwe]." She further alleges that' "[t]hey are now staying indoors. Their economies are screaming just like they did to our economy" (www.news24.com). The minister views COVID-19 pandemic as God's punishment for the US and Europe. She claims that the genesis of the coronavirus is traced to the Chinese labs where "botched experiments" resulted in the deadly virus (https://www.voanews.com/).

At the beginning of 2021, the minister also made further controversial comments about China accusing the Chinese for manufacturing the coronavirus in their labs. Muchinguri claims, "Isn't it that there is a serious upsurge of COVID-19 cases in China? It's them who had botched experiments. Now that's killing us. They can't reverse it anymore. Look at where the people we call friends have taken us to" (https://www.voanews.com/). In addition, the term "Chinese vaccine" captures scepticism among Zimbabweans about the genuineness of the Chinese government in donating the vaccine when WHO has sent the delegation to investigate the Chinese's involvement in alleged manufacturing of the coronavirus. WHO (2021) also warns Zimbabwean government against the use of "Chinese vaccine." Looking at languaging that projects linguistic understanding of COVID-19 pandemic, there is no agreement about the genesis of the disease and how its menace can be stopped. Each understanding is motivated by political, economic or religious concern. A Tanzanian President, John Magufuli posed that "coronavirus, which is a devil, cannot survive in the body of Christ...It will burn instantly...," (Mutahi 2020: 1). Although the Tanzanian president acknowledges the fact that the coronavirus is a deadly disease, his utterance suggests that the virus only infects non-Christians. Both Mnangagwa and Magufuli who are African presidents believe that the solution to COVID-19 pandemic should come from the spiritual realm, the ancestors for the former whereas the latter believes that Christians will be saved through their call to Christ.

As the coronavirus disease remains a grave danger to the public health across the globe, it is fundamental to contemplate the pertinent role of language in the COVID-19 discourse and how it influences the public understanding of the pandemic. The pandemic continues to be a great calamity to humanity which strives to grasp the nature of coronavirus and how it can be controlled. The COVID-19 discourse offers a salient linguistic site for the examination of language employed with regard to the public perceptions of the disease. This discourse is characterised by sea and war metaphors, risk tropes, and personification among other interesting linguistic strategies that deserve academic attention with the intention to explore how the pandemic metanarrative is framed linguistically.

Cognitive linguists such as Lakoff and Johnson (1980), Lakoff (2008) and Gibbs (2017) view metaphor as pervasive in everyday language. In this section, militant verbiage and warfare linguistic expressions employed in COVID-19 discourse by the global news outlets and WHO are scrutinised in an attempt to understand how language is used to construct different understandings and convey the meanings about the coronavirus disease. What messages do militarised metaphors convey and how may this potentially influence the public perceptions of COVID-19 pandemic? In the year 2020, *The Telegraph*, *Sky News*, *The New York Times*, *BBC News* among others mainstream media outlets presented militarised lexicalisation from the semantic domain of war such as "curfew," "self-defence," "healthcare workers are in the trenches," fighting the "lethal enemy," waging a war against the virus (BBC News 2020), "battle-ground," "battle plan," "winning a war, frontline soldiers" (Sky News 2020a,b) probably with the intention to elicit emotional response from the audience and gain public attention. For instance, *BBC News* (2020) reports that according to the Chinese President Xi Jinping, his country was confident and capable of "winning the war against the virus." For Shanapinda (2020), Molnar (2020) and Olimat (2020) assume metaphors generate fear, anxiety, panic at the same time meant to magnify and reinforce the idea of danger posed by the COVID-19 pandemic. The military lingo employed draws from war lexicon to associate the pandemic with war and achieve salience with regard to the virus. Healthcare workers are perceived as frontline soldiers in a war situation fighting the deadly virus that is threatening many lives. Metaphorisation of health workers and war metaphors carry an emotional valence which derives their function from tropes of human fragility in the context of COVID-19 pandemic. The risk posed by the coronavirus thereby justifies the war efforts against it. It could be argued that some metaphorised expressions are hyperbolic and they deform facts about COVID-19 pandemic (Olimat 2020).

In 2020, WHO issued a series of measures that deployed imperative terms such as "we will win the battle," "let us mask up," "let us exercise social distance," "the victory in this battle is ours," among others (WHO 2020: 2–3). The use of imperative language by WHO and top government officials across the globe compels and at the same time implores the public to take collective action against the coronavirus. The prominence and the affective values of such imperatives force on the public the urgency of observing the mitigatory measures (Rafi 2020). COVID-19 is depicted in the mainstream news media as a threat to public health systems worldwide. It is also demonised in personified metaphors like "killer disease," "an enemy that is tightening its grip, "attacking people," "causing mayhem" and "humanity is besieged" (Rafi 2020; Olimat 2020). Sea metaphors are used to describe COVID-19's behavioural stages. WHO (2021) also declared that the world has already gone through the "first" and in some countries the "second wave." Sea waves are life-threatening and destructive. The use of sea metaphors frames and foregrounds the risk posed by the pandemic. Coronavirus disease is further framed figuratively as "a monster," "Tsunami and storm" to foreground its destructive nature (Alvarez 2020).This hyperbolic description springs from the idea that the pandemic has disrupted many productive economic and social activities through imposed social distancing and shutdowns/closures that complicate the suffering of many (Olimat 2020), hence its associative semantic connotations with biblical "plagues" (Peters 2020). Thus, the term demon conveys emotional valence in conceptualisation of a disease that has greatly affected humanity's existential conditions.

Religious Conceptualisation of the Pandemic in Zimbabwe

The following sections examine COVID-19 pandemic discourse from three religions prominent in Zimbabwe: Christianity, Islam and African indigenous religion. The analysis of the religious responses to COVID-19 in Zimbabwe will be guided by the following questions: how are religions in Zimbabwe responding to the sociopolitical interventions of COVID-19 pandemic? What are religious and theological significance behind the causes of COVID-19? What are theological considerations on what could be done to do away with COVID-19 pandemic? This interdisciplinary approach to COVID-19 discourse resonates with Bakhtinian theorisation of the nexus between language and truth which is complex, multiple and conflictual.

Christian Perspective

The Christian and Islamic responses to COVID-19 in Zimbabwe are centred on the themes of eschatology and apocalypse. This is because Christianity and Islam are both Abrahamic religions with shared doctrines and teachings. Isiko (2020) defines eschatology as the study of the end times or the final destiny of humanity. Apocalypse also refers to "revelations of secrets of a spiritual nature" (Isiko, ibid: 83). Eschatology and apocalypse are two terms which have similar meanings that are associated with futuristic expectations about the end of the world. Sean (2020) observes that the outbreak of COVID-19 is portrayed by scholars such as Isiko (2020), Koire (2020) and Niringiye (2020) as a sign of the end of the world and humanity by Christians. Damir (2019: 7) also stated that a number of clerics are interpreting the outbreak of COVID-19 as an imminent sign of the end of the world. Niringiye (2020: 45) posits that:

> the human quest for meaning in the face of a monstrous and inexplicable natural disaster, catastrophe or plague, is a natural instinct. It is the way to cope or deal with panic, fear and uncertainty by the catastrophe; faith in the supernatural is an essential part of human arsenal to either fight or flight.

Some Christians have the view that the COVID-19 pandemic may have been caused by human sin evoking God's anger. Similarly, some Zimbabwean pastors of Apostolic Faith Church such as Madziva, Jinjika and Ndoni argued that inasmuch as there were pandemics in the past as a result of sin, a significant thing about COVID-19 pandemic has been preceded by a number of signs (D. Ndoni, personal interview, March 6, 2021). This end of the world signs that were experienced in Zimbabwe includes HIV and AIDS disease for about twenty years, Cholera for a period and now COVID-19. The argument here is that the tragic outbreak of COVID-19 pandemic does not mean the end of the world but rather serves a sign that the end is going to take place in the near future. It is viewed as God's punishment upon the sinful people. Since this study is informed by Bakhtin's (1981/1986) theorisation of language and human discourse, it is essential to recognise that each of the perspectives discussed is treated as a valid consciousness that contributes to the conceptualisation of COVID-19 as a complex reality that invites plurality of consciousnesses. In other words, Bakhtin disrupts any interpretive process that privileges absolutism in the understanding of human discourse.

Such understanding of the pandemic is contested in dialogic and polyphonic construction of COVID-19 narratives. Despite this understanding, it is evident that coronavirus is indiscriminate because both the faithful and unfaithful face the dangers of COVID-19 pandemic. Ignoring such valid reality has disastrous implications on humanity. The coronavirus is not selective whether one is sinful or not. In a different context, Sean (2020) made a claim that God was in charge of the Black Death which took place in the fourteenth century, he was angered by sinful acts such as indecent dressing, arrogance, promiscuity, immorality, among others. This argument is proffered in contemporary times by Stearns (2009) who states that God could have unleashed the coronavirus to humanity probably because people are no longer worshipping Him by legalising homosexuality.

The above views are supported by biblical texts which are made reference to explain the outbreak of COVID-19 by Christians; these are Numbers 16:1–35; 2 Chronicles 7:13–14; Jeremiah 17:14–18; Psalms 91:5–7; John 14:1; Matthew 17:14, among others. These texts attribute the source of disasters and pandemics to God's wrath against the disobedience of humanity. These scriptures indicate that pandemics are caused by sin and that humanity can only reconcile with God through prayer. In the present context of COVID-19, this argument suggests that humankind needs to repent and seek forgiveness as a solution to the pandemic problem. Reverend Mutume of Apostolic Faith Church in Zimbabwe remarked that verses such as Numbers 16:1–35 is a text which pastors can use in COVID-19 pandemic discourse to account for God's anger against the Israelites for their sinfulness and unfaithfulness in Zimbabwe (Reverend Julius Mutume, personal interview, February, 2021). The same text further alludes that God was prepared to destroy all Judeans because of the disobedience committed by the three families of Dathan, Korah and Abiram verse 21, and in the following verse 22, Moses' "intercession reversed God's" initial plan to kill only members of the three disobedient families. These biblical texts refer to the time of Moses, when he (Moses) interceded for the families of Dathan, Korah, and Abiram. The same God can reverse the pandemic which is wreaking havoc in Zimbabwe by killing thousands of people. This Christian understanding informs the view that Zimbabwean pastors should stand for the people of Zimbabwe pleading for God's forgiveness in order to be saved from COVID-19 pandemic. Furthermore, in the Zimbabwean context, it implies that the nation should have illustrious church leaders such as the Moses and Aarons of today who can intercede for the stressed and suffering people. This view is mentioned in an interview with an Anglican priest who said:

> Another verse which is being used by other pastors is 2 Chronicles 7:14 to imply that Coronavirus came as a punishment of sin and the anger of God. I don't think so. Nevertheless, the origin of COVID-19 is China. I would say it's a biological warfare but I disagree with the claim that the superior God is spanking humanity through coronavirus. (Edward Ncube, personal interview, March 12, 2021)

Whether the outbreak of the coronavirus disease is a punishment or not, the Christian perspective suggests that the solution to the current pandemic comes from prayer for divine intervention. This is so because in the New Testament, Matthew 17:14 discusses the importance of humility before God who has supreme power to offer total healing of any form of disease. In this text, prayer is again the key element in bringing healing to an individual. John 14:1 and Psalms 91:5–7 deliver a message of encouragement to the victims of disasters, afflictions and pandemics such as coronavirus. The cited scriptural texts would therefore be instrumental, according to the Christians, in bringing hope and encouragement in times of distress and suffering caused by COVID-19 pandemic in Zimbabwe.

The proponents of the Christian perspective are of the view that this was the reason that countries such as China, Europe and America experienced so many COVID-19 related deaths when compared to African countries. Basing on the Christian perspective, the differences in death statistics implies that the former countries are more sinful than the African states that had low fatalities. At the end of April 2020, there has been a world total of confirmed cases of 2, 667,526 which were recorded. The United States of America had the highest cases of 849,094, China had 82,798, Italy was third highest at187, 327 and Spain had 213,024. Yet Africa had a total of 26,870 confirmed cases (Worldometers 2020). It is against this background that scholars such as Isiko (2020) and Parsitau (2020) have given attention to the explanation of these fatalities from the perspectives of divine intervention. Page (2020) regards such perceptions as scapegoating and politicisation of the pandemic which ignore other explanations of the causes of coronavirus disease.

There is also the 5G issue as a possible cause of spreading coronavirus by radiation from the advanced technology of the mobile services. Radiation can come into contact with the skin for instance, when one puts a 5G mobile to their ear when receiving or making a call (Shanapinda 2020). It has been established that 5G is dangerous to humanity but its association with the outbreak of coronavirus disease is yet to be proved scientifically. Clearly, each of these perspectives has no monopoly to mean. This is in line with Bakhtin's (1981/ 1984) views which suggest that interpretation and comprehension of human discourses is an active and inherently responsive process. However, the critical question is that even within the Bakhtinian framework, how can one differentiate between the plausibly true statement and the pure nonsensical or even blatantly false ideas and arguments? Another problematic question is that does a purely stupid idea also find its way into the discursive framework that Bakhtin stipulates as potentially true? These are essential questions that trouble the Bakhtinian theorisation of truth. In other words, Bakhtin's arguments cannot be taken as the opportunity to consider all falsity and gibberish.

The existence of incompatible interpretations in COVID-19 pandemic discourse advances the notions of dialogism and polyphony and shows the constraint of a monologic reality. Regarding coronavirus disease as punishment from God could be valid and yet partial because there is semantic dissonance in a cacophony of voices, narratives and perceptions in the religious realm when debating the genesis of the pandemic. It is also incomplete to refute other angles of truths. Yet, further scholarly conversations are needful to address how to differentiate such angles of truth from unfounded claims. In another context but relevant to this discussion, Zuze, refuting the claim by a Zimbabwean high-ranking official that COVID-19 was a punishment for Western countries and the USA, states that the pandemic is not a disease for a particular race, religion, nationality or ethnicity. The monological stance of perceiving that coronavirus is a punishment from God is therefore insensitive to other possible interpretations thereby closing dialogic and polyphonic spaces of the pandemic discourse.

Islamic Perspective

The response of Muslims to COVID-19 in Zimbabwe is mainly based on the doctrines which are deduced from the Quran and the traditions Prophet Muhammad. From the Quran, there are well-tabulated Islamic guidelines which deal with pandemics. The Quran provides explanations about the occurrence, cause and prevention of natural disasters and pandemics. For Muslims, pandemics and natural catastrophes come from Allah. Mudhumi, a Muslim Imam said, "God is responsible for sending disasters and epidemics to humankind. All the good and bad originate from God. Muslims are admonished to accept God's wishes for humankind" (K. Mudhumi, personal interview, January, 12, 2021). Koire (2020: 20) argues that "the COVID-19 [pandemic] is not an accident but an incident which was predetermined by God, years before it struck humankind." There are three ways in which Allah expresses his anger to humanity: "God's resolve to make humanity realize his supremacy over the world through natural calamities beyond human control; Allah's attempt to test the faith of humanity; and finally, pandemics as a punitive measure to the disobedient" (Isiko 2019a: 103).

From the Islamic perspective, COVID-19 pandemic was sent by Allah to show his power over the whole universe. The fact that COVID-19 has crippled the world economies, while science is still scrambling to make a meaningful sense of the virus, seems to demonstrate the capitulation of humankind. The pandemic, according to the Islam, serves as a reminder to all humankind that Allah is in control of the universe. In spite of humankind's financial and social position and standing, humanity is powerless before Allah (Koire 2020). Isiko (2019b: 78) further argues that "weakness and helplessness of human beings amidst COVID-19 further demonstrate the unequivocal equality of humanity before Allah, the supreme leader, for the virus affects the rich and poor, the young and old, educated and the illiterate."

Thus, from an Islamic perspective, natural calamities and pandemics are meant to test humankind's faith in Allah. According to Isiko (2020), it is Allah who put people in panic, poverty, food shortage, fear and pandemics as trial for faith. Regardless of the predicament of the Muslims they required to go back to Allah for guidance. For everything that transpires in the Muslim's life Islam prescribes a solution to it. Allah allows troubles and sufferings on humankind. This is supported by what the Quran states:

"Allah touches you with harm, none can remove it but He, and if He intends any good for you, there is none who can repel His Favour which He causes to reach whomsoever of His slaves He will. And He is Oft-Forgiving, Merciful" (Quran10:107).

Based on the above Quranic quote, Muslims seem to believe that COVID-19 is one of the many natural calamities and pandemics that Allah had been sending to humankind for ages. Reference is made to the "... saints in paradise [who] experienced diseases of such a nature, but it was their endurance that made them able to have their way to paradise" (Isiko 2020: 90). This is reminiscent with what the Quran says: "No calamity befalls on earth or in yourselves but is inscribed in the Book of Decrees- (*Al-Lauh Al-Mahfuz*), before we bring it into existence. Verily, that is easy for Allah" (Quran 57:22). In addition, the Quran says: "No calamity befalls, but with the leave [i.e. decision and *Qadar* (Divine Preordainments)] of Allah, and whosoever believes in Allah. He guides his heart [to the true Faith with certainty, i.e. what has befallen him was already written for him by Allah from the *Qadar* (Divine Preordainments)], and Allah is the All-Knower of everything" (Quran 64:11). Allah will ultimately come and liberate those that have persevered the trying times and remain faithful to Islam. Thus, the Islamic belief requires perseverance, patience and faith in Allah as the spiritual ingredient that will enable Allah to deliver humanity from pandemics or other natural calamities. Lastly, pandemics are a form of punishment from Allah to the sinful. This is in agreement with what Mlambo an Imam said, "the sinful nature of humankind is responsible for epidemics like COVID-19" (Henry Mlambo, personal interview, January 13, 2021). From the Islamic perspective, the disobedience of humanity is responsible for epidemics such as coronavirus. In the case of China, such sinfulness will include the mass murder of Muslims through unjustified wars, violating human and religious rights against Muslims, and the prevention of freedom of worship (Isiko 2020). These views should be debated in the context of dialogic and polyphonic notions which displace rigid systems of thought and sense-making but rather support pluralistic nature of reality.

African Traditional Religious Perspective

The African indigenous religious' response to the outbreak of coronavirus can be understood from what traditional healers and diviners have said in Zimbabwe. According to African indigenous religious belief system, it is the Supreme Being and ancestors who are responsible for inflicting pandemics like the COVID-19 and natural disasters on humankind due to disobedience (Parsitau 2020). Such ideas from scholars of African Indigenous religious belief system are fundamental in the understanding of COVID-19 in Zimbabwean context. For instance, ancestral belief system does not agree with conspiracy theories which advance the claim that

COVID-19 pandemic is a result of a biological warfare between the United States and China. Shanapinda (2020: 12) argues that "conspiracists are suggesting that COVID-19 could have been a human error." Mwashita a traditional healer argued that COVID-19 pandemic did not come as a biological warfare but "it came as a result of the anger of the ancestors who are not happy with what Zimbabweans have done" (Daniel Mwashita, personal, interview, February 13, 2021). Unfortunately, African indigenous religious belief does not believe in conventional medicine, yet ancestors utilise people to achieve their will. African traditional belief does not subscribe to conventional medicine but rather advocates the traditional medicine (Adogame et al. 2015). Parsitau (2020) argues that ancestors may not bring any ailment without its cure. The implication of this argument is that the ancestors give the traditional healers and diviners' power to find medicine to heal all types of diseases, including COVID-19. Another diviner argued that the ancestors visit the traditional healers through dreams instructing them to get the type of medicine to give their clients (Sibanda, w, personal interview, January, 20, 2021). Although in the African traditional belief system the traditional healers and diviners use traditional medicine, they also venerate the ancestral spirits for healing.

In response to the coronavirus from an African traditional religious perspective, the current Zimbabwean President Emmerson Dambudzo Mnangagwa held a meeting with traditional and religious leadership apprising them on the COVID-19 pandemic. The religious groups that the President met include Zimbabwe Chiefs Council the Supreme Council of Islamic Affairs in Zimbabwe (SCIAZ) among others. Throughout the meeting, each religious leader submitted to the President what they want to do to lessen the effects of COVID-19.The President told the chiefs that traditionally every time there is a problem, the chiefs should be formally addressed being the guardians of the people and the land. He appealed to them to consult the ancestors for a solution to the pandemic in Zimbabwe Chief Charumbira argued that "it is our responsibility as chiefs to lead and protect our people from the COVID-19 disease by being able to standing on the gap" (Chief Fortune Charumbira, personal interview, December, 23, 2020). Fortunate Charumbira is a leader of the chiefs' council in Zimbabwe. In response to the president's plea, the chiefs in Zimbabwe visited Ematonjeni, a sacred place where traditional rituals are performed.

From the religious perspective, the genesis of COVID-19 pandemic is linked to offensive human behaviour to the Supreme Being (God for the Christians, Allah for Muslims and Ancestors for African Indigenous religion). Thus, it is perceived that coronavirus is a pandemic which has been unleashed by the ancestors to express their anger. Significantly, the three religions discussed in this chapter have a convergent point where they view COVID-19 as some form of punishment for disobedience. At the same time, there is a profound divergent point vis-à-vis the source that unleashes punishment on humanity. In addition, all the religions discussed above in the context of coronavirus disease are futuristic in the sense that what the adherents of each religion do in present time will shape their destiny. The intervention of the Supreme Being that comes as a result of the public outcry by the adherents provides a solution to the pandemic or the natural calamities.

Reflections

The chapter has explored how COVID-19 pandemic is understood from linguistic and religious perspectives. Unfortunately, each dimension falls short of a multidimensional framework Bakhtin advocates. Drawing from the linguistic construction and religious perspectives that explain and shape public understanding of COVID-19 pandemic, novel semantic avenues were highlighted in positions of conflict and convergence in dialogic and polyphonic spaces. Bakhtin's dialogic and polyphonic concepts problematise and unsettle traditional hermeneutical practices in both linguistics and religious studies that ignore multidimensionality and multiperspectivality in language and discourse. The discussion on languaging of COVID-19 pandemic discourse brought out a salient dimension of the pragmatic element in sense-making process. The pragmatic quality of language and religion is emphasised in principle of contextualism. Thus, Bakhtin's metalinguistics takes into cognizance the pragmatic dimension of language which is a shift from Saussurean langue/parole distinction. Furthermore, COVID-19 pandemic discourse is nuanced due to the presence of multiperspectivality and multidimensionality. In view of the arguments and observations proffered in this study, it is proper to claim that the dialogically and polyphonically constructed discourse is a complex site of meaning convergences and divergences which are embedded in languaging and religions. Language is instrumental in shaping the public conceptualisation of COVID-19 and the language users proffer their worldviews, beliefs and attitudes through languaging. It is apparent that the pandemic is perceived in various ways from both linguistic and religious perspectives. This is so because in Bakhtinian framework, attention is accorded to contextual embeddedness of language. Furthermore, the dialogic and polyphonic understanding of COVID-19 pandemic suggests that reality is complex and multiple.

Conclusion

The application of dialogic and polyphonic concepts has brought useful insights in linguistic and religious re-reading and reconceptualisation of COVID-19 discourse. The interface of linguistics and religious studies has demonstrated the importance of multidisciplinary approach in research in order to discover new sites of meaning-making. In view of the above reflections it is apparent that COVID-19 pandemic discourse is a terrain of different consciousnesses. It has been observed from the above submissions that dialogic and polyphonic concepts challenge and refute traditional claims about the monopoly to mean in discourse. Most essentially, reality cannot be limited to a single consciousness but is rather generated from a polyvocal or multiperspectival discourse by all social participants, religions because truth provisionally emerges from a point of touching of diverse consciousnesses. It has also been observed that COVID-19 pandemic discourse is constructed mainly through a militarised lingo, sea metaphors which heighten the gravity of the pandemic. Apparently, dialogism and polyphony unsettle traditional monologic interpretive practices in linguistics and religious studies because these Bakhtinian notions privilege the idea that semantic dissonance is ever present in human discourse since there are always conflicting views which call for re-reading and re-interpretation. Thus, it is relevant and appropriate to submit that linguistic and religious framing of COVID-19 provides numerous semantic entry points and diverse perspectives that are open to further scrutiny and revision in an ongoing interpretive process of COVID-19 pandemic.

References

Adogame, A., E. Chitando, and B. Bateye eds. 2015. *African Traditions in the Study of Religion, Diaspora and Gendered Societies*. Essays in Honour of Jacob Kehinde Alupona, Farnham-Burlington: Ashgate Publishing.

Agamben, G. 1998. *Homo Sacer: Sovereignty Power and Bare Life*. Translated by D. Heller-Rozzen. Stanford: Stanford University Press.

Aljazeera News. 2020. Outrage as Trump Calls Coronavirus 'Chinese Virus'. March 17. https://www.aljazeera.com/news/2020/3/17/outrage-as-trump-calls-coronavirus-chinese-virus.

Alvarez, R. 2020. An Alternative Approach to COVID-19: The Potential Language of SARS-COV-2. *International Journal Scientific and Engineering Research* 11 (4): 179–190.

Bakhtin, M.M. 1981. *The Dialogic Imagination*. Austin: University of Texas Press.

Bakhtin, M. M. 1984. *Problems of Dostoevsky's Poetics*. Translated by C. Emerson. Manchester: Manchester University Press.

Bates, B.R. 2020. The (In) Appropriateness of the WAR Metaphor in Response to SARS-CoV-2: A Rapid Analysis of Donald J. Trump's Rhetoric. *Frontier in Communication* 5 (50): 1–12. https://doi.org/10.3389/fcomm.2020.00050.

BBC News. 2020. Coronavirus: Ten Passengers on Cruise Ship Test Positive for Virus (Online). *BBC News*. Accessed March 3, 2022. https://www.bbc.co.uk/news/world-asia51381594?ns_source=twitter&ns_mchannel=social&ns_campaign=bbcnews&ocid=socialflowtwitter.

Chugh, A. and Sharma, A. 2012. Unfolding the Linguistic Features of Newspaper Advertisements in India, HOW (19): 157–168.

Crespo-Fernandez, E. 2013. Words as Weapons for Mass Persuasion: Dysphemism in Churchill's Wartime Speeches. *Text & Talk* 33 (3): 311–330.

Damir, H. 2019. Brief History of Pandemics (Pandemics throughout History), pp. 7–35. https://doi.org/10.1007/978-3-030-15346-5_2.

Flusberg, S.J., T. Matlock, and P.H. Thibodeau. 2018. War Metaphors in Public Discourse. *Metaphor and Symbol* 33 (1): 1–18.

Gibbs, R.W., Jr. 2017. *Metaphor Wars: Conceptual Metaphors in Human Life*. Cambridge: Cambridge University Press.

Isiko, A.P. 2019a. State Regulation of Religion in Uganda: Fears and Dilemmas of Born-Again Churches. *Journal of African Studies and Development* 11 (6): 99–117.

———. 2019b. The Nexus between Traditional Healing and Societal Organisation: Reflections on Busoga Society Socio-Cultural, Economic and Political Organisation. *Journal of Arts and Humanities* 8 (8): 71–88.

———. 2020. Religious Construction of disease: An Exploration Appraisal of Religious Response to the COVID-19 Pandemic in Uganda. *Journal of African Studies and Development* 12 (3): 77–96.

Koire, H. 2020. Coronavirus-an Islamic Perspective. *New Vision*. Accessed November 20, 2020. www.newvision.co.ug.

Lakoff, G. 2008. *Women, Fire and Dangerous Things*. Chicago: University of Chicago Press.

Lakoff, G., and M. Johnson. 1980. *Metaphors We Live By*. Chicago: University of Chicago Press.

Marcus, T. 2020. Coronavirus. US-China Battle Behind the Scenes [Blog Post]. https://www.bbc.com/news/world-52008453.

Mavengano, E. 2020. *A Comparative Stylistic Analysis of Selected Zimbabwean and South African Fictional Narratives (2000–2015)* Unpublished Ph.D. Thesis submitted to the North West University, Mafikeng.

Mavengano, E., Marevesa, T., and Dube, Z. 2020. A Bakhtinian Re-reading of the Resurrection Discourses. *Pharos Journal of Theology*, 101: 1–9. ISSN 2414-3324, http://www.pharosjot.com.

Moche, T. 2021. COVID-19 in Africa: Entire Zimbabwe Declared Coronavirus Hotspot. Sabcnews.com. www.sacoronavirus.co.za.

Molnar, A. 2020. Securitization of the COVID-19 Pandemic by Metaphoric Discourse During the State of Emergency in Hungary. *International Journal of Sociology and Social Policy* 40 (900): 1167–1182.

Mutahi, B. 2020. Tanzanian President John Magufuli: The Man Who Declared Victory Over Coronavirus. *BBC News*, Nairobi, 2 November, pp. 1–9.

Niringiye, D.Z. 2020. Faith in the Face of COVID-19 Pandemic. (Facebook Status Update). https://www.facebook.com/7844[illegible]111188/post/10158682919611189/.

Olimat, S.N. 2020. Words as Powerful Weapons: Dysphemism in Trump's COVID-19 Speeches. *The Southeast Asian Journal of English Language Studies* 26 (3): 17–29.

Page, C. 2020. Politicising Coronavirus Is Hazardous to Our National Health. [Blog post] https://www.telegraphherald.com/ap/commentary/article-58ffbb41-ob5d-5ac2-bfcl-bc590ad5a699.html.

Parsitau, D. 2020. Religion in the Age of Coronavirus. The Elephant.info. Accessed November 13, 2020.

Peters, M.A. 2020. The Plague: Human Resilience and the Collective Response to Catastrophe. *Educational Philosophy and Theory.* https://doi.org/10.1080/00131857.2020.1745921.

Rafi, M.S. 2020. Language of COVID-19: Discourse of fear and Sinophobia, Social Sciences and Humanities Open. Accessed January 30, 2021. http://www.papers.ssrn.com/so13/papers.cfm.abstract.

Sean, M. 2020. End of the World: Jesus Warned of Deadly Pandemic as a Sign of Apocalypse-Claim. https://www.express.co.uk/news/weird/1312791/end-of-the-world-coronavirus-pandemic-Jesus-prophecy-apocalypse-covid-19.

Shanapinda, S. 2020. No, 5G Radiation Doesn't Cause or Spread the Coronavirus. Saying It Does Is Destructive. *La Trobe University*, April 7.

Sky News. 2020a. Coronavirus More Deadly than SARS as Global Death Toll Reaches 910. [Online] *Sky News*. Accessed August 19, 2020. https://news.sky.com/story/coronavirus-wuhanvirus-death-toll-overtakes-sars-11928259.

———. 2020b. PM's Coronavirus 'Battle Plan' May Force Retired Doctors Back to Work. [Online] *Sky News*. Accessed July 28, 2020. https://news.sky.com/story/boris-johnsonannounces-coronavirus-battleplan-as-three-more-cases-confirmed-11946362.

Smith, D. 2020. Trump Talks Himself Up as 'Wartime President' to Lead America through a Crisis. *The Guardian*, March 22. https://www.theguardian.com/us-news/2020/mar/22/trump-coronavirus-election-november-2020.

Stearns, J. 2009. New Directions in the Study of Religious Responses to the Black Death. *History Compass* 7(5): 363–375. Accessed November 12, 2020. https://doi.org/10.1111/j.1478-054.2009.00634.x.

Su, Z. et al. 2020. Time to Stop the Use of 'Wuhan virus,' China Virus or Chinese Virus' Across the Scientific Community. *BMJ Global Health* 5 (9): 1–2: e003746. https://doi.org/10.1136/bmjgh-2020-003746.

The New York Times. 2020. China Spins Tale that the U.S. Army Started the Coronavirus Epidemic. *The New York Times*, March 13. https://www.nytimes.com/2020/03/13/world/asia/coronavirustheory.html.

WHO. 2021. What Is Risk Communication? January 15, 2020. Accessed January 20, 2021. https://www.who.int/news-room/q-a-detail/risk-communication-frequently-asked-questions.

Worldometers. 2020. Corona Virus Live Update. *Worldometers*. Accessed November 23, 2020. http://www.worldometer.info/coronavirus.

Part III

Representing COVID-19

15

Cartooning COVID-19 on Facebook

James Yékú

Introduction

In April 2021, fans and followers of the Nigerian political cartoonist Etim Bassey Asukwo (pen name Mike Asukwo) began sharing content about the 'arrest' of the artist who had allegedly violated an order by the Nigerian military restricting movement because of the pandemic.[1] Although the Army authorities eventually discredited the story and described it as fake news, the oppressive nature of state power in Nigeria and the fact of the visual resistance of state power in his cartoons left many legitimately concerned about Asukwo's safety. When the cartoonist later posted on his Facebook page and Twitter handle that he had been

[1] Kingsley Omonobi. 2020. Nigerian Army did not arrest me over COVID-19 lockdown—Asuquo. *The Vanguard*. Accessed February 8, 2021. https://www.vanguardngr.com/2020/05/nigerian-army-did-not-arrest-me-over-covid-19-lockdown-%E2%80%95-asuquo/.

J. Yékú (✉)
University of Kansas, Lawrence, KS, USA
e-mail: jyeku@ku.edu

F. Egbokhare, A. Afolayan (eds.), *Global Health, Humanity and the COVID-19 Pandemic*, https://doi.org/10.1007/978-3-031-17429-2_15

merely 'invited' based on his knowledge of an ongoing investigation, state actors were expectedly forceful in their denunciation of what they read as online misinformation. This episode demonstrates how social media, despite its extrative capture of profits from users, has emerged as an arena of tensions and contestations between state and society in Nigeria in the last decade. As the history of African cartooning has constantly thematized censorship in various ways, social media as the major outlet for Asukwo's most viral cartoons manifests as an invaluable space in which the artist balances "the barbed playfulness" of his art with the state power he constantly critiques (Limb and Olaniyan 2018: xix). But the Nigerian state has also asserted its presence and narrative authority on the social web through acts of interdiction as was evident with the Twitter ban of 2021 or by planting trolls through avenues such as the notorious Buhari Media Center to disrupt the activist expressions and activist speech of Nigerian netizens who produce contents that challenge or ridicule state power. This is besides several attempts to prohibit the voices of netizens through legislative modalities that proscribe or regulate social media platforms themselves. The most recent confrontation between the Nigerian state and citizens who encounter it both as a violent regime of coercion and a morbid "state of pathology" (Ebenezer Obadare and Wale Adebanwi 2010: 3) is the #EndSARS protest which foregrounded the power of young people to speak back against a culture of police brutality and the larger structural conditions that generate it. The #EndSARS movement also metaphorizes for protesters the viciousness of state domination and thuggery and, more broadly, Nigeria's culture of prebendal thievery that guarantees a gerontocratic hold on political and economic power. Although Asukwo produced several cartoons to document the #EndSARS protest, my analysis here attends to the pandemic-themed cartoons he posted on Facebook in the months leading to the protest.

Asukwo may not be the most popular social media influencer online,[2] but his cartoons, which make legible some of the most subversive representations of postcolonial domination in present-day Nigeria, are routinely encountered by anyone who pay close attention to the production and circulation of visual culture in the Nigerian digital ecosystem. Asukwo is one of the most viral cultural producers in Nigeria as his cartoons attempt to make sense of the interactions between state power and citizens. As Asukwo engages his artistic sensibilities in depicting the harsh realities of contemporary life in Nigeria, the strokes of his cartoons and other visual elements become "counter-narratives against dominant governmental narratives on sociopolitical issues," according to Ganiyu Jimoh (2019: 32), a leading scholar on Asukwo's works. Unlike Jimoh, and building on his several writings on the artist, my reading and approach to Asukwo's cartoons are specifically in the framework of social media as I contend that the archive of Asukwo's works in the last decade exhibits some of the most visually arresting documentation of the sociocultural and political history of Nigeria, including the political elite's relationship with the 2020 pandemic. Asukwo's skillful use of colors and graphic strokes demonstrate an awareness of network culture and what I describe in *Cultural Netizenship* as social media's "ontological visuality" (Yeku, 2022, 7), as the design and affordances of Facebook enable the seamless circulation of his craft. After years of drawing cartoons in black and white, his cartoons are draped in bold and beautiful colors that ironically and graphically bear visual witness to the precarious colorlessness of the postcolonial condition in Nigeria. In Asukwo's cartoons, the reality of a Nigerian postcolonial reality that lacks colors is well articulated! The eye-catching and almost born-digital works he produces in recent years are both evocative of the postcolonial drabness of Nigeria and fitting to a social media space in which his cartoons become circulated by friends, fans, and followers who easily encode the suggestions and underlying

[2] The figure of the social media influencer in Nigeria is one that deserves scrutiny, as more people perform prestige and symbolic power through the accumulation of followership and fame in the attention economy of social media. While there are *popular* social media cultural producers and/or netizens who are not influencers, to be an influencer means the ability to create cultural content that generate fame and is contingent on their capacity to 'brand' their digital lives and monetize their cult following.

assumptions of the images (Yeku, 2022). The notion of virality is especially important for this chapter. Significant for me is how the cartoons of Asukwo spread virally on social media in response to the state's engagement with the global outbreak of a virus. I will examine the conditions under which cultural netizens like Asukwo and his fans/friends make sense of the state's response to a viral outbreak, with the ultimate aim of showing how social media stages and documents the pandemic perspectives of members of the digital class in Nigeria. The chapter concludes on the note that social media is a digital public sphere ambivalently prone to uses and abuses.

Asukwo on the Social Media Stage

Social media technologies, as Jean Burgess et al. explain, include "those digital platforms, services, and apps built around the convergence of content sharing, public communication, and interpersonal connection" (2018: 1). My conception of social media as a digital arena of convergence and sociality enabling participatory politics can be read as disparate and performative voices appearing in a shared and networked space to discuss issues of public concern. Despite this democratizing potential of the participatory web, what Jodi Dean (2009) calls "communicative capitalism" continues to undergird social media as extractive and capitalist spaces that capture monetary value from the data of users, aside from its potential for the spread of hate speech and misinformation.

Despite its challenges, artistic practices and cultural productions on the platforms are some of the means of expressing voice and may reveal the ways in which those unconnected to state power tell their own stories and decenter the hegemony of previous cultural forms. As hinted earlier, the power of the social web consists in how it alerts citizens to the circulation of state-sponsored narratives in various media, print or online, and how it urges them to intervene as legitimate authorial actors. While the consumers of the traditional media are productive subjects able to encode media signs, they can now *actively* create and disseminate multiple media truths and identities, entering the realm of authorship as producers of meanings. Within the context of Nigerian political communication, social media enables a preponderance of individual narratives that challenge the hegemony of a highly regulated media environment. Social media users in Nigeria who protested online against the government's explanation of an austere crude oil policy in 2012, or the state's denial of the famous extrajudicial killings at Lekki during the #EndSARS protests were able, for instance, to produce their own counter narratives and alternative meanings both about the 'true' state of the energy sector, and in the case of Lekki, what happened at the toll gate. They were invested in this process not only through text-based status updates and tweets through which they organized rallies and protests, but also through visual self-representations such as cartoons and viral memes and videos, texts of cultural netizenship that offer oppositional meanings to the dominant narratives of government.

Writing in the context of postcoup Chile, Nelly Richard asserts that the production of contrary perspectives sometimes generates a radical questioning and overturn of official systems of thoughts and power. To have formulated meanings, Richard writes, "that were merely contrary to the dominant point of view, without taking aim at the larger order of its signifying structures, would have meant remaining inscribed within the same linear duality of a Manichaean construction of meaning" (2004: 4). Such view merely inverts the symmetry of what was represented, without questioning the topology of the representation. The personal tweets and Facebook posts of netizens, whether as visual popular arts or written forms, are not mere expressions of counter perspectives to the grand narratives of the Nigeria state. They likewise function to question and resist asymmetrical power relations and their narratives of dispossession. Cultural forms such as online cartoons and humorous images together with the political commentaries that emerge from them challenge what Richard refers to as "the fraudulent language spoken by the official power" (2004: 5). In Nigeria, official power perpetually circulates fraudulent speech, even creating on social media, as I have shown, structures among unsuspecting young people to co-opt dissenting voices and disseminate untruth. Produced and circulated online as dissident signifiers invested in the displacement of official knowledge systems, visual text such as the cartoons I examine here have the potential to rupture and counter the semantic force of such fraudulent narratives. I intend these illustrations to prove that signifying practices are always already modes of interrogating authority and resisting both state strictures and attempted monopolies on meaning. A semiotic component in my analyses is thus grounded in the way Nigerian social media enact and present selves through the staging of visual cultural forms like comics that signal the possibilities of engaging with state power in various productive ways. Social media expressions of resistance, it needs to be said, need not topple government but importantly it can emerge as a practice of radical speech against the impositions of power. This view is consistent with Francis Nyamnjoh's belief that we be critical of any suggestion that popular culture forms like cartooning have little impact simply because they have "failed to bring about a revolution or revolt against the status quo." (2009: 97). Nigerian digital subjects deploy social media like Twitter, Facebook, and even WhatsApp to re-encounter the state as an entity to be decentered and queried discursively. Although it may appear that the corrupt elite in Nigeria pays little attention to the potentially disruptive spaces enabled by the social web, a closer appreciation of the overarching picture reveals, as in the case of the Buhari Media Centre I mentioned above, an unsettled and suspicious governmental presence online bent on co-opting and disrupting dissident voices. Social media as digital networks of social relations illustrate new postmodernist performative dimensions of the self, expressed through visual culture. Whereas scholars, such as Manuel Castells and many other new media scholars, frame the discourse in terms of the way social media are used by netizens to *do and organize politics*, I signal attention to the social media users who *do things with images* as cultural texts of resistance to power.

To borrow Chinua Achebe's idea of the *Ilo*—a gathering place for play and deliberations—in his anti-colonialist novel, *Things Fall Apart*, social media exhibits the forms of a digital Ilo that envisions the possibility of a cultural and collective space which stages privatized narratives and individual subjectivity as a mode of public self-presentations and textual performances. With the social web, social activism and the questioning of traditional structures of power and nation-states take on a global intensification, manifest in the online reconstitution of the politics of dissent and resistance around the world. Platforms such as social media became the organizing mechanisms for coordinating and mobilizing protests activities of such notable social movements as the Arab Spring and Occupy Wall Street. In Nigeria, Occupy Nigeria was a local version of similar transnational movements around the world. From the #BringBackOurGirls Twitter campaign of 2014 to the recent 2016 #SacktheSenate or #OccupyNASS movements therefore, what is evident in the Nigerian political sphere is a new sociopolitical order constituted by a virtual public that counters the hegemonic designs of the state by mounting resistance through popular satirical texts and humorous images on social media. I have argued elsewhere that these hashtags are archives of Nigerian contemporary history, when considered in the sense that they serve, alongside popular images, as documentary monikers of citizens' digital engagement with power structures (Yeku 2018). Social media might have been effective within the context of the Arab Spring and indeed Occupy Nigeria, yet the inflections and particularities of its workings in different regions of the world need to be highlighted. As Paolo Gerbaudo frames the argument, the problem of a techno-optimistic narrative on social media becomes "a 'fetish' of collective action" (Gerbaudo 2012: 8) to the extent that social media becomes endowed with mystical qualities that only obscure the actors using the media. Within the Nigerian context, social media exerts a palpable influence on society, as much as society also shapes the kind of contents and genres that are evident on the platforms. Commenting on this point, Daniel Miller explicates the essential nature of social media in relation to its working in society by noting that it is not "that the world has made social media completely different, or that social media has changed the world. It's obviously always going to be dialectical. But in this case, it provides a new space for genres to occupy, which are not themselves particularly changed" (Borgerson and Miller 2016: 523). In other words, and this is particularly true of the social media culture in Nigeria, there exists a reciprocal influence between society and social media, with social issues supplying content for creative content producers whose work often serves to critique the country's political class.

Social media is central to the increasing role of Asukwo's political cartoons in expressing and conditioning a civic agency among Nigerians. His cartoons demonstrate how everyday media practices such as the decoding and duplication of popular culture texts online can challenge hegemonic structures. In Onookome Okome's (2007) reading of the popular audience of Nollywood, he underscores how citizens are forced to convert their vulnerability to state power into creative and artistic expression. Okome notes that "powerlessness in the roughly organized political and cultural spheres is converted into a peculiar narrative power in the realm of this existential disorder. What comes out of the various narrative acts of this ironic chorus is what we may refer to as "popular narratives" (2007: 9). Social media platforms likewise offer the opportunity for the production and distribution of popular narratives, mostly visual, through which netizens perform all kinds of subjectivities. Asukwo mainly distributes his works, as the editorial cartoonist of *Business Day*, on both Facebook and Twitter. His cartoons depict the abject conditions of urban life in Nigeria and are some of the most profound satires of the agonies and anguishes of postcolonial Nigeria. These visual texts are shared by the cartoonist and his many fans to comment on everyday life in Nigeria and push back against the hegemonic culture.

Covid Cartoons and Critical Infrastructure

Asukwo's works demonstrate how the semiotics of cartoons and comics on Facebook can supply insights into the infrastructural deficiencies of the state in the Covid era. Asukwo is among the most prolific political cartoonist in contemporary Nigeria, and his many viral images inform critical discussions online. His cartoons are disseminated both in digital and print avenues across Nigeria. Digital media have become an important location for the distribution of his works, as social media brings Asukwo and his audience into a shared space in which they converge to read, distribute and extend the political meanings and rhetoric of his cartoons. As the coronavirus forced a global lockdown, social media became the platform for another kind of viral circulation, that of creative productions such as Asukwo's cartoons. To illustrate, in Fig. 15.1, Asukwo offers a work that records the fatal consequences of Nigeria's iteration of the global pandemic lockdown on not only citizens but also on the state actors themselves. Entitled on Facebook as "The Death Trap," the cartoon signals the infrastructural predicaments both propelled by the

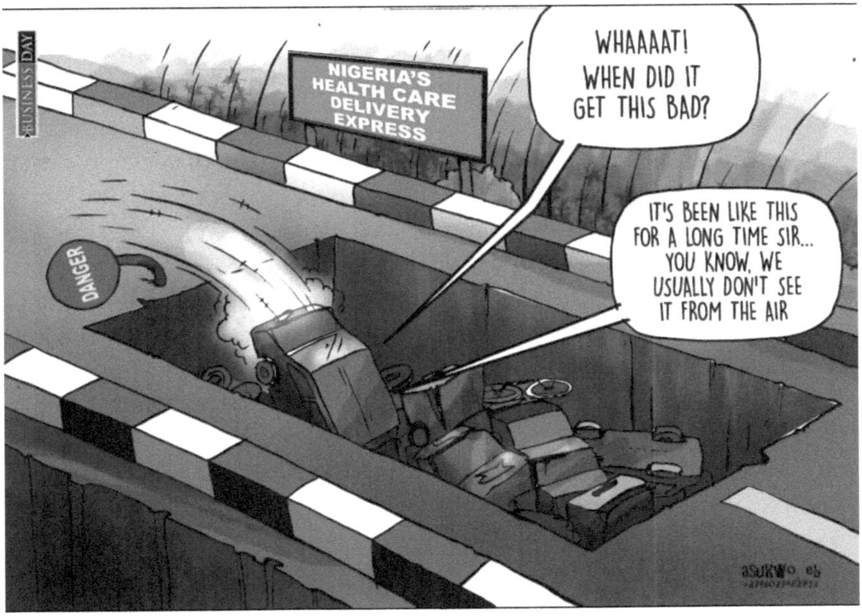
BUSINESS DAY
NIGERIA'S HEALTH CARE DELIVERY EXPRESS
WHAAAAT! WHEN DID IT GET THIS BAD?
IT'S BEEN LIKE THIS FOR A LONG TIME SIR... YOU KNOW, WE USUALLY DON'T SEE IT FROM THE AIR
DANGER
asukwo

Fig. 15.1 The Death Trap (*Facebook*)

political class in Nigeria and imposed on the public. Travelling on a pot-hole-ridden road, "Nigeria's Healthcare Delivery Express," a state official who travels mostly in airlines, and their surrogate have ended up in a ditch that swallows their vehicle. The official appears to be ignorantly alarmed that the express has become "this bad" but is quickly reminded by his accompanying passenger that their elite position as members of the ruling class who hardly ply the country's highway has blinded them to the true conditions of the road.

Asukwo's imagery is, of course, strategically ambiguous as it presents the "express" both in the context of Nigeria's healthcare crises and the country motorways and the dangers they pose to everyday people. While "It's been like this for a long time" is the voice of the non-elite class explaining a quotidian tragedy to a Nigerian state official, the statement connects more significantly to the anxiety across the country that the pandemic would sweep across a country whose porous social infrastructure and amenities are essentially a death trap. The discursive implications of this cartoon are even more dire when read in the contexts of the work of the sociologists Ulrika Trovalla and Eric Trovalla. In their work on the Nigerian city of Jos, the Trovallas note the ways in which the presence, absence, flows and non-flows of infrastructure shape urban character, becoming, and identity. Understood in this sense, infrastructure takes on important meanings in the everyday lives of people and cities. Whether it calls attention to itself or withdraws from awareness, "infrastructure," they write, "can assume a wide register of visibility" and connotations (2015: 44). This is essentially what Asukwo's cartoons unpack as they show the state of infrastructure in Nigeria as possessing divinatory possibilities in the manner outlined by Trovalla and Trovalla: "the wires, pipes, roads and signals, the water, electricity, transportation and phone networks that connect people to and disconnect people from society make up powerful instruments for analysing the nation" (2015: 54). Asukwo's cartoon is, therefore, a visual sign that encodes other signs, as it symbolizes an infrastructural code which itself signals other meanings.

The point here is to read infrastructure as a mode of interpretation that, at an institutional and material level, has social and political meanings. Understood this way, the representation of the absence and ruination of material infrastructure in the cartoons of Asukwo is made to reveal the workings of corrupt state power in all its articulations. In other words, infrastructure emerges in Asukwo's Covid cartoons as a trope that can be read critically to illuminate how material systems become implicated in the consolidation of hegemonic corruption in Nigeria. To put this in the words of a commenter[3] on Asukwo's Facebook page, the cartoon's narrative is "2 in 1. Bad Healthcare and Bad Road. If they are not forced to utilise the two now, they will never know how bad it is." We see that Facebook comments are pertinent as sources of cultural knowledge because Asukwo's network of friends and followers who share and comment on the cartoon are central to the constitution of his visual texts and their meanings on the social web. While it can be assumed, for instance, that the cartoon is suggesting that border and land closure has

[3] From the thread of the post on Asukwo's Facebook Timeline: https://www.facebook.com/asukwo/posts/10223010812879341.

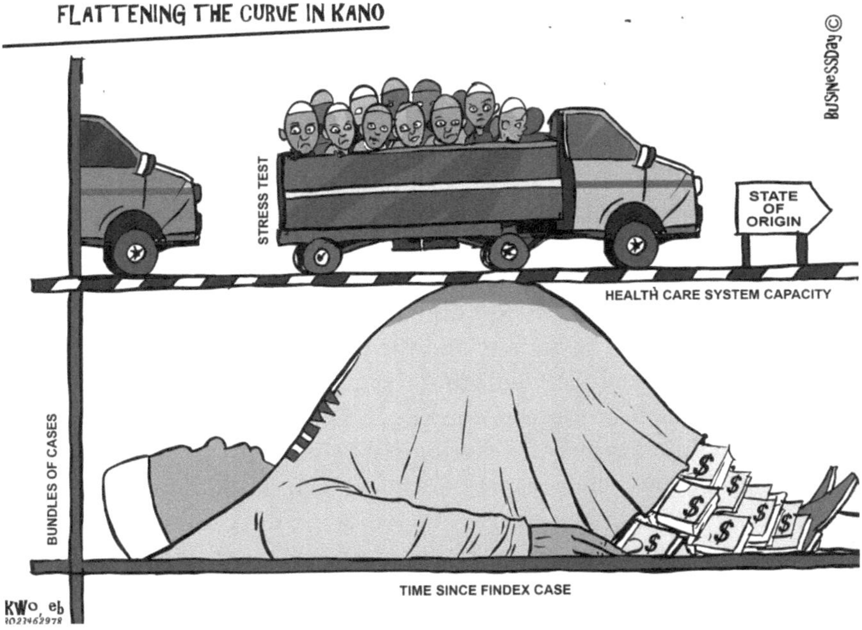

Fig. 15.2 Flattening The Curve in Kano (*Facebook*)

forced politicians to be on the ground to see things as they really are, another commenter reads the characters as being underground—a word that restates the cartoon's title and thesis.

A week after this cartoon was posted, Asukwo followed with a similar narrative that basically satirizes the politicization of the pandemic in Nigeria, again linking the pervasive theme of infrastructural deficiencies in his Covid cartoons (Fig. 15.1) with the state of corruption in Nigeria. "Flattening the curve in Kano" provocatively employs what became the dominant idiom of health officials around the world, as countries proposed different strategies like social distancing in addition to the initial lockdown to stop the exponential rise in the number of the infection globally. Figure 15.2 delivers a powerful message about ignorance—a theme in the first example—although in this instance, the lack of knowledge is on the part of the young residents in the Almajiri Islamic education system in Northern Nigeria. Without food, masking, and other protective measures, the children's precarious situation leaves them exposed to the pandemic as they roam about as beggars, or as people that are sent back to their state of origin because of the increase in COVID-19 cases, as this cartoon depicts.

What is more, the cartoon indicts the governor of Kano state as a state agent of corruption whose curvy and potbellied stomach embodies a culture of political corruption which hinders economic development and affect the health care capacity of the state. Asukwo's artful deployment of the mathematical elements of curves, straight lines, and graphs are ingenious representations that foreground the intersections he makes between the thievery of the political elite and the precarious conditions in which people like the Almajiri students find themselves. The curve in the image touches the straight line, intersecting in an unparalleled assertion that the governor's public history of diverting state funds, the dollars hidden in plain sight in his belly are the generating canvas of Kano's problem. Asukwo invites the reader to read the flattening of corruption's curve in Nigeria as a precondition for an effective campaign against the pandemic, inderstood here in in both its literal and figurative senses.

These cartoons are significant commentaries on the state of Nigeria in the age of Covid-19, and they graphically show the vulnerability of the masses to state officials whose endemic corruption are the conditions under which abjection is produced. As they spread online, Asukwo's cartoons disseminate rhetorical vitality, serving as consciousness-raising visual texts that render graphic material realities of decadent postcolonial leadership. This perspective is informed by the ubiquity of visual culture in Nigerian social media and suggests that we take social media more seriously as a new media space in which cultural productions become some of the most evocative and vital modes of performative engagements with power. The vitality of images is what W.J.T. Mitchell's alludes to in his suggestion that an image "is not merely a transparent medium for communicating a message but something like an animated, living thing" which has "feelings, intentions, desires, and agency" (2010: 27). There is implicit in this thinking the point that agential power in relation to visual culture extends to images, an idea that is the subject of Laurie Gries's *Still Life with Rhetoric*. In her new materialist analyses of how visual forms can be nonhuman entities that have rhetorical agency connected to the

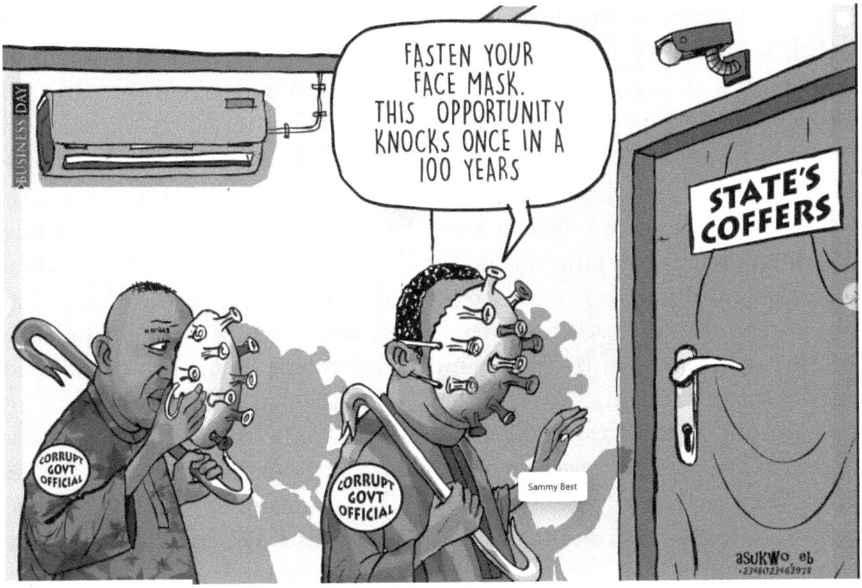

Fig. 15.3 Masks of The Beast (*Facebook*)

interior and external relations of meaning, Gries explores "how things (ideas, texts, images, people, capital, artifacts, etc.) move within and across and influence public culture" (2015: xix). One only needs to examine the viral images that make the Nigerian public sphere a vital location that accommodates anyone with access to an Internet-based mobile phone to see how images come alive and possibly impact resistance to the prevailing ruling norms and ideas. While resistance does not have to completely overturn power, it sometimes emerges in cartoons as a rhetorical challenge to a power structures.

Hence, resistance in this context need not topple government but importantly it can emerge as a practice of radical speech against the impositions of power. Figure 15.3 is one of many of Asukwo's viral images whose vitality potentially provokes an awareness of corruption.

In this cartoon, there seems to be the suggestion that the pandemic has been a metaphoric portal into Nigeria's prebendal politics, as it reveals not only infrastructural gaps and its morbid connection to corruption, but also, crucially, absurdities of the state officials who infect the body politic with misery and pain—much like the virus—through a patrimonial culture that claims economic benefits from state power. Richard Joseph (1987) calls this system prebendalism, writing that a prebendal system will be seen not only as one in which "the offices of state are allocated and then exploited as benefices by the office-holders, but also as one where such a practice is legitimated by a set of political norms according to which the appropriation of such offices is not just an act of individual greed or ambition" but concurrently the satisfaction of the short-term objectives of a subset of the general population (1987: 67). This practice is aptly demonstrated by the corrupt government officials in this text as they see the pandemic, as one that "knocks once in 100 years," as an opportunity to steal from the state coffers. While the irony here is that access to the state coffers is a regular reality for Nigerian state officials, the centennial reference probably accentuates the enormity of this particular thievery. It is also pertinent that Asukwo on his Facebook pages calls the face covering to be fastened "the mask of the beasts," which, as it plays into some of the various conspiracy theories about the pandemic among some religiously conservative Nigerians, basically frames the Nigerian political class as a horrid cohort of monsters who loot the country under the guise of fighting the coronavirus. They are the beastly virus that steals the health of the nation and the mask they wear gestures as nothing but a dance of corruption in the theater of power. The notion of the beast also evokes Fela Kuti's "Beasts of No Nation" in which the Afrobeat pioneer references apartheid South Africa's Pieter Willem Botha's remarks to anti-apartheid. Based on Fela's lyrics, "This uprising will bring out the beast in us,"[4] Asuwko appears to suggest through his cartoon that the Covid era brings out the beast in the ruling elite who mobilize the pandemic for political gains.

Again, an important element of this cartoon is how social media shapes its meanings through the multiplicity of users who share the post and add new narrative layers and connotations. One of the comments on Facebook suggests that the coronavirus in Nigeria "is different from what obtains in different parts of the world" since "the one we have is

[4] Fela Kuti, "Beasts of No Nation" (1989).

COVID-419."[5] This is a comment several others make in the discussion thread, suggesting that many people accepted the fact of government as an institution of scam that speaks to what Daniel Smith (2007) refers to as a culture of corruption in Nigeria.[6] As Smith writes, "Nigerians see themselves as complicit in corruption, and indeed it is this awareness of collective responsibility for corruption that fuels hopes for change, even as it paradoxically perpetuates cynicism and a sense of intractability" (2007: 6). As the #EndSARS movement and the Covid-relief palliatives looting that resulted from it later showed,[7] while the state is apparently a rogue regime of scam and corruption, the representation of state looting and thievery in cultural productions and spaces like social media expose close networks and solidarity between state and society. While Asukwo does not capture this idea in this cartoon, many symbolic and artistic practices online do, including several social media skits and comedic productions. What is, however, evident in most of the Covid cartoons is how they are implicated in the narratives of corruption—which "in its many valences in Nigeria, is a potent stimulus for cultural production, both as a means for corruption's pursuit and a method to combat its consequences." (Smith 2007: 6) As narratives about corruption dominate political and symbolic discourse in Nigeria, cartoons and other visual texts on social media become important as disseminating outlets.

To return to the Facebook audience, the various online comments that proliferate on social media threads as "narratives of complaint" generated by corruption become primary vehicles through which Asukwo, Etim Bassey fans and readers, like other Nigerians, visually imagine and create the relationship between state and society (ibid.). The importance of audience participation is signaled by the cartoonist in Fig. 15.2 when Asukwo writes on Facebook that "we can flatten the curve." The personal

[5] From a commenter on Asukwo's Facebook Timeline: https://www.facebook.com/photo.php?fbid=10222872928632321&set=a.2058448341395&type=3&theater.

[6] While not meant to be a homogenizing grid for the entirety of Nigerians, Smith's anthropological reading of culture here gestures at a practice that is both for and against the mechanisms of corruption in the country. While every day, non-state actors speak against corruption, they are also implicated in its production and circulation among members of the ruling elite who themselves have links and networks among ordinary people.

[7] Asukwo tackles the narratives of the palliative in this cartoon here: https://www.facebook.com/photo.php?fbid=10223078251805272&set=a.1451300003066&type=3&theater.

pronoun indicates a collective approach to the fight against the pandemic and emphasizes the general public's need to fight corruption. But the "we" is also a mode of address to his readers on social media who are invited to collaboratively engage the text and take it in different interpretive directions. The immediacy of responses and answers in the form of Facebook comments suggest that as Asukwo visually records the pandemic, many in his network become active participants in this documentary gesture to the coronavirus. What this implies is that Asukwo's cartoons provide an opportunity not only for his own challenge to power, but also a public arena in which the ordinary, everyday digital subject can appear in the public to share visual narratives as a form of performative speech against the exertion of power. But is social media really an effective space for oppositional public discourses, given what some read as the noise of its interventions? This is the final point I wish to conclude with.

The Liberty to Appear in Public

Despite social media's entanglements with data violations that serve neoliberal actors, people as rational agents convert the platform into a public sphere, producing political resistance that may be messy but not always noisy. Though constrained by underlying digital structures and protocols, agency on the social web may be conceived as the power to be heard and seen by others and often manifests as directed, meaningful, intentional, and self-reflective social action (Patrick Chabal 2009: 7). It is the individual capacity of everyday citizens to contribute to social processes with these institutional and structural restrictions limited. Social media in Nigeria often serves as a public sphere in which digital subjects and cultural netizens perform a culture of refusal to conservative and normative culture. Because the medium is ontologically visual, this resistance sometimes manifests as spectacles of outrage made visible in the performance of civic agency on the social web. While the potentials for civic engagements are potentially visible, there is also the obvious crude hostility engendered by these images and which often degenerate into banal ethnic exchanges that undermine the images themselves. Outrage is often a product of the realization that so-called democratic institutions do not represent the interests of citizens because the ruling elite have, as in the case of the Nigerian government, become "a self-reproducing cast catering mostly to their interests, and to the preservation of their monopoly over the state" (Manuel Castells 2012: 42). This idea of the state as a space in which elected actors encounter power as a performative site of buffoonery is apparent in several excellent works on postcolonial African states that tease out the problematic outlook of the state in contemporary African politics (Bayart 1993; Mbembe 2012).

My conception of the Nigerian digital public sphere as a realm constituted by visual culture circulated by young people on social media is based on the liberty of appearing in the public as a precondition for truth and justice in a nation. The liberty to appear and be seen or heard, which social media facilitates, is a mode of resisting a normative order that fosters silence and, sometimes, discursive erasure. Thus, the rehabilitation of cultural and political invisibility enabled by social media is itself a form of resistance. This claim can be appreciated more through Hannah Arendt's description of the public realm as an intersubjective and deprivatized space in which speech and visibility are major expressive principles. As Arendt puts it:

> everything that appears in public can be seen and heard by everybody and has the widest possible publicity. For us, appearance—something that is being seen and heard by others as well as by ourselves—constitutes reality. Compared with the reality which comes from being seen and heard, even the greatest forces of intimate life—the passions of the heart, the thoughts of the mind, the delights of the senses—lead an uncertain, shadowy kind of existence unless and until they are transformed, deprivatized and deindividualized, as it were, into a shape to fit them for public appearance...The presence of others who see what we see and hear what we hear assures us of the reality of the world and ourselves. (1989: 50)

It needs to be emphasized that the liberty of appearance often leads to the appearance of liberty, a point that resonates clearly in the above passage by Arendt. Her argument advances the notion of silence as an ineffectual mode of engaging in the public realm; it privileges speech as a productive and essential mode of appearing in public. This view is potentially problematic as silence itself can be an 'expressive' communicative form that can be profoundly political as a form of protest against the animating logic of the political milieu and its underpinning ethos (Ebenezer Obadare 2016: 103). In other words, silence and speech are not oppositional categories, but rather exist in a dialectic in which they enact each other.

Appearance in the public, as Jürgen Habermas reckons, is predicated upon a certain "kind of social intercourse that, far from presupposing the equality of status, disregarded status altogether" (1989: 36). According to Habermas, it is the force of argument and the content of public discourse that is more significant than the social or political status of participants in the public arena. This disregard of status is something the social web affords most netizens, especially minority groups such as women who, through groups like the Feminist Coalition, are now challenging patriarchal culture and politics in Nigeria. The increasingly vocal challenge to all kinds of authority is being facilitated partly by the access to social media platforms where people constitute counterpublics that standing in opposition to dominant culture. Without online gatekeepers, the authorial possibilities social media grants its users exist in a horizontal sense with few hierarchical constraints. Unlike the exclusion of particular sets of people that constitute the discourse of the Habermasian public (for instance, women), the digitally enabled public sphere in Nigerian social media includes anyone with access to the Internet, as citizens now possess the power of speech in the public arena. We see the manifestation of speech not just in the millions of social media posts and comments produced daily online in Nigeria, but specifically in cultural and visual forms like cartoons, humorous videos and memes that serve as the counter-hegemonic texts of cultural netizens.

To return to Arendt, the constitution of the politics in this public realm can be seen, for instance, in the ways social media enables networks and communities of individuals who, "in the presence of others," share reality at a differential, interactive, and multiperspectival level (Arendt 1989: 50). Even if their contributions in this public space are deindividualized, the interventions of social media users are individuated, bearing the persona, images of particular users, because of the ways in which user-generated media serves to articulate the authority and agency of the individual on social media. To critique this Arendtian framework of social

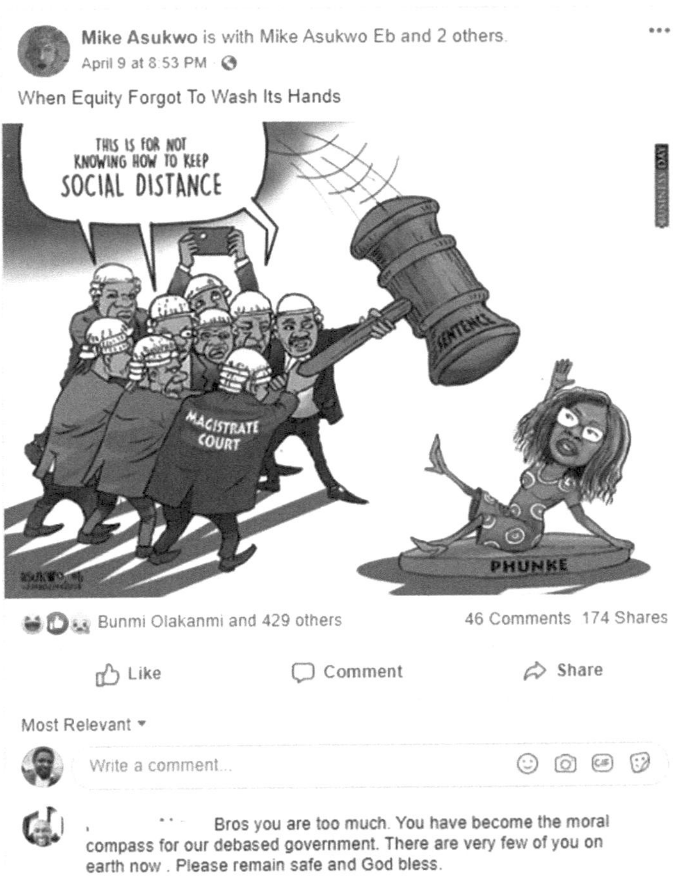
Mike Asukwo is with Mike Asukwo Eb and 2 others.
April 9 at 8:53 PM
When Equity Forgot To Wash Its Hands
THIS IS FOR NOT KNOWING HOW TO KEEP SOCIAL DISTANCE
SENTENCE
MAGISTRATE COURT
PHUNKE
Bunmi Olakanmi and 429 others
46 Comments 174 Shares
Like
Comment
Share
Most Relevant
Write a comment...
Bros you are too much. You have become the moral compass for our debased government. There are very few of you on earth now . Please remain safe and God bless.

Fig. 15.4 When Equity Forgets To Wash Its Hands (Facebook. https://www.facebook.com/photo.php?fbid=10222867151567898&set=a.2058448341395&type=3&theater)

media as a space of appearance, as do Nick Couldry and Jannis Kallinikos in a recent discussion of the sociology of social media's ontology, is to restate a popular skepticism about social media that erases the agency of users. They argue that that there is on social media platforms no appearance-in-itself but only ever appearance that is derivative of prior processes of [economic] calculation that challenge the basis of understanding the social (Couldry and Kallinikos 2018: 234). True, social media has the capacity to depoliticize radical voices and could serve as a performative space of play and plastic self-projection in which the digital labors of users are vulnerable to the neoliberal ideologies and values of its owners. However, to focus only on this perspective harbors a pessimistic approach to social media that occludes the meaningful social connections and political engagements that also take place on the platforms in many developing economies. It is useful to keep the ambivalence around technologies in mind. In my final example in Fig. 15.4, Asukwo is showing the proverbial miscarriage of justice by, again, drawing from the language of the pandemic to lampoon the Nigerian judicial system that is selective in its treatment of 'offenders,' even popular ones such as a Nollywood actress depicted.

A semiotic reading of this example uncovers the double standards women often have to publicly endure in Nigeria's patriarchal politics, but to return to the argument before now, my point is not whether algorithm itself cannot be an agent of subordination in their distribution of cultural meanings and voices; what I argue for, instead, is the possibility that the voice of everyday people also occasionally gets legible in the public disturbance of oppressive power and of tech companies themselves. This capacity to appear and register one's voice is vital in a country where people have limited avenues for democratic conversations and participation. Because of social media, subjects whose representation in a nation's public sphere is limited can now indeed appear in both the public arena and in the consciousness of the state and its actors. The Nigerian netizens who appear in such digital public spheres indeed exercise speech as a "performative power to lay claim to the public" (Butler 2015, 75) in a way that is not always sanctioned by the established cultural and political hierarchy in the country.

Conclusion

Many other cartoons have been specifically produced to capture the colorless realities of the Covid pandemic in Nigeria. The six-part cartoon, "National Immunization Rollout" reveals how Asukwo's works have evolved along with pandemic discourses worldwide while serving as local archives of the Nigerian situation.[8] The six cartoons in the series present Nigerian government officials being vaccinated, not with any of the major Covid vaccines that are still largely unavailable in the country, but with different popular elements of the country's culture of corruption. In another narrative in the series, a citizen's thoughts are on bread, rather than the jab itself, a pointer to the precarious conditions of many Nigerians who seem to be less concerned about vaccination than about the state of critical infrastructure, as well as the persistence of poverty and hunger in the country. In all of these cartoons, Asukwo is rhetorically narrating the Nigerian state in the age of the pandemic, using his works to document the response of the political class which he also excoriates. There is really no need, though, to romanticize the social media stage from which these critiques are mounted since digital technologies are far from perfect themselves. That said, the amplification of old popular culture forms like cartoons and the production of new digital genres and cultural productions on the social web makes digital and social media significant in understanding contemporary Nigeria. The Nigerian state as a beastly and corrupt entity that continues to impose abjection and despair on the masses contends with a digital public space in which politicized and radial voices now vehemently demand accountability of it. In numerous cartoons and other digital genres and performances online, many people with Internet access are producing and circulating narratives that challenge the structures and actors of power. The articulation of social media with new forms of popular culture online offers a rich archive of knowledge that ambivalently captures this tension.

References

Arendt, Hannah. 1989. *The Human Condition*. University of Chicago Press.

Bayart, Jean-François. 1993. *The State in Africa: The Politics of the Belly*. London: Longman.

[8] The first of the six-part series may be found here: https://www.facebook.com/photo/?fbid=10225937229397925&set=pb.1250241460.-2207520000.

Borgerson, Janet, and Daniel Miller. 2016. Scalable Sociality and How the World Changed Social Media. *Consumption Markets & Culture* 19 (6): 520–533.

Burgess, Jean, Alice E. Marwick, and Thomas Poell. 2018. *The Sage Handbook of Social Media*. Sage Publications.

Butler, Judith. 2015. *Notes Toward a Performative Theory of Assembly*. Harvard UP.

Castells, Manuel. 2012. *Networks of Outrage and Hope: Social Movements in the Internet Age*. Polity Press.

Chabal, Patrick. 2009. *Africa: The Politics of Suffering and Smiling*. Zed Books.

Couldry, Nick, and Jannis Kallinikos. 2018. *Ontology*. In *The SAGE Handbook of Social Media*, ed. Jean Burgess et al. Sage Publications.

Dean, Jodi. 2009. *Democracy and Other Neoliberal Fantasies: Communicative Capitalism & Left Politics*. Durham: Duke University Press.

Gerbaudo, Paolo. 2012. *Tweets and the Streets: Social Media and Contemporary Activism*. London: Pluto Press.

Gries, Laurie E. 2015. *Still Life with Rhetoric: A New Materialist Approach for Visual Rhetorics*. Utah State UP.

Habermas, Jürgen. 1989. *The Structural Transformation of the Public Sphere: An Inquiry into a Category of Bourgeois Society*. MIT Press.

Jimoh, Ganiyu Akinloye. 2019. Masked in Metaphors: Counter Narratives in the Works Nigerian Cartoonist Mike Asukwo. *African Arts* 52: 32–39.

Joseph, Richard. 1987. *Democracy and Prebendal Politics in Nigeria: The Rise and Fall of the Second Republic*. Cambridge: Cambridge University Press.

Limb, Peter, and Tejumola Olaniyan. 2018. *Taking African Cartoons Seriously: Politics, Satire, and Culture*. Michigan State UP.

Mbembe Joseph Achille. 2012. *On the Postcolony*. Berkeley: University of California Press.

Mitchell, William J.T. 2010. *What Do Pictures Want?: The Lives and Loves of Images*. University of Chicago Press.

Nyamnjoh, Francis. 2009. Press cartoons and politics: The case of Cameroon. In *Cartooning in Africa*, ed. J.A. Lent. New Jersey: Hampton Press.

Obadare, Ebenezer. 2016. *Humor, Silence, and Civil Society in Nigeria*. Rochester: University of Rochester Press.

Obadare, Ebenezer, and Wale Adebanwi. 2010. *Encountering the Nigerian State*. Palgrave Macmillan.

Okome, Onookome. 2007. Nollywood: Spectatorship, Audience and the Sites of Consumption. *Postcolonial Text* 3 (2): 1–21.

Richard, Nelly. 2004. *The Insubordination of Signs: Political Change, Cultural Transformation, and Poetics of the Crisis*. Duke UP.

Smith, Daniel Jordan. 2007. *A Culture of Corruption: Everyday Deception and Popular Discontent in Nigeria*. Princeton: Princeton University Press.

Trovalla, Ulrika, and Eric Trovalla. 2015. Infrastructure Turned Suprastructure: Unpredictable Materialities and Visions of a Nigerian Nation. *Journal of Material Science* 20 (1): 43–57.

Yeku, James. 2018. The Hashtag as archive: Internet memes and Nigeria's social media election. In *Art, Creativity, and politics in Africa and the diaspora*, ed. Adelakun Abimbola and Falola Toyin, 217–245. Cham: Palgrave Macmillan.

Yeku, James. 2022. Cultural Netizenship: Social Media Popular Culture and Performance in Nigeria. Bloomington Indiana: Indiana University Press.

16

"It's in Your Hands": Communicating a Pandemic to a Disengaged Public

Eyitayo Aloh

In a viral online video posted on Igbere Television's YouTube channel (2020), two elderly women, being interviewed on the subject of the coronavirus infection in Nigeria, boldly declared in Nigerian pidgin: "That corolla wey dem dey talk, no be for here e dey. Na for China e dey kill dem and na only the people wey get money go China, na dem go catch am. E no fit catch us for here". (Literally: The much-talked-about coronavirus is not here. It only exists in China, and it is only the rich and affluent who can afford to travel to China that can also be infected. Not (poor) people like us). In their repudiation of a global pandemic declared by the World Health Organisation (WHO) on 11 March 2020, the women call on their state of poverty as their immunity against the virus. That state of poverty is further enhanced by their seeming lack of formal education and a visible malnourished state and an unkempt environment. In another viral video circulated on social media, a line of school-aged children marched through the street of an unidentified Nigerian city

E. Aloh (✉)
Trent University, Peterborough, ON, Canada
e-mail: eyitayoaloh@trentu.ca

F. Egbokhare, A. Afolayan (eds.), *Global Health, Humanity and the COVID-19 Pandemic*, https://doi.org/10.1007/978-3-031-17429-2_16

singing: "Coronavirus, go back to China". And they were being hailed by passers-by who apparently also bought into the message of the children.

The two examples above demonstrate the impact that lack of proper communication and correct information can have on a population that is both misinformed and disengaged. Not only is it untrue that coronavirus as a disease cannot affect people who are living in poverty, it is also impossible to sing it away "back to China" in a denial that is premised on false information. It must be noted, however, that there is a reason why the population became disengaged to this point of denial and disavowal of a global pandemic that has fatal consequence.

When the news of a novel coronavirus first hit the media in Nigeria towards the end of January 2020, it was heavily laden with jargons such as "social distancing", "physical distancing" "communal transmission" and "social bubble". Even the name of the disease was confusing as the global health professionals could not agree on a name and as names such as "SARS-Cov 2" and "Coronavirus" made their way into the public domain and confused a lot of people. This led to a break in communication between the responsible agencies and the general populace who believe that such a disease can only be for the elite in society since the names are seen as elitist in nature. In the first example above, as at the time that the women believed in poverty as a sort of immunity to the virus, it did not help that patient "0" in Nigeria was identified as an Italian expatriate[1] and the first fatality was a former director in one of the elite government parastatal,[2] lending further credence to the false belief that it was a disease that can only affect the elite and foreign residence of the country. Unfortunately, initial communication efforts by government agencies were slow in coming out and when they did come out, there was no effort to break down the jargons for the majority of the people, which arguably, further alienated an already disengaged public. Understandably,

[1] Ironically, the first case in Nigeria was also officially confirmed on 11 March 2020 (though initial reports had surfaced around 27 February 2020), the same day that WHO declared Covid-19 as a global pandemic. The unidentified Italian expatriate, working in Nigeria, was said to have returned from a trip to his homeland in Italy, which at the time, was the epicentre of the disease in Europe.

[2] Engineer Suleiman Achimugu, a former Director at a subsidiary of Nigeria's State oil company, Nigerian National Petroleum Corporation (NNPC), was confirmed as the first fatality in Nigeria on 23 March 2020.

there was a whole lot to learn about the new disease and the governmental agencies were equally processing the information as they were coming out of WHO headquarters in Geneva, Switzerland.

It became obvious very quickly that to get the populace to take the virus seriously as a health risk and take preventive action, a novel approach must be made to communicate clearly to them the risks involved in being lackadaisical. And that exactly is what a charity organisation, Akin Fadeyi Foundation (AFF), did with the production of six 1-minute skits broadly titled "It's in Your Hands". So, how successful was the AFF campaign? What tools of communication did they use effectively and what lessons can be learned for future campaigns? This chapter will use cultural and communication studies lens to examine the AFF intervention in the communication of the risks involved with an emerging pandemic to a disengaged populace. My main argument will be that communicating with people in languages that they understand and using a medium that they are familiar with helps in making the message more impactful in the attempts to influence the actions of people.

First, I examine the theories that explain the lack of engagement with the messages on the coronavirus from government agencies. I draw broadly from cultural and Communication studies as both disciplines employ interdisciplinarity as part of their research tools in the analysis of social problems. Then, I apply the theories to my dataset, the six skits from AFF, and then provide an analysis of how the skits are designed to address some of the identified problems of disengagement. I conclude with preliminary results of how successful the campaign has been and point to probable ways that the message can be enhanced to further engage the populace in the quest to stem the spread of coronavirus and any other disease that may come after it.

Theorising Disengagement: Language, Culture and Communication

According to Kim Johnstone, "engagement is a socially responsive approach to communication practice with outcomes aligned with individual, community, civic and individual benefits" (2018: 19–20). This follows that any form of engagement must have clearly defined goals from the outset and call on the individuals and community to respond to the message as sort of connection with the message being proffered. In communicating a pandemic, therefore, the goal is clear from the beginning: get the population to take preventive action on a pandemic and help save lives. This should really be clear enough as engagement must also emphasise the "benefits" that come to the community from acting responsibly on the message. For this to happen, Johnstone identifies three levels of intervention: dialogue, advocacy and interaction.

However, the Nigerian condition presents its own set of unique challenges to communications in general and communicating a pandemic specifically. For one, Nigeria is a multilingual country with at least 250 ethnic dialects spoken within its borders. Therefore, to be able to communicate with the populace, there must be an effort to overcome the language barrier.

With English as a form of unifying language, it can reasonably be expected that this should not be a problem. However, according to a 2018 UNESCO report on Nigeria, 65 percent of the projected 180 million population do not have access to basic education. Therefore, this creates a form of disengagement in itself as it becomes a critical issue how to reach those not proficient in English.

Added to this is the problem of the pandemic itself. The virus was considered "novel" to indicate that it was not only new but more significantly that little was known about it beyond the fact that it can lead to fatality within days of infection. With communication defined as the "exchange of meaning" (Straubhaar et al. 2016: 21), it becomes a challenge to exchange "meaning" when meaning or a clear definition of the pandemic is unavailable. As Shannon and Weaver (1949) theorise in their linear communication model, the message from the source must be very clear for the receiver to decode appropriately. Barnlund (1968) builds on the arguments of Shannon and Weaver by stipulating that the communication process is never complete without feedback from the receiver, which then moves the communication from a linear to an interpersonal one that truly engages with the recipient (Corey 2019). It is the feedback from the receiver of a message that helps the sender to measure if the message being exchanged has been communicated and received correctly. In the case of the coronavirus disease, the meaning is unclear due to the unknown nature of the virus, and it naturally follows that the message cannot be clear and what follows will be the kind of feedback that we have in the opening examples which typifies a disengaged citizenry; a set of people who are unresponsive to messages and refuse to work along with the set goals and objectives that the message is out to accomplish.

The agencies of the Nigerian state with the primary responsibility of informing and responding to a pandemic were cautious in putting out information; perhaps in an effort to have adequate information. The National Centre for Disease Control (NCDC), Ministry of Information and the National Orientation Agency (NOA), charged primarily with dealing with and communicating with Nigerians, had nothing on their websites as at 1 February 2020. The caution exercised by these agencies meant that the social space was awash with misinformation such as "heat kills coronavirus" and "coronavirus cannot survive in a tropical climate". With Paul Watzliawick et al. (1967) already indicating that you "cannot not communicate", the silence and caution on the part of government agencies communicated misinformation. Attempts by these agencies to correct information via media releases on their various websites did little in the form of engagement. What could account for that?

For one, the releases put out were in English, and still using the jargons mentioned above that characterized the initial introduction of the virus to Nigerians. Understandably, English is the official language in Nigeria, but a UNESCO (2012) report puts the literacy rate of Nigeria at 61.2 percent with further disparity in the rural parts of the country where it is reported as low as 14 percent. The attendant outcome is a disconnect from the meaning, through the heavy jargons, which the government agencies sought to encode in English, and which Nigerians are expected to decode. What followed was disengagement and a population that was largely uninformed about a fatal disease despite the risk it posed to them personally.

Speaking further on social engagements and its drivers, Johnstone (2018: 20) postulates that social conditions "influence the outcome of the social and individual levels of engagement". With the poverty level at 45 percent and a further 40 percent in the lower rung of the middle class (AlJazeera 2020), economic survival becomes uppermost in the minds of the people as opposed to a pandemic.[3] The prevailing social condition of poverty makes it impossible for any form of engagement to take place and that proves true as the people would rather engage in improving their socio-economic condition than engage with a pandemic no matter how serious its consequence to their well-being may be. This fact is illustrated by a Nigerian citizen who told American broadcaster, CNN, that he would prefer to die of Covid-19 than hunger (CNN 2020).

Something further has to be said for the medium of communication, with most of the messages being in English and available only on website. Now, within a country that has only 35 percent power output for its entire population—a situation that leads to constant power outage and some areas not having access to any form of electric power for at least two weeks successively—hoping that the message will eventually get to the people was asking for too much on the part of the agencies. Simply put, it becomes impossible to reach majority of the populace using this medium. While the message is there from the agencies, it was not getting to the targeted audience, and hence, was not instigating the required action. This situation seems to hint at a negation of "biopower," a concept deployed by Michel Foucault (1978) who insists that it was possible for government to establish a form of control on the population through "an explosion of numerous and diverse techniques for achieving the subjugations of bodies" (1978: 140). It may just appear that the techniques were not as diverse and numerous as the philosopher prescribed to move the population to take action against the pandemic.

[3] In the *AlJazeera* report, the National Bureau of Statistics (NBS) puts the actual figure at about 82 million people living below the poverty line that they set at an income of ₦137,430/household in a given year.

With the seeming gap in communication leading to a rise in the number of cases in Nigeria, it became apparent that for there to be a shift in the perception of the disease amongst Nigerians, then there has to be a shift in the communication methods being employed. Many private individuals and corporate organisations decided to step in financially and through other social interventions. However, a charity organisation, Akin Fadeyi Foundation, decided to step in on the communications side of the engagement in order to better inform the people and hence get them to take responsibility for their own safety against the pandemic. First though, let us briefly look at the organisation and how its intervention was strategic in the communication of the pandemic to Nigerians.

Partnership for Communication and Engagement: Akin Fadeyi Foundation

When the Akin Fadeyi Foundation was launched in 2016, one of the organization's key statements is to engage and communicate with Nigerians at the grassroots as a way of rooting out conceived social problems (AFF website 2020). The major focus of the organisation at the time was corruption. According to the organisation's website, the campaign against corruption has been largely focused at the "top"—politicians and social elites who occupy the consciousness of the populace through media presentations. Yet, corrupt practices that are carried out at the grassroots and affect society more at the local level are largely ignored. Therefore, as a way of sensitizing the citizens of Nigeria on the corruption that takes place at their local level, AFF launched a campaign tagged *Corruption, not in my country*. The campaign employed regular and recognisable Nigerian actors, mostly from the Nollywood film industry, in short video skits that focus largely on specific acts of corruption: a taxi driver who lies to his customer in order to keep them waiting so as not to lose them; an artisanal trader who employs illegal means to ripen his fruits for quick sale; a student who tries to lure her instructor into sex for grades; etc. since Nigerians already recognize the actors from several Nollywood films, it becomes easier for them to identify with the messages the actors convey on anti-corruption.

However, all of these efforts by the AFF appears to be a mere act of simply dumping informational materials in the public domain. Yet, for a proper engagement to take place with an identified public, the feedback channel must be fully engaged. As already argued, engagement is part of a dialogue, the process of exchanging meanings between parties in a conversation (Taylor and Kent 2014), and if a society is to be fully engaged, then the channel for feedback must be open. In fact, Taylor and Kant argue that "engagement is both an orientation that influences interaction and the approach that guides interaction among groups" (2014: 384). Therefore, social engagement must allow room for social interaction, not just as a form of feedback but also as a form of interaction amongst groups who may hold divergent views. To fulfil this element of engagement, AFF partnered with one of the most maligned institutions of the Nigerian state,[4] The Nigeria Police in a public relations blitz under the "Corruption, not in my country" campaign. However, rather than serve as an image laundry exercise for the Nigeria Police, the campaign provided a platform for the police, and for Nigerians in general, to further engage in a dialogue that serves mutual benefit. A digital app, "Flag it," was launched as part of this dialogic process to make it easier and possible for any member of the society to report any act of impropriety on the part of Nigeria Police. An additional objective of this project was to attract another government agency, Federal Road Safety Corps (FRSC), to this program. These partnerships with agencies of the Nigerian state, with public engagement as the clear goal, enabled the AFF to facilitate a kind of social interaction between the state and the citizens. Nigerians were able to drop their concerns on the "Flag It" app and resolution has been reached for six cases at the last count.

With all the foregoing in place, it appears that when the coronavirus pandemic eventually hit the shores of Nigeria, the organisation was well placed with the manpower and infrastructure to engage the Nigerian

[4] In October 2020, in the midst of the pandemic, a youth-led protest engulfed Nigeria to protest police brutality especially by the subdivision of the police, Special Anti-Robbery Squad (SARS). The protest would crystallize under the digital movement, *#Endsars*.

public in an orientation process that will communicate the mortal dangers that the pandemic portends to any citizen who refuses to take the necessary precaution, with the goal of building social responsibility on the part of all Nigerians and non-Nigerians alike. And it is here that we must now turn to examine the things that they deployed in their communication and measure its efficacy.

"It's in Your Hands": The Dynamics of Engaging the Public

The AFF campaign addressed six key areas of engagement with the Nigerian populace which were identified as necessary to pass on the initial message of prevention against a global pandemic. These are denial, hygiene, social distancing, misinformation, panic buying, and "believe it or not". Rather than adopt a top to bottom communication model, something that has already been resisted by the majority of Nigerians, the AFF decided to bring the population into the campaign program with the theme "It's in Your Hands". The organisation produced six video information skits that were uploaded on the "Corruption, not in my country" YouTube channel, as well as the AFF official website, www.akinfadeyifoundation.org.

In adopting the theme, "It's in Your Hands", there is a deliberate attempt to engage the population and show that they are part of the entire process of preventing the spread of the pandemic. The theme is a specifically not only a creative play on the literal handwashing exercise that medical experts have identified as a crucial action in the fight against the disease, but also a figurative allusion to the responsibility that all the people must bear in the fight against the pandemic. What follows is an interrogation of each thematic skit to see how the message is encapsulated for the purpose of communicating the pandemic in a way that not only initiates a conversation with the Nigerian populace but also critically engages them in ways that instigate actions against the coronavirus.

Denial

This is one of the most potent issues that heralded the advent of the pandemic in Nigeria and in most African countries. And the denial of the coronavirus was heavily influenced by religious belief under the sway of Pentecostalism. The usual rhetoric, promoted by Pentecostal pastors, especially, is either that there was no coronavirus in Nigeria or that faith in God has the capacity to undermine the power of the virus.[5] It does not help that there were evangelical leaders who were peddling this kind of information that faith can make the pandemic disappear. One of such evangelical leaders, Pastor Kingsley Innocent of the Bible Believing Mission Inc., Abia State, Nigeria, told his congregation: "That Coronavirus cannot come here to Nigeria. What do you mean by 'Coronavirus' when there are corrosive anointing in Nigeria? I tell you, Coronavirus is not in this Nigeria" (Youtube Video 2020). Buoyed by rhetoric like this that are clearly based on insufficient information and evidence (since the coronavirus did get into Nigeria), it became necessary to tackle denial as part of the communication process. And it would appear that the "It's in Your Hands" campaigns of AFF have this kind of mixed messages in mind with the skit on denial.

The skit opens with a man calling his friend James on the phone for a regular chat, but the phone was answered by a nurse from the hospital where James has been hospitalised and diagnosed with Covid-19. The nurse tells the friend that the hospital was just about to call him so he can also self-isolate or get medical help if his case worsens. On hearing this news, the friend changes tact and claims he does not know James and had dialled the number in error, so he does not have Covid-19. He further puts a religious spin on his denial, claiming that the only James he knows "is in the bible" and so he cannot be infected with Covid. The skit then cuts to a direct message from the actor to the audience about the dangers of denial. He urges the people to take the disease seriously as "Coronavirus is real". He follows this with an exhortation to follow the safety protocols

[5] It should be noted that the late president of Tanzania, Mr. Magufuli supposedly died of the coronavirus. Before his death, Magufuli insisted that the "coronavirus, which is a devil, cannot survive in the body of Christ…. It will burn instantly". "John Magufuli: Tanzania's late president in his own words", BBC News, 18 March, 2021 https://www.bbc.com/news/world-africa-56441421.

required to stay safe. The skit shows a deep understanding of what is at the heart of the denial by most of the populace—a deep belief in supernatural spiritual powers and in Pentecostal leaders who appears to be more concerned about prosperity than the health of their adherents (Ayegboyin 2006), and addresses it without any form of condemnation.

Hygiene

Medical advancement has seemingly not replaced the key role of maintaining proper hygiene in the fight against a virus. Even the World Health Organisation (WHO) in its campaign tagged "*There's a Hero in All of Us*" (www.who.int 2020) encourages proper personal hygiene as the first line of defence against the pandemic. Therefore, it becomes one of the major areas of engagement in the fight against the virus. And it is this awareness that led to the second thematic focus of the AFF, and the skit on personal hygiene.

In the skit, a wife is busy preparing dinner for the household and the husband comes in from work and moves straight to get his meal directly from the pot. The wife stops him and reminds him of the need to wash his hands as part of the proper hygiene process required to combat the Covid-19 pandemic. The husband dismisses the wife's concern as unnecessary since he is immune. "Corona no dey catch Blackman" (corona does not affect a black person), he declares to his wife in Nigerian pidgin. The wife responds by wearing a facemask and gloves, applying hand sanitiser, and chasing the husband out of the kitchen with a spray sanitiser. The skit once again cuts to the husband addressing the audience directly on the need to take precautions. He emphasises the critical role of hygiene in the prevention of coronavirus and ends with the catchphrase, "it's in your hands".

Social Distancing

In a telephone conversation between two friends, one friend asks the other if he was still coming to a "meeting", a social gathering that is to be held in his enclosed living room. The other friend reminds him that such a meeting should not be taking place due to the pandemic. He further explains that it might actually be against the lockdown law in operation at the time. The friend hosting the meeting responds that it is in his living room and so no authority can arrest or apprehend them. The cautious friend suggests a viable alternative in the form of online platforms that will keep them all safe from the virus that does not respect people and can infect anyone. He proceeds to emphasise the message of maintaining "social distancing" as a preventive measure against the virus.

With this skit, there is a shift away from the punitive approach that underscores the dire consequences of underestimating the virus. The subtext of the skit is simple: even though we cannot overlook the often-fatal consequences of contracting the coronavirus, an emphasis on the personal benefits accruing from taking heed to the warning about the pandemic can lead to the willingness on the part of the citizens to be safety conscious. The fact that the campaign is designed to be citizen-centred, as opposed to law-oriented, is seen in the effort of the cautious friend in suggesting an online platform for meeting without putting themselves at risk. Interestingly, it is the careless friend who delivers the skit's direct message: "Not all infected persons show symptoms, but all infected persons are contagious". It further takes the message away from the punishment to the responsibility that is expected of everyone in the joint effort against coronavirus.

Misinformation

If anything can be described as a pandemic within a pandemic, then it has to be the wave of false unverified stories around the pandemic itself, mode of transmission, and prescriptive cures. This is what has been called *infodemic*. It does not help that such misinformation, especially around cures, are being propagated by eminent leaders, especially political and religious, with huge influence across a wide demographics. This has led to unsavoury outcomes such as the reported death of two people who ingested an overdose of a largely untested, yet highly touted medication by the President of the United States of America, Donald Trump (York

2020). There is also the case of the popular Nigerian Pentecostal leader, Pastor Chris Oyakhilome, making a spurious connection between the coronavirus pandemic and 5G. Therefore, it becomes very clear that tackling the pandemic also implies tackling misinformation about it.

In the skit on misinformation, a man keeps knocking on the door of his visibly disinterested neighbour with fabricated and unverified news. First, he knocks to tell him that a fumigation process in the neighbourhood will contaminate the air and everything around, and so he urges his neighbour to quickly go remove his clothes from the clothes line. The neighbour simply closes his door. Seconds later, he knocks again to tell his neighbour of a cure involving a multiple dose of "cough medication". Again, the neighbour closes his door. The camera shot on the neighbour tells the story of a disinterested individual who wishes the neighbour would stop spreading false and fake news around the virus. In making the neighbour silent throughout the one-minute skit, there is a clear message that silence is golden. In other words, it helps to be the stoic brick wall that prevents the spread of a rumour and false information than be a conduit. This is then reinforced in the direct message by the same neighbour to the wider audience to "shun fake and unverified information".

Panic Buying

One of the measures that governmental authorities across the world undertook to stem the tide of the pandemic was to impose a lockdown on all citizens, limiting their activities and keeping them at home. This gave rise to panic buying and some ugly scenes at supermarkets all over the world. The Internet was soon awash with videos of massive brawls over items such as toilet rolls, canned food and sanitary items. Nigeria was not exempted from the ugly scramble for household essentials as people punched their way through supermarket aisles to get their hands-on supplies to last them through the lockdown, which had no end date. It became necessary to engage the citizens of Nigeria on their shopping habits as part of the pandemic information drive.

To address the issue of panic buying, the "It's in Your Hands" skit spotlights a wife and her husband. The husband had gone to the store to get his wife a loaf of bread, only to come back home with a carload of stuff from the market. The surprised wife asks why the husband had bought so much stuff that the family apparently does not need at the time and he answers that it is because of coronavirus and the impending lockdown. The visibly unhappy wife chastises him and offers the wise nugget of message: "If you create scarcity, you create panic. Stock up on supplies, don't panic buy". A comic element is added when she asks for the bread that was his original reason for going to the store. His exclamation reveals that he forgot to get it! This skit demonstrates that the coronavirus as a disease wasn't just a health challenge; on the contrary, it has a fundamental impact on the collective psyche of the people. What else could have made a husband engage in the panic buying of less essential materials while forgetting the main reason he visited the supermarket?

Believe It or Not

The sixth and final skit will seem to be an all-encompassing message on the need to be vigilant against the virus. This can only happen if the people acknowledge the existence of the virus and take responsibility for stemming its spread. The skit opens with a customer at a newspaper vending stand trying to greet the vendor with a handshake. The vendor, on the other hand, extends his elbow for a bump as advised by WHO. The customer asks why he refuses not shake his hands as is customary and he says it is because of the virus that is spreading fast. "So, you believe that thing? Look, if you like, gather the whole Naija [Nigeria] make dem cough, the thing no go catch". The vendor simply shakes his head in astonishment at the denial of his customer. When the customer demands his change for the payment, the vendor calls on a bystander to help give the customer his change. To see if the customer believes in his denial of Covid, the bystander coughs on the currency note and extends it to the customer who declines in shock. The camera cuts to the direct message by the same bystander: "This virus no get leg, na we dey carry am. Protect yourself" [The virus has no legs; we are the one spreading it]. A simple and direct message for the people.

Analysis

In communicating the message of the pandemic to the populace, three elements were inserted to engage the citizens and instigate action: repetition, direct and simple messaging, and the deployment of a common language. I will now examine these three elements to demonstrate how they engage the population in a communication process.

As a cultural tool of communication, repetition helps reinforce a message and literally imprints it in the consciousness of the target audience. Henry Louis Gates Jr. states that repetition serves as a form of signifying for cultures in Africa, helping them achieve a form of cooperation (1988: 12).[6] If we extrapolate, cooperation is the goal of the message and a form of required action and as such, to ensure that a message is acted upon, it must not only be clear, but repeated. In the skits, the clear message of "denial is dangerous" is repeated across five of the skits. While denial gets its own themed skit, that message is reinforced in the skit on "hygiene", "misinformation", "social distancing" and "believe it or not". In fact, the same statement which most Nigerians understand—"Corona no dey kill Blackman"—is used in varying forms in all of the skits as a way of ensuring that Nigerians get the message and act on the reality that the virus exists and can affect all. Repetition also reinforces the message as one that requires the urgent attention of every audience, with a demand for immediate feedback which, again, comes in the way of action on the part of the audience.

The technique of direct messaging is noteworthy as all the skits cut to such messages from one of the actors to the audience. The message is simple, in clear language and directs attention to the overall theme of the skit. As stated above, the jargon-heavy approach that was initially used by government agencies failed with most Nigerians who were not educated enough to decode the meanings. In a way, there was no communication between the agencies and Nigerians on coronavirus. Therefore, it became necessary to package the message in a simple and matter of fact manner.

[6] The other strand of signifying in the book is oppositional and can help resist any form of hegemonic oppression. However, as the thrust in this chapter is "engagement", the oppositional strand of signifying is not required.

In any communication process that intends to engage, there must be "intentionality", which Frank Dance describes as "purposeful message sending and receiving" (1982: 9). It therefore becomes pertinent to make the message as clear as possible. And to achieve intentionality and purposefulness, it is best to directly address the audience and eliminate any sort of ambiguity. The lack of attention to ambiguity was how the messaging on the government websites lost all the people the government was trying to engage. On the other hand, by keeping the messages short and "intentionally" direct, the AFF was able to deliver their message straight to those who are required to act on it within one-minute video skits.

Closely linked to simple messaging is the language in which the message is presented. In a country as linguistically diverse as Nigeria, it is challenging to present a message in all the languages simultaneously. Yet, language plays a major role in communication as "talk is linked to prior talk, not only within turns but also to one's previous statement and those of other speakers" (Bonvillain 2014: 40–41). The breakdown in communication highlighted above came about because the jargons were like foreign language to a majority of the people and so the link required for communication to carry on was broken. There has to be a unifying language of communication for a proper "exchange of meaning" to take place. Nigerian Pidgin has been identified as an effective means of communication as it is widely used amongst Nigerians. Even religious groups have started translating their materials into Pidgin to have a wider reach (Ojomoyela 2018). Hence, it is not surprising that the "In your hands campaign" had a mix of pidgin elements in its original production. This helps in the process of facilitating a wider reach that increases the level of engagement in their quest to collectively combat the disease.

However, beyond delivering some of the original materials in Pidgin English, the desire to reach more Nigerians influenced the organisation to translate all six skits into pidgin language for effective communication with the Nigerian public. Further, with support from an international funding organisation, the MacArthur Foundation, all the skits were further translated into the three major Nigerian languages.[7] This further aided the spread of the messages to the furthest part of the country and to additional people who may not have the benefit of formal education.

These three key elements of repletion, direct messaging and language were effectively deployed so much so that the skits drew over four thousand positive comments within their first week of release. Other organisations, recognizing the efficacy of the approach that the AFF had adopted, quickly incorporated the skits and provided further evidence that the campaign is a success. While there is not enough data to make a pronouncement that the dip in the cases in Nigeria between July and November 2020 has anything to do with this campaign, it can be safely assumed that it contributed to getting Nigerians to take the disease serious and act to prevent its spread.

Conclusion

Though it started out as a public health crisis that engulfed the world, the novel coronavirus disease (Covid-19) soon became a social-political and economic crisis that required multiple levels of approaches in the effort to deal with it. One of the major challenges was communication: engaging the wider public in ways that they understand so as to take the requisite action to protect themselves and their community. In Nigeria, it became imperative that due to the diversity of the country, a novel disease demanded a novel communication approach. While the action of the governmental agencies was commendable, it became apparent very quickly that more needed to be done to fully engage the population in a way that will ensure their hearkening to the message with actions that match the spread of the disease. The "It's in Your Hands" media campaign of the charity organisation, Akin Fadeyi Foundation, provides a snapshot of the kind of extra push from the private sector that complemented government efforts at getting the people to take responsibility for

---

[7] I owe this information to a personal conversation with the founder/Executive Director of the organisation, Mr. Akin Fadeyi and I will like to acknowledge his cooperation in writing this chapter.

their actions in dealing with the coronavirus disease in Nigeria. It demonstrates how interventions, with humanities methodologies, can be a key process in communication that save lives.

That the National Orientation Agency (NOA), an arm of the federal Ministry of information, and the Lagos State Government can quickly endorse and co-opt the campaign into their plan of action is a proof that such a public-private partnership can work with proper orientation and direction. This for me also represents a level of success for the campaign approach that AFF adopted in communicating the pandemic to Nigerians as well as the method of engagement chosen.

And, as the deployment of the various vaccines continues to push the boundaries of the virus back, it will still require all the best kind of communication and engagement with the public to ensure that the populace take action and make themselves available for vaccination. This becomes even more imperative as not only the anti-vaxxers campaigns across the world has demonstrated, but news coming out of Nigeria reveals that many have become sceptical about taking the vaccines. It is at this level that keeping healthy and safe become a civic responsibility that keeps the entire Nigerian society safe.

References

AFF website. 2020. www.akinfadeyifoundation.com

AlJazeera. 2020. *Forty Percent of Nigerians Live Below the Poverty Line*. News Report. Abhu Dhabi: Al Jazeera News Agency.

Ayegboyin, Deji. 2006. A Rethinking of Prosperity Teaching in the New Pentecostal Churches in Nigeria. *Black Theology.* 4 (1): 70–85.

Barnlund, Dean C. 1968. *Interpersonal Communications: Survey and Studies*. California: University of California.

Bonvillain, Nancy. 2014. *Language, Culture and Communication: The meaning of Messages*. New York: Pearson.

Channel, Igbere Television. 2020. *Igbere Television Channel.* Youtube. April 18. Accessed 1 Nov 2020.

CNN.com. July 21, 2020. A country of 200 million has carried out just 212,000 virus tests. Accessed February 2021.

Corey, Amy M. 2019. Introducing Communication. In *The Evolution of Human Communication: From Theory to Practice, by Tess Pierce*. Oshawa, ON: Etre Press.

Dance, Frank E. 1982. *Human Communication Theory: Comparative Essays*. New York: Harper & Row.

Foucault, Michel. 1978. *The History of Sexuality*. London: Allen Lane.

Gates, Henry Louis. 1988. *The Signifying Monkey: A Theory of African American Literary Criticism*. Oxford: Oxford University Press.

Johnston, Kim A. 2018. Towards a Theory of Social Engagement. In *The Handbook of Communication Engagement*, ed. Kim A. Johnston and Maureen Taylor, 19–32. New Jersey: John Wiley & Sons.

Ojomoyela, Rotimi. 2018. Jehovah's Witnesses boost Pidgin language development. *Vanguard Newspaper*. Nigeria, December 24: 4.

Shannon, C.E., and W. Weaver. 1949. *The Mathematical Theory of Communication*. Urbana, IL: University of Illinois Press.

Straubhaar, Joseph, Robert LaRose, and Lucinda Davenport. 2016. *Media Now: Understanding Media, Culture, and Technology*. Boston, MA: Cengage Learning.

Taylor, Maureen, and Michael Kent. 2014. Dialogic Engagement: Clarifying Foundational Concepts. *Journal of Public Relations Research*: 384–398.

UNESCO. 2012. *Revitalizing Adult and Youth Literacy in Nigeria: Program Document*. Abuja: UNESCO Office. in Abuja.

Video, YouTube. 2020. Bible Believing Mission Inc. Abia State, Nigeria, February 22.

Watzlawick, Paul, Janet Beavin-Bavelas, and Don D. Jackson. 1967. The pragmatics of Human Communication: A Study of Interactional patterns, pathologies and paradoxes. New York: Norton.

www.akinfadeyifoundation.org. 2020. June 18. Accessed 18 June 2020.

www.who.int. 2020. February 2. Accessed 18 Aug 2020.

York, Geoffrey. 2020. Nigerians Poisoned After Taking Doses of Drug Praised by Trump. *The Globe and Mail World*, March 22: 3.

17

Musical Representations of COVID-19 on Social Media Among Young People in Nigeria

Toyin Samuel Ajose and Jeremiah Oluwadara Omotayo

Introduction

The outbreak of COVID-19 witnessed various human responses both scientifically and socially to the pandemic. Several medical and non-medical interventions were employed to manage and/or combat the virus. For example, personal hygiene like regular hand-washing with soap and water, the use of alcohol-based hand sanitizers and wearing of face masks were recommended as safety measures. Social distancing also became one of the most effective ways to reduce the spread of the virus that is easily transmissible through coughing and sneezing (Agusi et al. 2020; Melo and Sousa Soares 2020; Quian and Jiang 2020). Social

T. S. Ajose (✉)
Department of Music, University of Ibadan, Ibadan, Nigeria
e-mail: ts.ajose@ui.edu.ng

J. O. Omotayo
Department of Political and Governance Policy, Nigerian Institute of Social and Economic Research (NISER), Ibadan, Nigeria
e-mail: jo.omotayo@niser.gov.ng

F. Egbokhare, A. Afolayan (eds.), *Global Health, Humanity and the COVID-19 Pandemic*, https://doi.org/10.1007/978-3-031-17429-2_17

distancing is described as a set of methods for reducing frequency and closeness of contact between people in order to decrease the risk of transmission of disease (Centre for Disease Control [CDC] 2020). Social distancing further facilitates "remaining out of congregate settings, avoiding mass gatherings and maintaining distance from others where possible" (Agusi et al. 2020, 2). In this chapter, social distancing and physical distancing are used interchangeably.

The effects of social distancing, amongst other measures in managing COVID-19 pandemic, have been discussed (Agusi et al. 2020; Kalahikhina 2020; Melo and Sousa Soares 2020; Quian and Jiang 2020). On a positive note, social distancing offers, among other benefits, one of the safest ways of minimizing disease infection rate, and consequently reducing death rate (Jacobson et al. 2020), alleviates the burden on medical facilities, and allows for ample clinical time for health workers to respond to infected patients (Quian and Jiang 2020). Conversely, loss of livelihood, domestic violence and poor mental health have been associated with social distancing as occasioned by the lockdown directives of the government in many countries (Kalahikhina 2020; Melo and Sousa Soares 2020; Santiago and Smith 2020). With the lockdown orders, economic activities were severely affected as offices and businesses were shut down. Many businesses had to migrate to the digital space to continue transactions. In order to mitigate the severe effects of the social distancing strategy, many people including young and old, sought for alternative and viable means to contact and connect socially in the face of the extreme difficulty with physical interactions. Hence, the social media offered such opportunity for people of the world irrespective of distance to seamlessly communicate and interact during the heat of the pandemic. The reason for people to find a means at all cost to socialize is not far-fetched: humans are social beings who must interact irrespective of the dangers.

The importance of the social media during the COVID-19 pandemic cannot be underestimated. It serves as an active tool for different social engagements among various people in different societies (Obi-Ani et al. 2020). Also, it offers a space for information gathering and sharing especially as it relates to the pandemic. Besides the use of social media for socializing, we should also note its complementary roles in healthcare services, including spreading of public health awareness and advocacy during the pandemic (Obi-Ani et al. 2020; Sahni and Sharma 2020). In India, for example, Sahni and Sharma (2020) found that the social media was used as an effective means of disseminating COVID-19 health-related issues because of its rapid and wider access by the citizens. Since proximate physical interaction is strongly discouraged, the social media served as an effective alternative for health workers to access patients under a regulated situation. The UK Nursing and Midwifery Council operates a Facebook page in sharing health information to members of the public. In Nigeria, the Lagos State government set up a telemedicine initiative to help people access medical care using a toll-free line. Globally, many of the CDCs have and manage their social media platforms in an up-to-date method for the dissemination of information on the state of the pandemic in their countries.

Scholars have discussed the merits and demerits of social media during this global pandemic. While extant studies agree that the social media provided a quick time information access to a wide spectrum of social media users, the credibility and reliability of the information generated and circulated are of great concern to many (Ahmad and Murad 2020; Obi-Ani et al. 2020; Sahni and Sharma 2020). In their observation of the social media space during the pandemic in Nigeria, Obi-Ani et al. (2020) argue that social media was used largely to disseminate wrong information about COVID-19. They also found that social media was used as a space for propaganda and misinformation among the citizens. The widespread dissemination of wrong and misleading information about the pandemic made the World Health Organization (WHO) declare that social media has precipitated an "infodemic" that have to be combated if there must be a headway with dealing with the COVID-19 pandemic.

Not only was infodemic a "virus" that was spreading so fast, cybercrimes also spiked during the pandemic. As Mahadevan notes, "as the virus spread, so did the scale of cybercrime exploiting it" (Mahadevan 2020: 7). The stay-at-home orders and the increase in remote work space led to the rise in the number of online users for both economic and social purposes. The shift to the virtual space is reportedly accountable for the increase in cybercrimes globally (Hawdon et al. 2020; Mahadevan 2020; Naidoo 2020). In America, for example, while physical crimes such as burglaries, murders, robberies and assaults were declining, cybercrimes were reported to be on the increase during the COVID-19 pandemic (Hawdon et al. 2020). In other words, "as we spend more time online, our cyber-routines change, and we would anticipate that these changes would alter cybervictimization rates" (Hawdon et al. 2020, 547).

Cyberfraudsters did not only take advantage of the influx of the digital space users during the pandemic, they also used COVID-19 themes in reaching out to those that Hawdon et al. described as "suitable targets" (Hawdon et al. 2020, 549). For example, Mahadevan (2020) found that cybercriminals used phishing emails to reach out to people on COVID-19-related matters including soliciting for funds to aid medical assistance or provide welfare supports to communities ravaged with the pandemic. He explains,

> The sophistication of internet-enabled scams directed at non-government entities, such as private companies and individuals, varied considerably. Several reports have mentioned phishing messages spoofed to look as though they originate from national healthcare authorities, such as the Centers for Disease Control (CDC) in the United States. These messages solicit donations for COVID-19 vaccine development. In other cases, internet advertisements have offered face masks and hand sanitizer, and occasionally even 'cures' for COVID-19. Buyers are required to make full payment in advance, but the product never arrives. (Mahadevan 2020, 7)

While the negative activities of the social media during the pandemic is replete in extant literature on COVID-19, the positive and creative engagements of its users especially in coping with the psychological and physical stress associated with the pandemic during the lockdown is yet to be fully examined particularly among young people who are arguably the largest users of the social media. This is particularly so with the exploration of the place and space of music as a site for social interaction in a pandemic. Only few studies exist on the agency of music to inspire hope, resilience and solidarity among young people in Nigeria during the pandemic. The big question here is: if the social media is a viable means for spreading public health awareness and advocacy especially about COVID-19, how did young people in Nigeria joined in the conversation through the deployment of music as an expressive form of art?

As earlier mentioned, social distancing provides a life-saving strategy during the pandemic; however, its attendant negative psychological consequences including loneliness, panic and restlessness abound (Gupta 2020). As a coping strategy during quarantine and stay-at-home period, the creative arts—music, dance and visual arts—proffer a suitable and therapeutic alternative to the negative psychological effects of the pandemic. Gupta notes that "art is available for all people to participate in as a tried-and-true 'vaccine' of sorts, working its therapeutic magic to protect the physical, social, and mental health of the human species as we struggle together to confront COVID-19 with simultaneous distance and solidarity" (Gupta 2020, 2–3). Suffice to say, then, that the various artistic undertakings by different people during the lockdown has been described as "quarantine arts" or coronavirus art (Gupta 2020). These art works provide some sort of psycho-social empowerment for many people while positively shaping their reaction to the pandemic. The arts possess the capacity to transform worrying experience by turning collective anxiety into collective support and action (McNiff 1998).

With reference to music as an art form, its therapeutic character has been well established in literature (Sheppard and Broughton 2020; Macdonald 2013; Mofredj et al. 2016). Across different cultural and geographical contexts, music helps people to "remain motivated, resilient and united in the face of collective challenge" (Gupta 2020, 3). In spite of the isolation occasioned by the social distancing regime, music offers social bonding and solidarity. Thus, "musical solidarity has the therapeutic ability to puncture the isolation of social distancing, to foster resiliency by lifting the collective spirit, and to move people's emotions toward spirited action—even if that action, in these circumstances, means staying home to save the lives of others" (Gupta 2020, 3–4).

Globally, music-making was experienced in diverse manners in physical and virtual spaces during the pandemic. Physically, people who were fed up with the boredom of staying locked down in their homes turned to making music, as well as singing and dancing, from the balconies of their homes. Digital forums and platforms—Facebook, YouTube, Tiktok, Instagram and Twitter—became the preferred site for creative performances that replaced concert halls, worship centres and clubs. These platforms thus became the combustible spaces that brought the lockdown energies of bored youth into contact with the creative dynamics of music. Music plays an important part in the lives of young people; it influences their thoughts, preferences and aspiration (Arnett 1991; Brown 2006; Ross 1994). As Arnett observes, "it is not just a music preference to them, but intense avocation that shapes their view of the world, their spending habits, their moods, their friendship, their notion of who are what is admirable, and their hopes for what they might become" (Arnett 1991, 445). Young people engage with music more often than other structured activities in the society including education and religion (Mickel and Mickel 2002 cited in Brown 2006; Ross 1994). And they deploy music in a number of ways—social, religious, political, economic, linguistic and psychological. For Roberts and Christenson,

> music can relieve tension; provide escape or distraction from problems; relieve loneliness; fill the time when there is nothing much to do; ease the drudgery of repetitive, menial tasks and chores; fill uncomfortable silence; provide topics of conversation; make parties more lively; teach new vocabulary; articulate political attitudes; and perform many other uses for listener. (2001, 134)

As a representational art form, music presents a most suitable form for representing COVID-19. Music can represent and be represented as a subject or an object (Berenson 1994; Bohlman 2005; Scruton 1976). Bohlman notes that "when music serves 'as representation,' we are witnessing its subjective potential; when music is a 'representation of' something, we recognize its objective functions" (2005: 206–207). Scruton also agrees that "if music is to be representational, then its subject must be not only picked out, but also characterized" (1976, 276). For Berenson, "as long as music conveys something/anything to us then that something is represented. … If we can talk about something in the music, then we have a subject-matter the representation of which is in some way there, in the music" (Berenson 1994, 65).

In this chapter, we examined how COVID-19 was musically represented among young people on social media in Nigeria. This study seeks to contribute to the growing scholarship on COVID-19 pandemic by exploring the interdisciplinarity of musicology, media studies, public health and social sciences. We purposively sampled six music videos from Facebook and YouTube. Globally, Facebook is one of the leading social network sites and YouTube is a known online video-sharing platform. In a survey by NOIPolls, Facebook is the most widely known social networking site in Nigeria and more than 90 percent of Nigerians who have access to the Internet know of Facebook (NOIPolls 2019). Some of these music videos created were uploaded on YouTube channels and then shared on Facebook to reach out to a larger audience. The music videos selected (a) are replete with COVID-19-related themes, (b) are performed by young Nigerians, and (c) were shared between March 30 and July 31, 2020 (which spans the peak period of the stay-at-home order by the Nigerian government). In selecting the six music videos, search filters were used, including trending hashtags such as #covid19music, #covid19songs, #coronanigeria, #coronavirusmusic, #coronaija, and #covid9ja. Furthermore, the online engagements—views, likes and comments—generated from selected music videos were analyzed.

Music-Making, Social Media and COVID-19

Music, like other forms of art, offer the space for creative expressions among people including young people. Music, vocal or instrumental or combination of both, can be experienced through "live" or recorded performances in mediated forms such as cassette tape, compact disc, DVD and the Internet. The advancement in the world of Internet technology has opened up a plethora of opportunities for music-making, production and circulation. Digital streaming platforms which allows for seamless access to music videos are increasing daily. These platforms have significantly transformed the ways whereby musicians negotiate musical performances. For example, musicians can reach a much wider audience with their performances outside the conventional performance spaces. Listeners alike now have access to a broad range of musical performance across styles from the comfort of their homes whenever they choose to do so. Beyond providing information about and on the coronavirus pandemic, the social media also engendered different creative activities such as skits, comedy and music videos.

Studies have explored the connection between social media use and creativity in different settings. The negative impact of social media on creativity including cyber-bullying, reputation risk and information security threats have been established (Aula 2010; Everett 2010; Whittaker and Kowalski 2015). However, the numerous potential benefits of social media for creativity has been examined. As a "platform for the creation and exchange of user-generated content" (Kaplan and Haenlein 2010: 61), social media offers the site for participation and collaboration in various creative expressions. It provides the market space for creative transactions where "anyone can access and share ideas at low or no cost to gain acceptance and support" (Acar et al. 2019: 40). Due to accessibility and affordability social media and other digital platforms provide their users, young people were motivated to put forward their creative ideas or projects to the virtual audience which they believe will appreciate the ideas. Acar et al. (2019) believe that one good reason people are creative on the social media is that they know that some people will see, read, watch or test out their work. It therefore implies that social media users may be more creatively productive since they know they will get recognition in such spaces.

Acar et al. (2019) explored the relationship between social media and creativity from three perspectives: time spent using social media, frequency and nature of SM use and purpose of social media use. They found out that time spent using social media has positive relationship to ideational behaviour and the creative activity and accomplishment. In order words, the more time people spend on social media, the more creative ideas they are likely to generate. This confers on social media a kind of currency for negotiating creativity among humans. As earlier noted, the lockdown necessitated human interactions largely through the use of social and digital platforms thus increasing the amount of time people spend on the social media. As Acar et al. argue "the use of social media for a longer time, and more frequently, fuels user's ideational capacity" (p. 48), it therefore suggests that young people who spent most of their time on the social media during the lockdown must have increased their creative abilities through the use of social media. This explains why many creative activities including music increased during the lockdown. Despite the negative accounts about the use of social media during the lockdown, the creative opportunities it provides for young people remains novel.

Whether or not the passive or active use of social media also has correlation with creative behaviour in people have been probed. Robinson et al. (2019) investigate the effect of social media on human creativity by discussing how exposure to social media can enhance creative thoughts among girls in university setting. While the study reveals that there is no correlation between use of social media and creativity, the authors argue that passive social media use may have negative impact on psychological functions such as creativity. In their study, Acar et al. (2019) found that frequency of social media use improves creative activities. They observed that the higher frequency of passive and active use of Twitter and active use of Facebook and YouTube were positively related to creativity measures. Little wonder why many of the creative activities among young people during the lockdown were on Facebook and YouTube.

People use social media for various purposes which affects their creative-related activities. For example, "those who use social media primarily for 'expressing their ideas and opinions,' 'gleaning topics and information to talk about,' and 'self-education and learning' had higher creative-related variables than those whose primary purposes were 'entertainment' or 'relaxation'" (Leung and Kier 2008; Acar et al. 2019: 47). Young people in Nigeria employed social media to express their ideas and opinion especially about the coronavirus on one hand and to serve as a tool for entertainment or relaxation during the lockdown on the other hand.

Given the creative potentialities it offers, young people in Nigeria explored the various social and digital media platforms that provides them with unlimited access and uncensored content. Unlike the traditional media platforms with control processes, social media created the space for personal expression where "individuals have almost complete freedom in posting and reading what they want" (Acar et al. 2019: 48). As observed in this study, young people found social media as performance sites where they can create and circulate their music from their local context to a global audience. Social media provides an "ongoing 'audience' for creative expression at any moment of the day" (p. 48), which the lockdown would not have allowed in a physical setting. So, music-making comes almost at a cheaper rate in reaching a wider audience on social media given its affordability and accessibility. Young people, individual or groups creatively and affectively deployed social media in communicating their messages—through music—to the world using their local narratives about and around the coronavirus.

Music-making provided the arena for solidarity among young people in the heat of the pandemic by creating and sharing their music on social media. The connection between music and solidarity is known. Nicholls (2014) believes that music has the emotional ability to bind individuals together in solidarity and to build alliance for a course. And for Laurence (2011, 5), solidarity is "the harmony of interests and responsibilities among individuals in a group, especially as manifested in unanimous support and collective action for something". As creatives, music enables young people to come together as individuals to form a group thereby showing their collective resolve to survive the stress associated with physical isolation and to express their concerns during the lockdown.

Musical Representation of COVID-19

As earlier mentioned, music can represent and be represented. Critical observation of the selected music videos on social media with COVID-19-related themes reveals that various representations were given to pandemic by different the young people. COVID-19 was represented in three prominent ways: public health awareness, spiritual/religious and sociopolitical. In what follows, we shall discuss the representations.

Public Health Awareness Representation

The role of public health awareness in managing the pandemic is considered a vital one. It helps in containing the spread of the virus and reduces mortality rate (Ali and Bhatti 2020). In managing the virus, several stakeholders employed various information modes in disseminating health tips among the populace. Like other forms of communication, young people used songs to complement the efforts of these stakeholders in passing messages related about the pandemic on the social media. An example is "Stay at home" by the Oyedeles:

> Stay at home, stay at home
> Corona dey for road o [Corona is out there]
> stay at home
>
> Stay at home, stay at home
> Corona no dey look face [Corona respects no one]
> stay at home
>
> Stay at home, stay at home
> For you to live a long life
> stay at home

Call	*Response*
No wedding	stay at home
No school o	stay at home
No go church	stay at home
No visit	stay at home
No hangout	stay at home
Just prayer	For your house
Only prayer	For your house
Serious prayer	stay at home
For you to live a long life stay at home	

The music video performed by a quartet, —two females and two males inside a motionless car, was posted around April 13, 2020, a period when the stay-at-home order and the social distancing rule followed by many countries including Nigeria were strict. The song, performed in a four-part—soprano, alto, tenor and bass (SATB)—western choral style, articulates the public health awareness on the need for self-quarantine and stay-at-home as viable measures in flattening the curve of the virus. This information is captured in warning phrases such as "corona no dey look face" (corona respects no one), "corona dey for road" (corona is in the public space), and "for you to live a long life", listeners are therefore admonished to "stay at home". Listeners were reminded to avoid large gatherings including religious events.

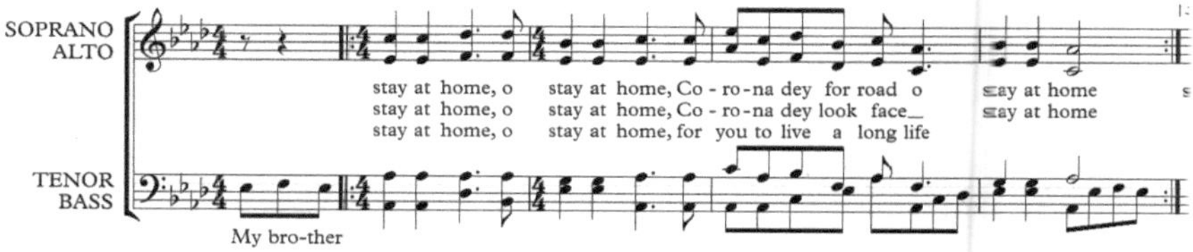
SOPRANO
ALTO
stay at home, o stay at home, Co - ro - na dey for road o stay at home
stay at home, o stay at home, Co - ro - na dey look face stay at home
stay at home, o stay at home, for you to live a long life
TENOR
BASS
My bro-ther

Music example: Stay at home (SATB transcription by the first author)

As social actors, the Oyedeles seem to have flouted the government's directive of stay-at-home and the use of face masks in the public during the making of the music video. As seen in the video, none of the singers wore a face mask and they sat in a very close range to each other. Research have examined the ignorant or defiant attitude of people towards the social distancing orders during the lockdown. In Nigeria, for example, Agusi et al. (2020) observed that social distancing directives was partially or not observed at all both at individual and cooperate level. One important question to ask is: how effective can the public health awareness efforts of the Oyedeles be if they themselves are seen as deviants in the music video?

Another song that offered public health awareness, while highlighting the various COVID-19 protocols as recommended by health practitioners, is "Covidus 1 vs 9" by the Kabusa Oriental Choir—a popular music group on Facebook known for imitating the indigenous-choral style common among church choirs, particularly in South East, Nigeria. Their music employed Igbo choral dance style with instrumental accompaniments such as keyboards, drums, guitars and few Igbo percussion instruments as well as the use of parody. With the use of digital recording tools, the three-man singers were able to produce a kind of large choral performance. Besides their sonic representation, the music video also presented some Christian visual aesthetics such as choir robes and clergy dress.

The song started with a note of caution to Okoro (a name of a person) to be careful of not getting infected by Coro (colloquial form for the coronavirus in Nigeria). It expresses the concern that the virus cannot be facially identified but can be prevented by taking necessary hygiene procedures such as regular hand-wash and avoiding physical bodily contact.

> Okoro be careful make you no catch Coro
> Okoro be careful make you no catch Coro
> Corona, e no dey show for face
> Go wash your hand and say hello
> No more hand shake, no more hugging
> No more until further notice
> Corona e no dey show for face
> Cover your mouth when you are coughing
> Even when you're sneezing, when you're yawning

The song employs satire in its bid to attract listeners to its message. In the second section of the song, the coronavirus is represented as something that stigmatizes whosoever contracts it, and such person(s) may have "Coro" added as a suffice to their name(s):

Aunty if you catch am o,	Aunty if you contract the virus
Your name go change to Aunty Coro	You will be called "Aunty Coro"
Iya if you catch am o,	Mother if you contract the virus
Your name go change to Iya Coro	You will be called "Mother of Coro"
Baba if you catch am o,	Daddy if you contract the virsu
Your name go change to Baba Coro	You will be called "Daddy of Coro"
Mama if you catch am o,	Mama if you contract the virus
Your name go change to Mama Coro	You will be called "Mama Coro"

Research has shown that humour is associated with stigma creation and reduction (Corrigan et al. 2014). A closer examination of the second section of the song text above reveals a form of stigma that Mahmud and Islam (2020) refers to as humour-prone stigma. In a study on the effects of social stigma in responding to COVID-19 in Bangladesh, they identified "humor-prone stigma, residential stigma, organizational stigma, community stigma, and apathetical stigma" (Mahmud and Islam 2020: 1) as the various forms of social stigma associated with COVID-19. Furthermore, they found out that "health-risks, harassment, discrimination, life-insecurity, psychological disorder, loss of social capital and emotion capital, shattering family bond and social solidarity that work as barrier to community well-being" are many of the effects of social stigma. Although Mahmud and Islam did not explain what exactly a humour-prone stigma is, we consider it as a kind of stigma resulting from jocular or funny conversations or commentaries. The use of humour/satire by the Kabusa Choir in the song above is significant in two ways: first, it signals the subtle expression of societal perception of the virus as a capable of causing stigmatization. In the music video, for instance, a clergyman held a water hose at a distance for someone to wash his hand. Second, it provides the creative "hook" to attract listeners while disseminating the necessary information. This is evident in the part where they satirized about how illegal collection of money on the road by Nigerian Police men could be a potential way of them being infected. The last part of the song is even more poignant:

> Protect yourself and protect Africa
> Coronate yourself and coronate Africa [Infect yourself and infect Africa]
> Simple!

Religious/Spiritual Representation

Beyond representing COVID-19 as a public health matter which the populace needed to be sensitized, it was also given religious/spiritual representation. The reason for such spiritual representation demands some explanation. In the African ontological worldview, sicknesses and diseases are linked to both natural and spiritual factors. Medical imbalances are believed to be caused not only by transgressing certain hygienic requirement, but also a result of some supernatural forces. This makes it necessary therefore to seek divine intervention that undermine the sicknesses. This ontological perspective on diseases and the spiritual well-being of humans also crept into the musical representation of COVID-19. The Holy Trinity Church Youth Choir, Mushin, Lagos, represented COVID-19 as a matter of religious/spiritual concern:

> Lord we ask for your mercy and grace
> Heal the nations of this world
> Show us your glory and loving face
> Let your love direct and lead
> COVID-19 who art thou?
> Ravaging this sinful world
> By the name of Jesus Christ
> Surely we shall overcome

The music video, which was posted on Facebook on April 10, 2020, was presented in a four-part choral style. The performance venue, genre and text of the song have both religious and spiritual representations. The song, performed by a group of five singers dressed in choral robes in front of the chancel (altar) area in a church, is an adaptation of a Christian hymn—"Pleasant are Thy courts above" written by Henry Lyte with the tune "Maidstone". The song text above presents a prayer of penitence, direction, healing and resilience during a time of crisis. It therefore highlights the significance of religion in responding to and coping with epidemics. The foregoing corroborates research findings that religious explanations thrive during natural disasters and that religious practices including prayer offers coping strategy during adversity (Bentzen 2019; Dein et al. 2020). During the COVID-19 pandemic, many people sought for divine intervention through prayers especially when there was no vaccine to cure the virus. Coppen (2020) observed that the number of people who prayed increased during the pandemic.

The phrase, "COVID-19, who art thou? Ravaging this sinful world", signals the intrusion of apocalyptic reference which has been the response of some Christians to coronavirus disease. While some believe that the virus is part of God's plan as earlier prophesied by John in Revelation 6:1–8, others see it as divine punishment for an erring world. For example, Dein et al observed that "recently fundamentalist Protestants and radicalized Catholics have taken to the internet to propagate the views that the pandemic is a punishment for a variety of sins ranging from gay marriage, abortion, blasphemy, environmental pollution, paganism and witchcraft…." (2020: 5). The phrase "by the name of Jesus Christ, surely we shall overcome" in the song corroborates findings in previous studies on the role of religion as coping strategies during the coronavirus pandemic.

In another music video titled "Just one plague" by Esther Igbekele—a renowned Nigerian female gospel musician, coronavirus was represented as a spiritual plague. During the instrumental intro to the song, the musician instructed her listeners to make some declaratory statements: "Can somebody say after me, I dwell under the shadow of the Almighty and I possess divine immunity against all plagues and infirmities … Amen and amen!" Furthermore, Esther Igbekele narrated how the COVID-19 pandemic brought the whole world to a standstill. In the chorus section of the song, she sings:

> Just one plague, only plague
> Just one plague and world stood still
> They call am [it] coronavirus
> They call am [it] coronavirus
> Just one plague and world stood still

In the video, the artist, with the aid of motion and still images, narrated how global activities were halted by the pandemic:

> The world government was humbled
> The world powers got confused
> Everyone scampers for safety
> All economies shut down
> Mecca sent down worshippers
> Jerusalem sent back their tourists
> Vatican City was closed down
> All churches are shut down
> All mosques at closed door
> All sports are postponed

All clubs are sealed o
And the entertainment industry groaned for peace
Olympics is shutting down

The musician reminded her listeners of how several civil unrests and protests in different countries were put on hold by the coronavirus. According to her, COVID-19 is a plague that is beyond the efforts of medical scientists, hence the need for divine intervention. She prayed:

We need Divine intervention
because of this deadly disease
Them [they] call am [it] Coronavirus
O Lord, we don't want it again

After singing the first and second stanzas of the hymn "Thy Kingdom Come O God", she continued by citing a portion of the Bible, Psalm 18:45, wherein she reappropriated the virus as a "stranger" that should be expunged from the society—the world. She submits:

Psalm eighteen verse forty-five o
Na em [it] tell me say [that]
"The strangers shall fade away and
Be afraid out of the close places"
Coronavirus common hear the word of God
Na stranger you be for our land
Na stranger you be for the world
Pack your load, come dey go!
We don't want you anymore
We need our peace, Covid-19!
Coronavirus, pack your load oo dey go!
Coronavirus, pack your load oo dey go!

The personification of coronavirus by Esther Igbekele calls our attention to the correlation between religion, culture and personification of human and non-humans. Cohen (2011) argues that conferring the status of "person" on human or non-human is largely psychological and is influenced by the religious and cultural dispositions of the individual. For

Esther, the virus is anthropomorphic in nature with sensory components—of sight, touch, taste and ear thus attributing personhood to the virus which can be instructed to "pack and go". In Christianity, particularly in Charismatic settings, it is beleived that the spiritual world controls the physical reality. Little wonder why the musician believed that the virus is a physical manifestation of the spiritual and should be communicated with has a human entity. Rendered with a mix of English and the Nigerian Pidgin English, the song featured Nigerian-calypso style with some caller-response patterns. Like the Kabusa choir, Esther Igbekele realized almost all the musical instruments through digital sampling. Although she is from the south-western part of the country, she imitated the Igbo vocal style in her song. We encountered three-part voices in harmony at the chorus section and during the verses.

Sociopolitical Representation

For many people, the COVID-19 disease was not just a public health concern, it also facilitates some sociopolitical commentaries, especially about the infrastructural deficit in postcolonial African states. The pandemic exposed the bad politics that remains the bane of the underdevelopment predicament on the African continent. In Nigeria, the government's response to the outbreak of the virus was at best lukewarm. For example, it took the government a long time to shut its borders even when many countries had earlier taken such vital decision. Instead, top government officials travelled out of the country to attend functions in countries with very high infection rates. The pandemic also exposed the poor medical infrastructure that could have made a difference in the clinical management of the virus. This is the context which M-Josh's song "Coro Dagbo" is meant to represent:

When coro never show	Before the coronavirus was discovered
Dem say e don show	It was already announced
Say Italian man enter Lagos	That an Italian man entered Lagos
Country get plenty doctors	The country has many doctors
Money come fly	There was no money

Doctors con cure	Doctors can cure
When coro con show	When corona was eventually discovered
Hospitals close	Hospitals were closed
Everybody run, church shut down	Everybody run, churches were shut down
Professional doctors enter ghost mode	Professional doctors are nowhere to be found
Gbege con show for the Bigi man house	There is trouble in the big man's house

M-Josh reports the state of affairs of the nation which the pandemic has further exposed. He decries the poor state of the health sector "which has plenty doctors," but with hospital where even "professional doctors were nowhere to be found". Like many others, M-Josh believes that the virus has revealed deficiency in the nation's healthcare system that lacks qualified medical personnel and inadequate specialized hospitals to manage epidemics and pandemics. Isolations centres required to admit and treat infected persons were either moribund or non-existent. The outbreak of the pandemic from the first confirmed case by an Italian man in Lagos, the economic capital of the county, necessitated the efforts by both the federal and state governments to build new or in some cases renovate existing isolation centres.

The efforts by the government to compulsorily respond by providing necessary medical facilities in managing the pandemic, such as construction of isolation centres, have received criticism by some social commentators who believed that the interventions were mainly in the interest of the political class than for the masses. To better understand these critics, a brief survey of the healthcare system of the nation will be necessary. In Nigeria, the political class very often seek medical help outside the country, thus paying little or no attention to the healthcare system of the nation. The Nigerian political class is noted for its medical tourism, a state of affair that constitutes an open indictment of the country's policy incapacity. A news report notes:

> In terms of time spent abroad getting medical help, Nigeria's President Muhammadu Buhari, 74, is the first among equals, but in the past year all these heads of state have travelled overseas for health reasons. In many cases they are leaving behind poorly funded health services, which most of their citizens have to rely on. As for Nigeria, the public health system is "terrible" because of poor funding. ... A health insurance scheme for government workers and some private employees has given some people access to private medicine, but most people have to rely on government-funded services. In both countries, good private healthcare is available to those with money but in some cases there is a feeling that things are better abroad. The Nigerian president has spent more than four months in London this year getting treatment for an undisclosed illness, causing considerable disquiet at home. Unlike one of his predecessors, Umaru Musa Yar'Adua who went to Saudi Arabia to see a doctor, Mr Buhari did leave his deputy in charge, but this has not dampened the criticism. (BBC 2017)

The logical deduction from this political insensitivity is that the political class has no sense of governance direction, especially in terms of infrastructural development that Nigerians can benefit from. For M-Josh therefore:

Hospital na dagbo	Hospitals are fake
Facilities dagbo	Facilities are fake
Education na dagbo	Education is fake
Power supply na zero	Power supply is zero

The infrastructural deficit of the Nigerian state speaks to a development situation where what is available is not what is expected. And the pandemic has further made that reality starker. Following the declaration of the virus as a global pandemic by WHO, many countries suspended international flights, and this made travelling extremely impossible for whatever purposes, including medical tourism. This restriction left many top government functionaries with no choice than to seek medical services in private health facilities. For example, the death of the Chief of Staff to the President, Abba Kyari, followed a string of incidences that speak to the government's lackadaisical attitude to the pandemic. While other countries were frantically closing their borders and putting measures in place, Nigeria was slow to do the same. Kyari was reported to have been on an official trip to Germany sometimes in April 2020, where, according to the Garba Shehu, the senior special assistant to the Nigeria's president, he possibly contracted the virus. And because there was no possibility of traveling for medical treatment abroad, he lost his life. His demise caused lots of consternation in political circles. In an Afro hip-hop accompaniment style, this is how M-Josh represents it:

Now coro don show for area	Now there is corona in the community
News headline don talk am	It is reported in news headline that
Say Chief of Staff don carry am	The Chief of Staff has been infected
Say Governors don carry am	Governors have been infected
Say Ministers don carry am	Ministers have been infected
Say Senators don carry am	Senators have been infected
E be like President don carry am	It's like the President too has been infected

The unsubstantiated news of possible infection arguably can be linked to the social media space where information goes viral without any significant attempt at verifying their authenticity. However, the insincerity on the part of the Nigerian government in informing its citizens about the infection status of its official was also accountable for the "fake news" which circulated the social media.

For young people like M-Josh, the coronavirus pandemic was not just a matter of public health concern but also an urgent call for the complete overhauling of the social, economic, educational and the political systems of the country. For instance, when schools reopened in many countries of the world, they remained closed in Nigeria for long time. The reason is because the necessary tools to facilitate remote learning such as effective Internet broadband, electricity and computers are non-available or inadequate and obsolete where available. In addition, traditional classroom pedagogy is still widely practiced in Nigeria even when others in developed climes have migrated to virtual learning spaces.

M-Josh employed Afrobeat style in his music. Afrobeat, an urban popular music in Nigeria which developed in the late 1960s, is characterized by African percussion rhythms with a blend of jazz and funk. This style is reputed to be popularized by Fela Anikulapo-Kuti and scholars have observed how contemporary popular musicians in Nigeria appropriate

Fela's sound, text and symbols in their musical work (Osiebe 2020). Through electronic recording technology, M-Josh invoked the sonic components of Afrobeat style-groovy percussion and bass line with brass riffs. Using *yabis*, an abusive epithet of Fela's artistry through which he interrogates the socio-economic scandal of Nigeria governance (Salawu 2019: 14), M-Josh, like many of the performers sampled in this study, used Nigerian Pidgin English in his commentaries on the pandemic. As seen in his music video which is captured in figure 4, M-Josh performing almost half naked calls our attention to Osiebe's (2020) discussion about how Afrobeats musicians not only appropriate the text and sounds of Fela but also manifest his appearance in proliferating their art.

Conclusion

This chapter contributes to the growing corpus of scholarship on COVID-19 pandemic through its focus on the musical representation of the virus by young Nigerians on social media. In the face of public health crisis, young people found music-making not only as a form of entertainment but also as a means of coping during the lockdown. It was evident from the music videos analyzed that the coronavirus was musically represented under three prominent themes: public health, spiritual/religious and sociopolitical themes. Western choral and Nigerian choral dance as well as Afro hip-hop styles were creatively employed in these instances. Nigerian Pidgin English with code mixing featured prominently in the text of many of music videos selected for this study. As way of drawing viewers' and listener's attention to the message contained in the songs, the authors employed parody/satire in their music. Music for young people during the lockdown contributed to quarantine arts in Nigeria on one hand, while also offering public health awareness in curbing the spread of the virus on the other hand. Therefore, we assert that young people made music not just as entertainers, they equally served as health educators in public awareness on COVID-19 disease. The musical representation of COVID-19 by young people on the social media not only offered a space for social solidarity and resistance, but also served a sustainable means for public health advocacy in Nigeria.

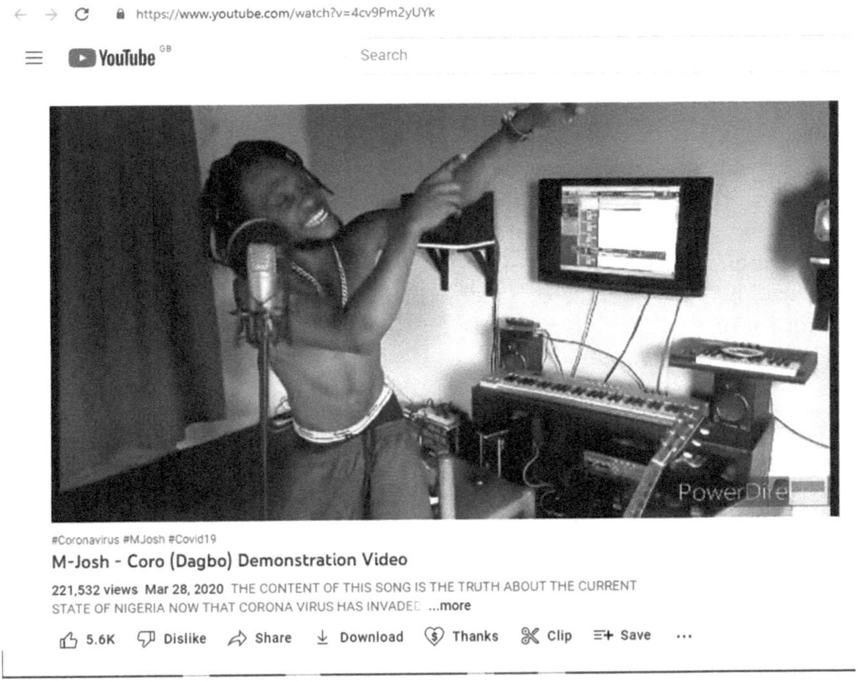

References

Acar, S., M. Neumayer, and C. Burnett. 2019. Social Media Use and Creativity: Exploring Influences on Ideational Behavior and Creative Activity. *The Journal of Creative Behavior* 55 (1): 39–52.

Agusi, E.R., S.I. Ijoma, C.S. Nnochin, N.O. Njoku-Achu, C.I. Nwosu, and C.A. Meseko. 2020. The COVID-19 Pandemic and Social Distancing in Nigeria: Ignorance or Defiance. *The Pan African Medical Journal* 35 (2): 52. https://doi.org/10.11604/pamj.2020.35.2.23649.

Ahmad, A.R., and H.R. Murad. 2020. The Impact of Social Media on Panic during COVID-19 Pandemic in Iraqi Kurdistan: Online Questionnaire Study. *Journal of Medical Internet Research* 22 (5): 1–11. http://www.jmir.org/2020/5/e19556/.

Ali, M.Y., and R. Bhatti. 2020. COVID-19 (Coronavirus) Pandemic: Information Sources Channels for the Public Health Awareness. *Asia Pacific Journal of Public Health* 32 (4): 168–169.

Arnett, J. 1991. Adolescents and Heavy Metal Music: From the Mouths of Metalheads. *Youths & Society* 23 (1): 76–98.

Aula, P. 2010. Social Media, Reputation Risk and Ambient Publicity Management. *Strategy and Leadership* 38 (6): 43–49.

BBC (British Broadcasting Service). 2017. Why do Buhari, Dos Santos and Mugabe Go to Hospital Abroad? Accessed 20 October 2020. https://www.bbc.com/news/world-africa-40685040.

Bentzen, J. S. 2019. Acts of God? Religiosity and Natural Disasters Across Subnational World Districts. *The Economic Journal* 129 (622): 2295–2321. https://doi.org/101093/ej/uez008.

Berenson, F. 1994. Representation and Music. *British Journal of Aesthetics* 34 (1): 60–68.

Bohlman, P.V. 2005. Music as Representation. *Journal of Musicological Research* 24 (3–4): 205–226. https://doi.org/10.1080/01411890500233924.

Brown, V. 2006. Guiding the Influence of Hip-Hop Music on Middle-School Students' Feelings, Thinking, and Behaving. *The Negro Educational Review* 57 (1–2): 49–68.

Centre for Disease Control (CDC). 2020. What is Social Distancing? *Centre for Disease Control.* https://www.cdc.gov/coronavirus/2019-ncov/videos/social-distance-people/social-distance-people.pdf.

Cohen, A. 2011. Religion, Culture, and the Personification on Non-human Entities. https://metanexus.net/religion-culture-and-personification-non-human-entities/.

Coppen, L. 2020. Will Coronavirus Hasten the Demise of Religion—or Herald its Revival? *The Spectator*, April 11. Accessed May 6, 2020. https://www.spectator.co.uk/article/will-coronavirus-cause-a-religious-resurgence-or-its-ruination.

Corrigan, P.K.J., K. Fokuo, and K. Kosyluk. 2014. Does Humor Influence the Stigma of Mental Illness? *The Journal of Nervous and Mental Disease* 202 (5): 397–401.

Dein, S., K. Loewenthal, C. A. Lewis, and K. I. Pargament. 2020. COVID-19, Mental Health and Religion: An Agenda for Future Research. *Mental Health, Religion & Culture* 23 (1): 1–9. https://doi.org/10.1080/13674676.2020.1768725.

Everett, C. 2010. Social Media: Opportunity or Risk? *Computer Fraud and Security* 6: 8–10.

Gupta, N. 2020. Singing Away the Social Distancing Blues: Art Therapy in a Time of Coronavirus. *Journal of Humanistic Psychology* 60 (5): 1–11. https://doi.org/10.1177/0022167820927807.

Hawdon, J., K. Parti, and T.E. Dearden. 2020. Cybercrime in America amid COVID-19: The Initial Results from a Natural Experiment. *American Journal of Criminal Justice* 45: 546–562. https://doi.org/10.1007/s12103-020-09534-4.

Jacobson, T. A, L. E. Smith, L. R. Hirschhorn, and M. D. Huffman. 2020. Using Implementation Science to Mitigate Worsening Health Inequities in the United States During the COVID-19 Pandemic. *International Journal for Equity in Health* 19 (1): 170. https://doi.org/10.1186/s12939-020-01293-2.

Kalahikhina, I. 2020. Demographic and Social Issues of the Pandemic. *Population and Economics* 4 (2): 103–122. https://doi.org/10.3897/popecon.4.e53891.

Kaplan, A. M., and M. Haenlein. 2010. Users of the World, Unite! The Challenges and Opportunities of Social Media. *Business Horizons* 53 (1): 59–68. https://doi.org/10.1016/j.bushor.2009.09.003.

Laurence, F., and O. Urbain. 2011. *Music and Solidarity*. Taylor & Francis.

Leung, A., and C. Kier. 2008. Music Preferences and Civic Activism of Young People. *Journal of Youth Studies* 11 (4): 445–460. https://doi.org/10.1080/13676260802104790.

Macdonald, R.A. 2013. Music, Health, and Well-Being: A Review. *International Journal of Qualitative Studies on Health and Well-being* 8 (1): 1–13. https://doi.org/10.3402/qhw.v8i0.20635.

Mahadevan, P. 2020. Cybercrime Threats during the COVID-19 Pandemic. Global Initiative Against Transnational Organized Crime. www.globalinitiative.net.

Mahmud, A., and M.R. Islam. 2020. Social Stigma as a Barrier to Covid-19 Responses to Community Well-being in Bangladesh. *International Journal of Community Well-Being*: 1–7. https://doi.org/10.1007/s42413-020-00071-w.

McNiff, S. 1998. *The Arts and Psychotherapy*. 1st ed. Charles C Thomas Publishing.

Melo, M.C.A., and D. Sousa Soares. 2020. Impact of Social Distancing on Mental Health during the COVID-19 Pandemic: An Urgent Discussion. *International Journal of Social Psychiatry*. https://doi.org/10.1177/0020764020927047.

Mofredj, A., S. Alaya, K. Tassaioust, H. Bahloul, and A. Mrabet. 2016. Music Therapy, a Review of the Potential Therapeutic Benefits for the Critically Ill.

Journal of Critical Care 35: 195–199. https://doi.org/10.1016/j.jcrc.2016.05.021.

Naidoo, R. 2020. A Multi-level Influence Model of COVID-19 Themed Cybercrime. *European Journal of Information Systems* 29 (3): 306–321. https://doi.org/10.1080/0960085X.2020.1771222.

Nicholls, T. 2014. Music and Social Justice. *Internet Encyclopedia of Philosophy*. http://www.iep.utm.edu/music-sj/.

NOIPolls. 2019. Social Media Poll Reports. Retrieved November 2019. https://noi-polls.com/social-media-poll-result-release/

Obi-Ani, N.A., C. Anikwenze, and M.C. Isiani. 2020. Social Media and the COVID-19 Pandemic: Observations from Nigeria. *Cogents Arts and Humanities* 7 (1): 1–15. https://doi.org/10.1080/23311983.2020.1799483.

Osiebe, G. 2020. Methods in Performing Fela in Contemporary Afrobeats. *African Studies* 79 (1): 88–109. https://doi.org/10.1080/00020184.2020.1750349.

Quian, M., and J. Jiang. 2020. COVID-19 and Social Distancing. *Journal of Public Health: From Theory to Practice*. https://doi.org/10.1007/s10389-020-01321-z.

Roberts, D.F., and P.G. Christenson. 2001. Popular Music in Childhood and Adolescence. In *Handbook of Children and the Media*, ed. D.G. Singer and J.L. Singer, 395–413. Thousand Oaks, CA: Sage.

Robinson, L., J. Streuli, and A. R. Fidalgo. 2019. Social Media's Impact on Creative Thought. In *2019 11th International Conference on Knowledge and Smart Technology (KST)*, January 23–26. https://doi.org/10.1109/KST.2019.8687632.

Ross, A. 1994. "Introduction." In *Microphone Friends: Youth Music and Youth Culture*, edited by A. Ross and T. Rose, 1-13. New York: Routledge.

Sahni, H., and H. Sharma. 2020. Role of Social Media During the COVID-19 Pandemic: Beneficial, Destructive, or Reconstructive? *International Journal of Academic Medicine* 6 (2): 70–75. https://doi.org/10.4103/IJAM.IJAM_50_20.

Salawu, O.M. 2019. *Abami Eda:* "Personhood and Socio-political Commitment in Fela's Music". *Muziki* 16: 4–21.

Santiago, A.M., and R.J. Smith. 2020. Community Practice, Social Action, and the Politics of Pandemics. *Journal of Community of Practice* 28 (2): 89–99. https://doi.org/10.1080/10705422.2020.1763744.

Scruton, R. 1976. Representation in Music. *Philosophy* 51 (197): 273–287. https://doi.org/10.1017/S0031819100019331.

Sheppard, A., and M.C. Broughton. 2020. Promoting Wellbeing and Health through Active Participation in Music and Dance: A Systematic Review. *International Journal of Qualitative Studies on Health and Well-Being* 15: 1–19. https://doi.org/10.1080/17482631.2020.1732526.

Whittaker, E., and R.M. Kowalski. 2015. Cyberbullying via Social Media. *Journal of School Violence* 14: 11–29.

Online Discography

1. Kabusa Oriental Choir., 2020. https://www.facebook.com/watch/?v=208059203856663&external_log_id=70daef3f293f37345e8877e21c7eb4e3&q=kabusa%20oriental%20choir%20coro retrieved March 10, 2021
2. The Oyedeles., 2020. https://www.facebook.com/tosin.oloyeoyewole/videos/10222549495824986/ retreived March 20, 2021
3. Holy Trinity Church Youth Choir, Mushin, Lagos., 2020. https://www.facebook.com/chidubem.onyesoh/videos/4022017841149184/ retrieved April 10, 2021
4. What is Social Distancing?, 2020. *Centre for Disease Control*, https://www.cdc.gov/coronavirus/2019-ncov/videos/social-distance-people/social-distance-people.pdf.

18

COVID-19, Food and Freedom to Worship: An Analytic Approach to Nigeria's Religioscape

Benson Ohihon Igboin

Introduction

In late December 2019, the first experience of the novel coronavirus, later code-named COVID-19, was announced by the Chinese government. The first instance was in Wuhan province, in a market where different kinds of meat were sold. The World Health Organization (WHO) declared COVID-19 a pandemic in January 2020 and announced preventive measures such as social distancing, wearing of face mask, regular washing of hands, use of alcohol-based sanitizer, avoiding crowded places and so on. In February 2020, an Italian man from Milan brought the coronavirus to Nigeria, and the eventual spread resulted in the initial lockdown as a measure to curtail further spread and to trace those who had contracted the disease. On 29 March, President Muhammadu Buhari announced the total lockdown of Lagos, Ogun, and Abuja, the Federal

B. O. Igboin (✉)
Department of Religion and African Culture, Adekunle Ajasin University, Ondo, Nigeria
e-mail: benson.igboin@aaua.edu.ng

F. Egbokhare, A. Afolayan (eds.), *Global Health, Humanity and the COVID-19 Pandemic*, https://doi.org/10.1007/978-3-031-17429-2_18

Capital Territory, for two weeks in the first instance. The president announced that all public and private establishments including religious worship centres should observe the lockdown. Only those on essential duties like medical personnel, the police, journalists and so on should cautiously go about their assignments. Markets were partially locked down in the sense that first, some were relocated to places considered to be more spacious and safe, and second, they were to operate on certain days of the week and within specified hours (Olukoya and Mohammed 2020; Bishi et al. 2020).

The reason for the partial lockdown of markets was to enable citizens have access to food. The government believed that it would be unreasonable to completely lock down the markets as other public and private spaces since people would not have access to food. Food was essential to human beings; in fact, without it, many people would die despite the coronavirus. As Agatha Chikelue, the Executive Director of the Cardinal Onaiyekan Foundation and Coordinator of Religious for Peace's Interfaith Women's Network observed, "people are afraid of dying of 'Hovid'—the hunger caused as a result of loss of livelihoods from the lockdown" than COVID-19 itself (Karam and Ali 2020). Bolarinwa (2020: 32) shares the same observation: "the resistance of people against the government directives on lockdown was predicated upon lack of means of survival as someone warned that the government should ease the lockdown so that after the Pandemic, people will not suffer 'hunger pandemic.'" Both Chikelue and Bolarinwa raised concern on the immediate and post-COVID-19 effects of COVID-19 on food and its accessibility in the country such as deaths and increased rate of criminality. Their interest apparently lies heavily on human survival rather than human freedom. But implicitly, their position reifies freedom because freedom of movement to places or sources of food has been tampered with by the order of staying at home. Nothing else sharply brought it to people's consciousness than the lockdown when everyone could feel the very presence taken for granted in pre-COVID era (Zizek 2020). In the same vein, the presidential order also brought the stark realization that freedom of, or restriction on, corporate worship can be tampered with by the government

The argument or reaction of some of the religious leaders, particularly some Pentecostal pastors, which forms the fulcrum of this chapter, is that not only would government have considered them as essential workers as those who minister to human souls (like medical personnel who minister to human body), but also the churches should not have been closed down because they are the 'theaters' for ministering to the souls. Bishop David Oyedepo, the founder of the Living Faith Church Worldwide (aka Winners' Chapel), is one of the most vociferous voices against the lockdown. Oyedepo questions the continued lockdown of churches whereas the markets are open. According to him, there is no evidence that people who congregate in market places observe the COVID-19 protocols such as washing hands, keeping social and physical distancing, wearing face masks and so on. Oyedepo satirically reacts thus: "Everyone is in the market running over each other every day of the week and there is no outbreak but there is now outbreak, perceived outbreak from the church.... Now, freedom of worship is no longer a constitutional right but now determined to buy some individuals" (Royal 2020). Oyedepo further maintains that by shutting the churches, the government has infringed on the fundamental human right of the Christians to worship. Oyedepo believes that the lockdown is 'anti-church' rather than a measure to stop the spread of the coronavirus. He adds: "the church is God's banquet hall where we are fed with spiritual food to keep us alive and strong. So, whatever stops the church from fellowshipping is out to destroy what God is building. There must be a devil behind it. It is not virus, it is demon" (Olukoya and Mohammed 2020). Oyedepo further posits that healing does not take place in the markets but in churches. Thus, allowing the markets to be opened was to tacitly ensure the spread of the disease, whereas if the churches were not shut, the disease would have been curtailed more effectively because of the healing power of God.

Oyedepo holds that closing the church is synonymous with closing hospitals. Since hospitals and markets were not closed during the lockdown, he proceeded to hold Sunday service in defiance to the presidential lockdown order. Curiously, while the police prevented some churches from holding services, arrested some pastors during the worship, Oyedepo was neither prevented from holding services nor arrested (Ogundipe 2020). This raises critical questions about the relations between church and state, which will be considered shortly. Interestingly, Oyedepo's reconsideration of his position on holding services during the lockdown was not essentially due to the fear of government enforcement of the lockdown order, but apparently due to the fear of losing his clientele, most of whom, though believed in him, were afraid of being either arrested for violating the order or actually contracting the disease in the church (Ogundipe 2020). However, in apologizing for flouting the lockdown order, Oyedepo carefully argues that the church could be a veritable medium for the dissemination of information to the public about the pandemic. He submits that the church complied substantially with the directive as its universities and other schools immediately shut down.

> There has (sic) been diverse responses varying from well-meaning concerns to uncharitable insinuations, misinterpretations, and unfounded allegations that the service was held in deliberate defiance of Ogun State Government ban on high-density gatherings, in the wake of COVID-19 pandemic. Nothing can be further from the truth. For avoidance of doubt, as stakeholders and as a responsible organisation, the Living Faith Church fully supports and encourages compliance with all initiatives of government to combat the spread of this dreaded virus. However, information has to be strategically disseminated to the grassroot, noting that the Church is a family and not an industry, it is for this reason that enlightenment and sensitization from the church platform is a most effective way to get people involved in playing their part in terms of prayers and intercessions and not just staying away from Church without knowing what to do.... To show how law abiding our organisation is and in compliance with government directives, all our primary and secondary schools across the nation have been directed to close down. Also, our students at Landmark University... were sent back home, while Covenant University Students (sic)... were instructed to stay back at home.... (PM News 2020)

For many of the pastors, the Nigerian markets, unlike the grocery stores in Europe and America, are not as organized as the churches. To be sure, a typical Nigerian market scene cannot effectively ensure the observance of social and physical distancing just as some rituals (e.g. praise and worship, dancing and thanksgiving) in many Pentecostal churches. In other words, according to these pastors, churches are more organized and could meet the standard of physical distancing than any local market during the lockdown. It is for these reasons that a few of them (initially) resisted and defied the presidential order, which resulted in the questions whether food or freedom to worship was more essential and beneficial to the citizens at the time of the lockdown or whether the pastors who disobeyed the order were forming an alternative state. While many Pentecostal churches criticized the government for the lockdown, they also donated food and gave financial support to their members, government and general public (Irekamba and Taiwo 2020). The resort to donate food, Ayeni (2020) argues, is to find alternative way of feeding their congregations. Many Pentecostal churches offer food to members, especially new entrants every Sunday. This practice has kept many people in the church as they are sure that, at least, a meal awaits them on Sundays. The lockdown was therefore a move to take away their free meal, a reason among others, the congregation supported their leaders in opposing the lockdown order in addition to the benefits they derive from corporate worship.

In what follows, we shall conceptualize food and freedom: the relationship between food and freedom and how one affects the other in choice-making and how food as an instrument defines one's position in the polity. The following section will espouse theological issues bordering on food and freedom within specific context; the context of exodus because it clearly depicts contexts in which a person or group of people may prefer food to freedom or vice versa, or even both. But the exodus experience is placed with a somewhat theocratic government where rules are dictated by a divine authority other than man. This thus leads to the discussion on the nature of Nigeria's secularity. It is argued that Nigeria's secularity is a peculiar one because of the influence of different religious traditions that have impugned on it. Thereafter, we will examine how food and freedom played out during the lockdown, and the last part will be the conclusion.

Conceptualizing Food and Freedom

Food is important for the survival of all living things from birth to death. Thus, food is a basic human need. Akanji (2002: 13) defines food as "all substances or mixture of substances both solid and liquid which are intended for human consumption or ingestion for nutritional and/or pleasurable benefits." He argues that it is not just to eat at a point that makes a person healthy, but the continuous availability of food gives psychological and physiological satisfaction. According to Aktas-Polat and Polat (2020: 280), food is "a glorious thing in the center of biological and social life, [which] expresses that we eat for days, seasons and years to satisfy our physical hunger, our emotions and to feed our bellies." Apart from the biological and social meaning of food, Albala (2013: 1) asserts that "Feeding people has always been the primary concern of our species, and more than any other factor, finding, growing and trading food products has been the prime catalyst in human history." Albala traces the historical and cultural development of foods across different continents. Briley and Jackson (2016) conceive food as medicine as well as poison. They add that food has historical, social, cultural, religious, spiritual and political dimensions and roles it plays in human society. For Chinea et al. (2020), "the meaning of food is determined by learning and cultural transmission." Thus, food carries cultural, identity, symbolic and moral import, which varies from culture to culture. Aktas-Polat and Polat (2020) further posit that food has correlation with human rights.

The issues of food and freedom have been sources of conflicts in history. Sen's (1987) seminal thought on food and freedom as social ethical issues presses home the significant roles food plays in human freedom. According to him, even though food and freedom may seem not to have a relationship at first, a deeper study will reveal that both do affect how humans relate with the consequences of availability and lack of both. Sen holds the view that

> The provision of food is indeed a central issue in general social ethics, since much in human life does depend on the ability to find enough to eat. In particular, the freedom that people enjoy to lead a decent life, including freedom from hunger, from avoidable morbidity, from premature mortality etc., is quite centrally connected with the provision of food and related necessities. Also, the compulsion to acquire enough food may force vulnerable people to do things which they resent doing, and may make them accept lives with little freedom. The role of food in fostering freedom can be an extremely important one. (Sen 1987: 1)

Sen further avers that freedom is critical to food accessibility and healthy life. He argues that freedom can be conceived in different ways such as negative and positive freedom. In its negative form, freedom means independence or non-interference from other people, agencies, institutions and so forth. Positive freedom is thought of as what "a person is actually able to do or to be" (Sen 1987: 3). These two forms of freedom are interrelated in practical ways. For instance, if an individual lacks food, there is the tendency that he may not be able to enjoy positive freedom. In other words, to be negatively free does not automatically guarantee achieving positive freedom. Sen again elucidates this point as follows:

> If a person is not free from hunger and lacks the means and the practical opportunities to feed himself or herself adequately, then that person's positive freedom must be seen as having been thoroughly compromised. On the other hand, his or her negative freedom may be completely unviolated, if this failure to acquire enough food is not a result of his or her having been stopped by interference from others. (Sen 1987: 3)

Sen's view can lead to conceptualizing freedom as both intrinsic and instrument; in the former, freedom has value in itself and it is constitutive of what it achieves. Instrumental freedom implies that it is a means to an end. Although food has been a tool for power and empowerment, it is also an instrument for control and negotiation. As a political instrument, food has been used to manipulate the will and wishes of people who would have acted otherwise. The widespread use of food as political bait during elections in Nigeria is a case that elicits a systematic study. Staples such as garri, rice, beans and so on in ridiculously small quantities are always being offered to electorates by politicians to secure their votes (Olu-Adeyemi 2018). Joanna Macrae and Anthony Zwi (1992: 299) argue that "the use of food as a weapon of war by omission, commission and provision has contributed to the creation of famine in recent decades" in Africa. By omission, they mean occasions deriving from government's refusal or inability to monitor food and plan for food security for the country. Commission implies acts of direct or indirect attacks on the sources and means of production and procurement of food. In addition, provision speaks to situations where government deliberately supplies food to those who support it to the detriment of those who oppose it, especially in a conflict or war situation.

Many scholars have interrogated the role that food played in the determination of the Nigerian Civil War (1967–1970). Iwuagwu (2012: 284), for instance, posits that the Nigerian federal troops' continuous bombardment on sources of food for the Biafran soldiers and people was a tactical and decisive strategy that, among other factors, led to the surrender of Biafra. "By the end of 1968, virtually all the major food producing areas of Igboland have come under the federal troops…. It has been argued that it was the loss of major food producing areas … to the federal troops in fact, more than any other factor that led to the collapse of Biafra." Starvation therefore became a veritable weapon of war. William Schanbacher (2010: vii) expresses the view that the weaponization and politicization of food by such powerful institutions as World Bank and International Monetary Fund have generated many global reactions. According to him, "riots protesting the World Trade Organization (WTO) on the streets of Seattle in 1999, global demonstrations against the World Bank and the International Monetary Fund (IMF), and civil unrest around the world due to rising food prices … all speak to a growing global awareness of and discontent with the fact that the basic necessity of food is not reaching hundreds of millions of people around the world each year." Schanbacher emphasizes that fighting for food is synonymous with fighting for freedom as these institutions' policies on food are geared toward actual denial of food to millions of people, while making huge profits.

In her "Food for Freedom," Potorti (2015: vi) argues that hunger in the midst of superabundance of food in the US during the civil rights era was the cannon fodder for the proponents of black freedom who aptly recognized "the capacity of food to perpetuate oppression and to promote human equality." Potorti further stresses that food is inherently political, and it has the propensity to change political action and narrative depending on how it is utilized. The politics of food, defined around whether to eat or deliberately refuse to eat, is a powerful tool for political organizing and negotiating. Accordingly, "the politics of food—here defined as personal, local, organizational, and national power struggles driven by fundamental concerns of who can eat what and under what conditions—came to be viewed by movement activists as both a means of social control and, conversely, as a call to arms to recruit the hungry for political organization at its most basic level" (Potorti 2015: 2). Food, she avers, has political, cultural, racial, social and religious dimensions, all of which have impact on personhood and identity. Food does not only define personhood and identity; hunger not only defines one's place in the social order, it also marks one's exclusion from the polity.

Theology of Food and Freedom

Theologically, the relationship between food and freedom is a complex one. It can be argued that human beings, as free moral agents, are prone to making critical moral choices depending sometimes on exigent or ultimate considerations. This applies to freedom and food in the case of the Israelites before, in Egypt, and shortly thereafter. The biblical account posits that there was famine in Canaan where Jacob and his family had settled for a period of time. As shepherds, they tended their animals and lived "freely." The freedom enjoyed in Canaan weaned and waned when there was famine in the land and critical decision had to be made whether or not to remain in Canaan and die of hunger or migrate to Egypt and lose their freedom. Jacob really had his fear, especially the safety of his son Benjamin. But the ultimate decision was taken in favour of migrating to Egypt where there was food in order to survival. It would appear that the Israelites at the time of migration to Egypt did not contemplate the place of freedom in their existence (Gen. 41–46). In any case, the children of Israel lived in Egypt for 430 years. At Goshen, where they settled in, they had access to fertile land where they catered for their cattle. Considering where they were coming from and the exigent reason—famine—for their migration, freedom was not a premium to them. In fact, right from their arrival in Egypt and their settlement in Goshen, it is clear that they were segregated. By their very occupation—shepherding—the migrant Israelites could not be fully integrated into Egypt. "So it shall be, when Pharaoh calls you and says, 'What is your occupation?' that you shall say, 'Your servants' occupation has been with livestock from our youth even till now, both we and also our fathers,' that you may dwell in the land of

Goshen; *for every shepherd is an abomination to the Egyptians*" (Gen.46:33–34 Emphasis added).

What this implies is that during the time of Joseph, the Israelites apparently sacrificed freedom on the altar of food. Their freedom was completely lost when Joseph, who had facilitated their migration from Canaan where there was famine to Egypt where there was access to food, died and a new regime was instituted in Egypt that did not take cognizance of the contributions of Joseph to Egypt's economy (Ex. 1:8). The resultant treatment meted out on the Israelites made them to realize that they needed their freedom rather than food. With this realization came the fundamental question of whether they would continue eating in bondage. This is not only a normative question, but also a political one. Here, the Israelites would later be faced with a dilemma: should they return to Egypt and eat or to go to Canaan and live freely? The decision was taken in favour of the latter, at least while still in Egypt. This decision was activated by the struggle for liberation, hence the exodus. But not long thereafter, the Israelites were faced with the vicissitudes of life in the wilderness. The reality of the newly gotten freedom was put to test when there was attack, lack of water and food. Again, decision had to be taken: whether to go back to Egypt, that is, bondage and yet enjoy food or hold on to freedom without food and possibly die. At this point, there was a division among the people: some believed strongly that food was better than freedom while some held that freedom was better than food, yet another small group believed that food without freedom was vain and freedom with food was tempting. Rijneveld (2003: 11–12) sums up the Israelites' experience thus:

> The problem was the attack of the Egyptians, the second was the water problem in Mara, now a food problem, the fourth will be a water problem again at Refidim and the fifth attack again. This is a chiasmic structure (attack—water—food—water—attack), in which the middle element is often meant to receive emphasis: the food problem.... They remember Egypt obviously with rose-tinted glasses.... Egypt is to be seen as the pot with meat. They did not really get so much meat every day, but the security of food being present for the day and morrow was what they longed after. The security stands for comfort, brick quotas are forgotten. This is the essence of salve mentality.... God delayed to assist them, 'because he will first try their fortitude and the pleasure they take in their freedom, that he

may learn whether they have souls great enough to bear the want of food or whether they rather love to be slaves.'

From the narrative above, it can be suggested that freedom and food dialectics has some contextual underpinning. In other words, different contexts determine whether food is more important than freedom. In Egypt, the value of freedom seemed not to be initially realized and prioritized; it was an ideal that was anticipated without actually contemplating the price and hardship that would be endured to gain and sustain it. Of course, the Israelites were all happy leaving Egypt, with hope of a better, freer and prosperous future. The enthusiasm of freedom was almost completely lost in another context where there was no water or food: "they preferred the fleshpots of Egypt above their newly gained freedom" (Rijneveld 2003: 1). In the wilderness, food seems to be more profitable and valuable than freedom for the Israelites. In fact, they seemed to suggest that you have to live in order to have freedom. What is the value of freedom to a dead person anyway? The absence of food at the moment greatly contrasts with freedom from the oppression in Egypt (Igboin 2018).

The second thought has to do with the management of freedom. Freedom is not free; it has responsibilities. The Israelites most clearly undermined the struggle that culminated in their freedom. They did not estimate the full realities and dimensions of the values and benefits that freedom could and would afford them afterwards. How do we gauge this? Despite the colossal losses and the nation-wide pain and mourning in Egypt, Pharaoh and his cabinet understood what freedom for Israel meant for the economy of Egypt. Pharaoh must have compared the amount of food consumed by the Israelites against the economic values that they generated. For Pharaoh, the political economy of food is critical to the sustenance of his country. He came to the astute decision that it was more profitable to keep the Israelites in bondage with food than to allow them enjoy their freedom and its prosperity, which, of course, was not immediately visible to the Israelites (Igboin 2018).

What we can possibly infer from the foregoing is that food is critical in freedom discourse and vice versa. But different contexts made the Israelites to make different choices. Shortly, it will be shown how context affects the government decision to open markets and close churches and how the reactions of the latter impact on the secularity of the country. In so doing, it is important to undergird our thought by realizing that the exodus experience took place within a theocratic order where instructions were given by a divine authority—Yahweh—the same theocratic order Pentecostal churches have recourse to in their conception of secularity. But that does not also preclude human free choice. As we have seen, despite the divine order, the Israelites still attempted to make decisions on the basis of what they believed best suit their condition. It would therefore seem that divine authority does not completely rule out human moral agency.

Secularity in Nigeria's Religioscape

According to Onishi (2018: 4–5), while "secularism is an ideology that adheres to the idea of a modern project of emancipation based on the strict regulation of religion in the public sphere," secularity "is not an ideology to enact, but a mode of comportment to the world." In this sense, secularism implies that religion should be consigned to private practice. Secularism theory states that religion constitutes an obstruction to order, truth, meaning and so on in society. Casanova (1994: 1) argues that secularization thesis is founded on three fundamental components, namely; decline of religion generally, privatization of religion and increase in institutional differentiation of modern society. Warner lays it out more clearly when he states that secularization is "understood to be both a process of social change, closely intertwined with the evolution of the modern world, and also a theory of increasing religious marginalization not only descriptive of present and past transitions, but predictive of a future society where religion would have little or no public influence, social utility or plausible claim to a revelatory authority that in any sense transcended reason" (Offiong and Ekpo 2020: 151). Scholars like Peter Berger, Thomas Luckmann, Harvey Cox, Jose Casanova among others have at one time or the other maintained that religion would decline from the public sphere and secularism would take over. However, Cox (1995) sprang a surprise when in 1995 he published his *Fire from Heaven: The Rise of Pentecostal Spirituality and the Re-shaping of Religion in the Twenty-first Century*. Cox seems to have converted from the 'death of God' thesis to the abundance of God's presence in a secular world. In 1999, Berger also reversed his thesis to accept the reality of a flourishing religious influence in the public sphere. He states: "My point is that the assumption that we live in a secularized world is false. The world today, with some exceptions… is furiously religious as it ever was, and in some places more than ever" (Onishi 2018: 3). In fact, Jeffrey Hadden would add that "secularization theory had not been subjected to a systematic scrutiny because it is a doctrine more than a theory" (Onishi 2018: 4).

Although the secularization thesis once predicted that religion would fade out of the public sphere, the events of 9/11 have resurged interest in the study of the influence of religion in politics at both national and international levels. In fact, Toft, Philpott and Shah (2011: 2) describe the twenty-first century as "God's Century." What this means is that religion is as furiously present in the public sphere as it was in the pre-Enlightenment era. There is hardly any news item today that is not coloured with religious sentiment, motivation, belief or idea. In the case of Nigeria, Obadare (2018) argues that the rise and influence of Pentecostal Christianity poses a challenge to the dominant argument hitherto held about the relationship between the state and religion. The Pentecostal Christianity appears to be a militant wing of Christianity at the turn of democracy in 1999.

The nature of secularity in Nigeria is complex because of the different opinions Christians and Muslims have maintained about it. For the most part, some Muslims view the concept of secularism as godlessness or atheism. Lateef Adegbite, one of the prominent and articulate Muslim scholars, vehemently rejected secularism as connoting godlessness and atheism. According to him, "No Moslem will support a secular state. I want to say it with all the emphasis at my command because as far as we are concerned, secularity means 'godlessness', and Moslems will never support it" (Ogbu 2014: 5). Some Muslim scholars have expressed that Adegbite's view is an extreme one. Abdulrasheed Muhammad, for instance, argues that rather than conceive secularism as godlessness and atheism, it should be thought of as an ideology that promotes the view that the state should not be concerned about religion in the public sphere. The political authority is to be seen as instituted independently from religious or supernatural forces. The state does not have recourse to extraneous authority beyond the provisions of its constitution (Ogbu 2014: 5). Some others who do not align with either of the two positions canvassed above describe Nigeria simply as multi-religious country, a term they consider most appropriate since the Preamble of the constitution and the National Anthem have recourse to God (Igboin 2014). At the heat of the sharia crisis in 2000, President Olusegun Obasanjo had to cautiously avoid the use of the term—secularity—preferring to describe Nigeria as a multireligious state. For him, the sharia was purely a political one, which he argued would fizzle out naturally after some time (Igboin 2014).

Although Christianity has been figured as originating and spreading secularism, Christians do not conceive it as depicting godlessness. Ogbu's (2014) etymological exploration of the term unravels the context within which Christians conceived it: it was used to differentiate the divine from the mundane, the time-bound values and eternal values. Therefore, Christians conceptualize secularism as pertaining to the world rather than being godless. But with time, the application of the term extended to sharp boundaries between eternal and mundane values. By the time of the Enlightenment, secularism had assumed a radically different meaning that appropriated godlessness within its borders. Thus, there was to be a dichotomy between the supernatural and the mundane, the state and church. But in Nigeria, one of the most telling differences between the Christians and Muslims is that whereas the former see secularity as not occluding God, but that the state should be neutral with reference to religion, the latter hold that any sovereignty that contradicts the Islamic faith is tantamount to godlessness. Nkwoka (2006: 328) puts it succinctly: "whereas the Church is basically demanding for a secular state in Nigeria so that the double citizenship can be maintained by Christians, Muslims especially in Sharia states contend that the best is a theocratic state."

This is clearly brought to the fore during the implementation of sharia in 1999–2002 in the northern part of Nigeria. The sharia issue complicates the positions both Christians and Muslims hold in secularity discourse. In fact, Fox (2011), Ogbu (2014) and Offiong and Ekpo (2020) conclude that the constitution of Nigeria is a peculiar one in the study and exercise of secularity because it both bans and approves of state and federal governments adopting religion. Ogbu apparently maintains that constitutionally Nigeria is a secular state despite the praxis of sharia and government involvement in religion. For Fox, such a straightforward declaration of Nigeria's secularity is difficult because the paradox (of not approving a state religion and yet allowing a sharia court to an appellate level) needs to be resolved in the constitution, which, of course, requires a great deal of political will. Offiong and Ekpo (2020: 168) assert that Nigeria cannot be regarded as a secular state but a "theocratic diarchy," that is, "a dual religious state with clear canons on what constitute the state, the Gods, the law, the people, the checks and the balances."

As noted earlier, the rise and influence of Pentecostal movement is redrawing the map of secularity argument in the country. Pentecostal churches, particularly the megachurches, have traversed the 'split' or gap between the state and church. Obadare (2018), Marshall (2009), Vaughan (2016), Ukah (2020) among others have explored how Pentecostal faith is challenging the hitherto religious terrain dominated by Islam and orthodox Christianity. In fact, rather than maintain some distance from the state, the Pentecostal Christians are pushing to the center of political authority and trying to dominate and use it to their advantage, on the one hand. On the other, they hold tightly to their churches as the base for their public or political interest and influence (Igboin 2020). Igboin argues that many Nigerian Pentecostal pastors attempt to form an alternative state within the nation-state. They tend to build a state that more or less allows participation of members in their communitarian unity. He observes that

> This kind of political theology thinks of a contrastive parallel to the secular political ideology that births and fosters injustice and oppression. In conceiving its political theology, Pentecostalism is actively engaged in setting up an alternative state, though one without a physical military.... This form of contrastive politics is borne out of the realisation that the church cannot effectively manipulate the power structure of the secular politics for its advantage, especially in a multi-ethnic and religious country like Nigeria. (Igboin 2020: 10–11)

This is not without resistance, and/or parallel from Islamic religion, especially the rise of Nasrul-lahi-li Fathi Society of Nigeria (NASFAT), which is adopting similar Pentecostal strategies in their spiritual and public engagement (Obadare 2016).

The vision of 'converting the world for Christ' and dominating it as a Christian mandate tends to blur the line of demarcation between the church and state. Pentecostals, as Togarasei (2015) observes, have not only fought against secularism but are secular themselves in many ways. He states that "secularisation in Pentecostal churches is seen in how they have undermined the traditional values in favour of modern, secular values" (Togarasei 2015: 60). Acolatse (2021) shares a similar opinion when she argues that rather than secularization being a bane of Pentecostalism, it has become an instrument or partner in imagining the acts of God. The dichotomy between the other-worldly and this-worldly is collapsed because of the belief that both dimensions are not only composite, but also belong to the same divine being and/or order, which they, the Pentecostals mediate. It is the same God that animates the secular and the religious and as such, the Pentecostal believes that rugged separation means ceding apart of creation to God and the other to man. Borrowing from Nimi Wariboko's thought, Acolatse believes that Nigerian Pentecostalism focuses more on the material, secular goal than spiritual, even though spiritual capital plays an important role in achieving the former. The political and the spiritual are embedded in one: "Pentecostalism and secularization in Nigeria have found a happy medium in the soil of the penchant for the commodification that drives both…. We are hard press to follow the optimistic voice that leads through the terrain especially when it comes to civil society and the claim of Pentecostal theology in preaching and teaching about what sometimes sounds like a return to theocracy" (Acolatse 2021: 234). The Pentecostal recourse to God's imprimatur in the public sphere is quintessentially a theocratic flair. It is this theocratic penchant that is exuded during the lockdown.

The Lockdown, Food, Worship and Secularity

Availability and accessibility to food are important to any population. This is more acute during the lockdown occasioned by the COVID-19. With the coronavirus and second recession in five years in Nigeria, food prices have risen astronomically. PwC (2020: 11) sums it up thus:

> Prior to COVID-19, Nigeria's agricultural sector is affected by several challenges ranging from drought and flooding occasioned by climate change, and widespread instabilities including Boko Haram crisis, cattle rustling in the North and farmer-herder clashes across the South and Middle Belt.... By the end of the first half of 2020, the number of people from the 16 Northern states suffering from acute food insecurity is projected to increase to seven million people. In March 2020, Nigeria was enlisted among 44 countries globally that require external food assistance.

Of course, with COVID-19, the rate of depletion of food reserves will definitely accelerate faster than its replacement. Partial effect of COVID-19 on food resonated in October 2020 when hoodlums across many parts of the country invaded warehouses and charted away COVID-19 food palliatives allegedly hoarded by the government. The rising rate of criminalities and civil unrest may give vent to the old Chinese proverb: "you cannot lead a people you cannot feed" (Igboin 1997: 57). The government must have considered this when it decided to open markets so that people could access food and also provided some palliatives meant to ameliorate the effects of the lockdown.

Even though the Nigerian government claims that there was sufficient food to cater for the food demand during the lockdown, the Economic Community of West African States (ECOWAS) states that with the COVID-19, there could be "increase in the number of people at risk of food insecurity and malnutrition from 17 million to 50 million people between June and August 2020" (Olukoya and Kamara 2020). Although government offered some palliatives to the people, apart from the corrupt practices that surrounded the distribution such as hoarding and diversion, the manner of distribution could lead to hundreds of people contracting the disease. The rowdiness and the scrambling for food resulted in stampede in some instances. According to Folashade Samuel, "We were scrambling for food when my sister with a young baby was pushed away, and she had to give up" (Olukoya and Kamara 2020). For most of the people, according to Benjamin Jeje, a resident in Lagos state, "food is more important than corona.... We are running away from the virus, but lack of food must not kill us. We must not go hungry" (Olukoya and Kamara 2020). This resolve not to go hungry resulted in many contravening the lockdown order.

The opening of markets by the government became necessary, not because the government did not know the nature of the markets, but because it considered food and access to it as critical in indirectly maintaining the lockdown order. In not allowing the churches to reopen when the markets did, it can be argued that the government was not frontally flouting the rights of freedom of worship. On the contrary, the government weighed the implications of access to food vis-à-vis access to corporate worship. As Wild-Wood et al. (2021) note, the COVID-19 is not first and foremost a medical issue; it is indeed a political health issue that requires political decisions to address its health effects on the population. In their own words, "the pandemic is not simply a health matter, nor is it being managed or controlled by health leaders. It is a geopolitical phenomenon where the authority to act is determined not just by medical knowledge but by the political and societal influence" (Wild-Wood et al. 2021: 66). The implication of this is that opening markets and closing places of worship is part of the political decision to manage and control the spread of the disease. Thus, the medical personnel and facilities that were functioning then were indeed at the service of both secular and religious spaces.

Worship is central to Pentecostal ethos and practice. In fact, Warrington (2008) and Asamoah-Gyadu (2021) describe worship in Pentecostalism as an encounter with the divine. It is a place, an event, an experience, a suspense, an intervention, a sacrament, or a contact zone that produces a tension and a meeting between God and humans. Through worship, a worshipper can be at once with God and other worshippers. Wariboko (2018) brings out the essence of worship more effectively when he states that worship makes grace tangible, material, concrete, visible, experiential, a feeding on the word of God; and it also makes it a possibility for "all other practices integrate and cohere as a crazy quilt of pulsating divine-human relation" (Wariboko 2018: 15). The mood of worship elicits the intervention of the supernatural in human world; it makes "the power of Jesus Christ come alive" in concrete form (Asamoah-Gyadu 2021: 198). This simply captures the importance Pentecostals place on corporate worship and why they believe that the churches should have been reopened as markets and hospitals. Truly, corporate worship provides an opportunity for worshippers to learn the word of God. After all, "One does not live by bread alone, but by every word that comes forth from the mouth of God" (Matt. 4:4 The African Bible).

Commenting on this verse (Matt. 4:4), *The African Bible* states that humans cannot devote all their energy toward the struggle for material bread alone, but they must counterbalance it with the word of God; and in fact, "the word of God should be 'eaten' within the church." This is pertinent to the call by the Pentecostals for the reopening of the churches. Maritain brings this out in a philosophical tone when he writes: "Men do no live only by bread, vitamins and technological discoveries. They live by values and realities which for their own sake; they feed on that invisible food which sustains the life of the spirit and which makes them aware not of such or such means at the service of their life but of the very reason for their living and suffering" (Olu-Owolabi 2011: 11). In this sense, one can appreciate the position of the Pentecostals who called for the reopening of the churches in order for the members to be fed spiritually. But that does not seem to vitiate the legitimacy and authority of the government given its role in human society and the theological basis for its existence as well as the command to obey it (Rom. 13:1–7).

The COVID-19 pandemic created a nuanced context for further examination of the secularity of Nigeria. Interestingly, for most part of the lockdown, there was no virulent religious divide among the competing religious traditions in Nigeria, especially Christianity and Islam. In other words, unlike previously when adherents of these religions would either support or kick against a certain government policy, the lockdown was 'unanimously' resisted by religious leaders to a large extent. In the north, however, many Muslim leaders flouted the government order and conducted services. In fact, some of them went to praying grounds for prayers at the end of Ramadan. A pocket of violence erupted between some Muslims and the police, and in the process a police station was torched (Yusuf et al. 2020). According to Al-Amin Albarra, a Muslim worshipper, Muslims "observed the prayer according to the Islamic teachings and the teachings of the Holy Messenger of Allah and were not observing any social distancing which was not recognized by the teachings" (Yusuf et al. 2020). Yusuf, Brisibe and Bello report that in Ughelli, Delta state, the police did not stop or disrupt the Islamic prayer because they did not want violent reaction from the worshippers. However, in Yola, Adamawa state, attempt by the police to prevent the prayer resulted in violence from the worshippers.

Among the reasons for the resistance is the nature of Nigeria's secularity. Most Muslims believe that Nigeria's secularity means that Islam is placed second to government whereas it should have been the other way around. "Muslims also feel threatened by perceived attempts by secular powers to regulate their religion. Some even think that this is a conspiracy to prevent Muslims from praying" (Olukoya and Mohammed 2020); that Western powers (often associated with Christianity) were plotting "to stymie the practice of Islam" (Hoechner 2020). Hoechner notes that the contravention of the lockdown order was also due to the eschatological belief of an imminent end of the universe. Many Muslims believe that since the world was going to suddenly end, imposing a lockdown would prevent them from living "extra-righteously" (Obiezu 2020), particularly during the holy month of Ramadan. However, Nasir Umar, a Muslim, who finds it difficult to make ends meet as a result of the lockdown, avers: "Food is basic for life and important during fasting, but without food, [I] cannot fast" (Obiezu 2020). Sharafadeem Abdulsalam, a Muslim scholar, expatiates: "There's nothing like online Jumat, you can't do that. You can't ask people to form a row in their respective homes and follow you while you lead them in prayers. No, you can't do that. The Jumat service has to be physical" (Obiezu 2020).

The greatest resistance to the lockdown order seems to have come from the Pentecostals. In his *Pentecostal Republic*, Obadare (2018) views the second coming of President Olusegun as either coinciding with the rise of political Pentecostalism or the impetus for the flourishing of a Pentecostal politics. Obasanjo's overly romance with the 'big' leaders of Pentecostal movement engineered a Pentecostal bloc that came powerfully into the political stage with a strong voice. Vaughan (2016) also recognizes the kind of revolutionary ascendancy of Pentecostal movement in the Nigerian body politic. The emergence and growth of megachurches that dot the Lagos landscape has made some to refer to the city as "the Pentecostal capital of the world" (Moyet 2020), which capital is now being harnessed for political influence. In the context of COVID-19, Moyet (2020) argues that it is only where a state has failed or is weak that religious authorities like the Pentecostal movement can almost perfectly resist government order as witnessed in Nigeria. For instance, Oyedepo's response to public outcry that the church is a more effective mechanism of disseminating information suggests that the church can do better than the state in circulating information about COVID-19. This is not only audacious, but also an attempt to indict the government as incapable of rendering effective services.

Ukah (2020) describes Oyedepo's response as "proud and arrogant" just as his claim to possess "prophetic power and anointing above political leaders" is false. He adds that Oyedepo's apology for flouting the lockdown order demonstrates that government still has the powers to enforce its order. "COVID-19 has shown that there are no 'pentecostal republics' in Africa" (Ukah 2020: 459). Moyet (2020) also concludes that "this might suggest that the state, although weak, has not completely collapsed, and that Nigeria has not entirely become a 'Pentecostal republic' after all." Although there were instances of flouting the lockdown order, it is true that the government substantially maintained the order. It was an emergency situation that required some strict action. After all, "a strong state is needed in times of epidemics since large-scale measures like quarantines have to be performed with military discipline" (Zizek 2020: 10). If the government had grant more freedom as demanded by the religious bodies generally, there probably might have been an escalated number of infections.

In conclusion, the lockdown was a litmus test for church and state relations, especially as it relates to Nigerian secularity. Although food and freedom of worship are important to religious adherents, many worshippers preferred food to corporate worship. The religious leaders preferred freedom of worship to food. However, their provision of food to their members is a good evidence to suggest that food was critical at that time—in the context of the lockdown. It cannot be said that right to worship was completely eroded; only corporate or congregational worship was seriously affected. In order to exercise this right, that is, right of corporate worship, and also to reconnect with their members, church leaders embraced e-worship model. Despite the pressure on government to reopen churches, its refusal to give in is indeed a huge demonstration of strength and secularity of the country in the context of the COVID-19 lockdown, and that Pentecostal theocracy has not been established.

References

Acolatse, Esther E. 2021. Pentecostalism and Secularization in the Philosophy of Wariboko: The Logic of the Spirit in the Formation of African Civil Society. In *The Philosophy of Wariboko: Social Ethics, Economy, and Religion*, ed. Toyin Falola, 223–239. Durham: Carolina Academic Press.

Akanji, Musbau A. 2002. *Eat and Die by Little*. 67th Inaugural Lecture, University of Ilorin, 24 October.

Aktas-Polat, Semra, and Serkan Polat. 2020. A Theoretical Analysis of Food Meaning in Anthropology and Sociology. *Tourism* 68 (3): 278–293.

Albala, Ken. 2013. *Food: A Cultural Culinary History*. Virginia: The Teaching Company.

Asamoah-Gyadu, J. Kwabena. 2021. In *The Philosophy of Nimi Wariboko: Social Ethics, Economy, and Religion*, ed. Toyin Falola, vol. 'God is Split'. Really? Nimi Wariboko and the Reshaping of Pentecostal Studies in the Twenty-first Century, 185–208. Durham: Carolina Academic Press.

Ayeni, Tofe. 2020. Religion in Nigeria Despite Coronavirus Measures. *The Africa Report*, April 3.

Bishi, Hakeem, Shelby Grossman, and Meredith Startz. 2020. How COVID-19 Has Affected Lagos Traders: Findings from High-frequency Phone Survey. https://pedl.cepr.org/publications/how-covid-19-has-affected-lagos-traders-findings-high-frequency-phone-surveys. Accessed May 22, 2021.

Bolarinwa, Josiah A. 2020. The Place of the Church in a Changing World—COVID-19 and Its Attendant Challenges. *Spectrum: Journal of Contemporary Christianity and Society* 5 (1): 22–41.

Briley, Julie, and Courtney Jackson. 2016. *Food as Medicine Everyday: Reclaim Your Health with Whole Foods*. Oregon: Nunm Press.

Casanova, Jose. 1994. *Public Religions in the Modern World*. Chicago: University of Chicago Press.

Chinea, Cristina, Ernesto Suarez, and Bernardo Hernandez. 2020. Meaning of Food in Eating Patterns. *British Food Journal*. https://www.emerald.com/insight/0007-070X.htm.

Cox, Harvey. 1995. *Fire from Heaven: The Rise of Pentecostal Spirituality and the Re-shaping of Religion in the Twenty-first Century*. Reading: Addison-Wesley.

Fox, Jonathan. 2011. Separation of Religion and State and Secularism in Theory and in Practice. *Religion, State and Society* 39 (4): 384–401.

Hoechner, Hannah. 2020. In Northern Nigeria, Distrust Jeopardises the Response to Coronavirus. *The Conversation*, April 15.

Igboin, Benson O. 1997. *The Doctrine of Ahimsa (Non-violence) in Indian Religions: Impact and Relevance in Contemporary Society*. Unpublished Long Essay, Edo State University, Ekpoma, Edo State.

———. 2014. 'The President of Nigeria has no final say': Sharia Law Controversies and Implications for Nigeria. *Politics and Religion* 8 (2): 265–290.

———. 2018. *When Food Speaks a Higher Language than the Ordinary*. Presented at the Philosophy of Food Conference organised by the Department of Philosophy, Adekunle Ajasin University, Akungba-Akoko, Ondo State, between 7th and 10th March.

———. 2020. Nigerian Pentecostalism, Alternative State, and the Question of Accountability. *Studia Historicae Ecclesiasticae*. https://upjournals.co.za/index.php/SHE/index.

Irekamba, Chris, and Isaac Taiwo. 2020. COVID-19: How Churches Make Life Easy for Members. Sunday Magazine, *The Guardian*, May 31.

Iwuagwu, Obi. 2012. Food Shortages, Survival Strategies and the Igbo of Southeastern Nigeria During the Nigerian Civil War. *The Journal of International Social Research* 5 (22): 280–289.

Karam, Azza, and Mustafa Y. Ali. 2020. Religion & Its Discontents: Considerations Around Covid-19 & Africa. http://www.ipsnews.net/2020/05/religion-discontents-considerations-around-covid-19-africa/Languages. Accessed November 19, 2020.

Macrae, Joanna, and Anthony Zwi. 1992. Food as an Instrument of War in Contemporary African Famines: A Review of the Evidence. *Disasters* 19 (4): 299–321.

Marshall, Ruth. 2009. *Political Spiritualities: The Pentecostal Revolution in Nigeria*. Chicago: The Chicago University Press.

Moyet, Xavier. 2020. Pentecostalism, Public Health, and COVID-19 in Nigeria. https://religioninpublic.com/2020/04/03/pentecostalism-public-health-and-covid-19-in-nigeria/#more-1586. Accessed November 19, 2020.

Nkwoka, Anthony O. 2006. The Nigerian Nation and the Christian Church in the Context of Jesus' Dictum in Mark 12:13–17. In *The Humanities, Nationality and Democracy*, ed. S. Akinrinade, D. Fashina, and D.O. Ogungbile. Ile-Ife: Faculty of Arts.

Obadare, Ebenezer. 2016. The Muslim Response to the Pentecostal Surge in Nigeria: Prayer and the Rise of Charismatic Islam. *Journal of Religious and Political Practice* 2 (1): 75–91.

———. 2018. *Pentecostal Republic: Religion and the Struggle for State Power in Nigeria*. London: ZED.

Obiezu, Timothy. 2020. Nigeria Muslims Adapt to New Ramadan in Age of Coronavirus. https://www.voanews.com/covid-19-pandemic/nigerian-muslims-adapt-new-ramadan-age-coronavirus. Accessed November 28, 2020.

Offiong, Ekwutosi E., and Charles E. Ekpo. 2020. Nigeria: The Paradox of a Secular State. *Politics and Religion Journal* 24 (1): 149–172.

Ogbu, Osita N. 2014. Is Nigeria a Secular State? Law, Human Rights and Religion in Context. *The Transnational Human Rights Review* 1: 135–178.

Ogundipe, Samuel. 2020. Coronavirus: Oyedepo Holds Service, Vows to Keep Winners Chapel Open. *Premium Times*, March 23.

Olu-Adeyemi, Lanre. 2018. *Edibo, ke se Obe*: 'Vote for Cash' as an Emergent Paradigm of Electoral Corruption in Nigeria. In *Corruption: A New Thinking in the Reverse Order*, ed. Benson O. Igboin. Oyo: Ajayi Crowther University Press.

Olukoya, Sam, and Karim Kamara. 2020. Severe Hunger Threatens Africa during COVID-19 Lockdowns. https://www.dw.com/en/severe-hunger-threatens-africa-during-covid-19-lockdowns/a-53212565. Accessed November 27, 2020.

Olukoya, Sam, and Zainab Mohammed. 2020. Nigerian Religious Leaders Demand Lifting of COVID-19 Lockdown. https://www.dw.com/en/nigerian-religious-leaders-demand-lifting-of-covid-19-lockdown/a-53499533. Accessed November 25, 2020.

Olu-Owolabi, Kolawole A. 2011. *My People Perish for Lack of Philosophy*. Inaugural Lecture, University of Ibadan, August 11.

Onishi, Bradley B. 2018. *The Sacrality of the Secular: Postmodern Philosophy of Religion*. New York: Columba University Press.

PM News. 2020. Oyedepo Begs Ogun State for Flouting Ban on Large Gathering. *PM News*, March 24.

Potorti, Mary E. 2015. Food for Freedom: The Black Freedom Struggle and the Politics of Food. http://open.bu.edu. Accessed November 19, 2020.

PwC. 2020. Responding to the Impact of COVID-19 on Food Security and Agriculture in Nigeria. www.pwc.com/ng. Accessed November 21, 2020.

Rijneveld, Wouter. 2003. The Slave Mentality of the Israelites Before and After Their Delivery from Egypt. https://www.researchgate.net/publication/316108218.

Royal, David. 2020. Nigeria: What Some Nigerians are saying about Oyedepo's 'Anti-Church Virus' Statement. *Vanguard*, June 29. https://allafrica.com/stories/202006290761.html. Accessed May 22, 2021.

Schanbacher, William D. 2010. *The Politics of Food: The Global Conflict Between Food Security and Food Sovereignty*. San Barbara: Praeger.

Sen, Amartya. 1987. *Food and Freedom*. Sir John Crawford Memorial Lecture, Washington, DC, October 29.

Toft, Monica D., Daniel Philpott, and Timothy S. Shah. 2011. *God's Century: Resurgent Religion and Global Politics*. New York: W.W. Norton and Co.

Togarasei, Lovemore. 2015. Modern/Charismatic Pentecostalism as a Form of 'Religious' Secularisation in Africa. *Studia Historicae Ecclesiasticae* 41 (1): 56–66.

Ukah, Asonzeh. 2020. Prosperity, Prophecy and the COVID-19 Pandemic: The Healing Economy of African Pentecostalism. *Pneuma* 42: 430–459.

Vaughan, Olufemi. 2016. *Religion and the Making of Nigeria*. Durham: Duke University Press. https://doi.org/10.1215/9780822373872.

Wariboko, Nimi. 2018. *The Split God: Pentecostalism and the Critical Theory*. New York: State University of New York Press.

Warrington, Keith. 2008. *Pentecostal Theology: A Theology of Encounter*. London: T & T Clark.

Wild-Wood, Emma, Liz Grant, Babatunde Adedibu, Alan Barnard, Aloys Ojore, and Yossa Way. 2021. The Public Role of Churches in Early Responses to COVID-19 in Africa: Snapshots from Nigeria, Congo Kenya and South Africa. *Studies in World Christianity* 27 (1): 65–84.

Yusuf, Umar, Perez Brisibe, and Bashir Bello. 2020. Covid-19: Muslim Faithful Ignore Social Distancing in Kano, Yola, Ughelli, Observe Juma'at Prayers. *Vanguard*, April 4. https://www.vanguardngr.com/2020/04/covid-19-muslim-faithful-ignore-social-distancing-in-kano-yola-ughelli-observe-jumat-prayers/.

Zizek, Slavoj. 2020. *Pandemic: Covid-19 Shakes the World*. New York and London: Or Books.

19

Analysis of COVID-19 Risk Communication and Community Engagement on Social Media in Nigeria

Abiola I. Odejide and Olayinka A. Egbokhare

Introduction

On 30 January 2020, the World Health Organisation (WHO) Director-General determined that the outbreak of Coronavirus disease (COVID-19) constitutes a Public Health Emergency of international concern (WHO 2020). Unlike other SARS, MERS and influenza, COVID-19 is distinct and has a high case fatality especially among older age groups and people living with disability (Ohia et al. 2020). Many features of COVID-19 are novel or unknown, such as its community spread, severity and impact. At the time this study was conducted in 2020, there was no universally approved treatment. Information about preventive measures was constantly evolving and vaccines were in the developmental stage. Consequently, the belief was that the coronavirus had come to stay and would likely cause more flu-like epidemics after the initial epidemic (Kissler et al. 2020). Since the threats to public health are

A. I. Odejide (✉) • O. A. Egbokhare
Department of Communication and Language Arts, University of Ibadan, Ibadan, Nigeria

F. Egbokhare, A. Afolayan (eds.), *Global Health, Humanity and the COVID-19 Pandemic*, https://doi.org/10.1007/978-3-031-17429-2_19

rooted in human behaviour (WHO 2009), a major problem is not in the pandemic itself but how humans respond to it. Given the gradual development of vaccines and tentativeness of proven treatment regimes, individuals' preventive measures such as wearing of face mask, handwashing and physical distancing are essential for reducing the speed and extent of the virus' spread (Sleator et al. 2020; Sunjaya and Jenkins 2020).

Although governments play a central role in combating pandemics, individual actions are also crucial to the success of efforts to prevent the spread of infectious diseases and limit their transmission. Thus, the social and behavioural sciences, as well as communication models, can provide valuable insights for managing the pandemic. Access to accurate information via appropriate channels, adequate knowledge of its causes, mode of spread and containment, advocacy for the benefits of taking action and agency of individuals are key. Health promotion is therefore fundamental to disseminating clear messages about the virus, as is the recognition of the fact that one-size-fits-all communication campaigns that do not acknowledge the social and political contexts will fail. Thus, collaborations among health care professionals, communication experts, linguists, anthropologists and other researchers can provide the technical basis and content for the behaviour change campaign.

In a multilingual and multicultural country like Nigeria, with 38% record of illiteracy, it is essential to develop home-grown messages on COVID-19 so as to reach the masses with the right message in the right language. Since indigenous knowledge is well preserved in the historical, social and cultural domains such as the languages, oral literature, folklore, traditional practices and beliefs, health promotion messages that take cognisance of these are likely to resonate more with the target audience. Globally, the media have played a critical role in creating attention about the pandemic although an evaluation of the nature of its impact is still evolving. Some scholars have suggested that while the true risk from COVID-19 might be low, the broad mainstream media attention as well as the social media discussions may have induced more perception of risk among people (Lennart 2000; Huynh 2020). In effect, the higher the frequency of using social media, the higher the risk perception of the pandemic.

Health promotion messages often focus on how to reduce risky behaviour and promote healthy living by influencing what people know about diseases. Media framing of the messages may determine the success or otherwise of health interventions since the audience may underreact or overreact to information. Thus, survival may be determined by the access to information, sufficient knowledge and skills and adherence to suggested behaviour (Reuben et al. 2021). Effective communication between message provider and consumer ensures the success of health services and is affected not only by the contents, but by the encoding process and choice of communication channels. Community leaders, persons of influence, medical experts are significant encoders who have interpersonal influence on receivers. Their messages may limit the chances of misunderstanding and misinformation, especially when they are well guided or knowledgeable about the issue. Media effects research suggest that any effect of media content is enhanced or reduced by what the recipients make of it (Valkenburg et al. 2016).

Statement of the Problem

The Nigerian public has been exposed to myriads of information about COVID-19 in terms of formats and sources. However, the volume of information appears not to have translated to desirable attitude, practice or compliance, if people's behaviour in public places and their denial of the existence of coronavirus in Nigeria are indicators. The proliferation of conspiracy theories about the pandemic has been counterproductive. People have pushed and spread political, economic and religious postulations and beliefs about the pandemic especially because of the involvement of China and the USA (BBC News April 25, 2021). Some of the beliefs are that: it is the fulfilment of Biblical prophecies about the end times and the beginning of the new world order; it is borne out of China's apparent quest for global economic and political dominance; it is the after effect of the launch of the 5G network and an attempt at global depopulation through the mass administration of genetically produced vaccines. Also prominent are several claims about the superiority of local treatment options over western medicine, especially, the efficacy of self-cure with home-made potions and remedies. The capacity of the pandemic to generate dangerous infodemic constitutes a major challenge.

The Nigerian government's pronouncements about COVID-19 came at a time of intense societal distrust of the nation's leaders and the political elite which manifested in the people breaking the rules of curtailment and isolation. While many regarded the daily statistics on COVID-19 released by the Nigeria Centre for Disease Control (NCDC) as an alarmist measure, others believed that the figures were fabricated to deceive organisations and philanthropists to donate money and provide Public Preventive Equipment (PPE) and palliatives. The economic hardship caused by the lockdown, coupled with lack of transparency in government's provision and distribution of palliatives, increased the scepticism.

Running a successful communication campaign against such a complex political and social background demands expertise in message development. This study attempts a content analysis of a representative sample of COVID-19 messages to assess their thematic structure and message development elements. The study is driven by the Health Belief Model and the agenda setting theory and the following research questions:

1. To what extent do the selected messages present salient issues on COVID-19, drawn from the Health Belief Model and Agenda Setting Theory?
2. What appeals are employed in the selected messages?

Literature Review

Health Belief Model (HBM) suggests that a person's belief in the personal threat of an illness or disease together with a person's belief in the effectiveness of the recommended health behaviour or action will predict the likelihood that the person will adopt the behaviour (Sijbesma 2010). According to Carpenter (2010), HBM is one of the most influential and widely used theories to explain health conditions and health-related behaviour. Reviews and countless applications of the theory abound to explain and predict a variety of behaviour associated with positive health outcomes and many successful health communication interventions. HBM suggests that a person's beliefs in both a personal threat of an illness or disease, and in the effectiveness of the recommended health behaviour or action, will predict the likelihood that the person will adopt the behaviour. It is a value-expectancy model developed to explain an individual's health actions under conditions of uncertainty (Maiman and Becker 1974). The expectancy can be the individual's estimate of personal susceptibility to, and the severity of, an illness as well as the likelihood of being able to reduce that threat through personal action (Tatyana and Jim 2015).

The major constructs that predict why people would take actions to prevent or screen for disease are perceived susceptibility, perceived severity, perceived benefits, and perceived barriers (Orji et al. 2012) and are categorised into two main aspects of an individuals' representations of health and health behaviour, namely perceived threat and behavioural evaluation. In addition to these constructs, diverse variables like demographic, sociopsychological, and structural factors may indirectly influence health-related behaviour and improve adherence and encourage cue to action and self-efficacy. Knowledge of these enables public health professionals to provide training and guidance in performing action, use progressive goal setting, give verbal reinforcement, and demonstrate desired behaviours (Glanz and Rimer 2005). Critiques of the HBM focus on its perceived high level of abstraction (Fitzpatrick et al. 1984 cited in Tatyana and Jim 2015), the influence of non-health-related factors (the environment, the economy, societal beliefs and the degree of access to information) on adoption of desired behaviour and the fact that beliefs do not necessarily lead to action (Sijbesma 2010). Notwithstanding these limitations, HBM still provides the most appropriate theoretical framework for this study.

The second theory is the Agenda Setting theory which explores how the mass media attempt to change the pattern of political behaviour during elections, colour events for audiences (Matsaganis and Payne 2005, Schultz 2005, McQuail 2010, Arowolo 2017), promote change (Pierce et. al 1987), and set public agenda for healthcare reforms (Hacker 1996). The argument is that the mass media not only influence how audiences think but also what they think about. Many scholars (Zain 2014; Zhang

2020; Msughter and Phillips 2020) affirm that the mass media is proven, through research, to be influential in setting up audiences on what to think, especially when they believe the information to be credible. Some scholars conclude that the new media is more influential in setting the agenda in comparison to old media (Zhang 2020; Msughter and Phillips 2020).

The agenda setting theory suggests that how an issue is presented to the audience influences the choices about processing the information. Framing, the second-level agenda setting, contributes to shaping the audience's perception for events covered in the media (Scheufele 1999). Media organisations adopt framing not only to select and present content but also to produce various perspectives for the purpose of enhancing the important issues and events (Msughter and Phillips 2020). Social media have become an integral part of public health as a tool for mass message dissemination to audiences and for multiway interaction with sizeable audience segment (Neiger et al. 2012). In view of the way news about COVID-19 broke, the role played by the social media was pivotal to building a block of knowledge around the virus.

As Korda and Itani (2013) contend, the social media enable anonymity, social networking, easy and cost-effective access to a large number of people across geographical distances. This may lead to information overload and the spread of fake news. In fact, Wakefield et al. (2010) point out that there is strong evidence which indicates that public health social marketing campaigns conducted through mainstream media can have a direct and positive effect on behaviour. In addition, even though the tools of public health are changing, and older models of health communication are becoming inadequate, public health needs a strong, effective voice to be successful in the world of social media (Teutsch and Fielding 2013). Thus, despite the social media's broad reach and inexpensive platforms, the message must be customised and tailored to the needs and preferences of different audiences (Korda and Itani 2013). For social media messages to command attention, the encoder must be thoroughly briefed on the objective of the communication.

A cautionary note is that the deployment of social media must be integrated with traditional public health communication channels. In that way, the interactivity of social media has to be explored for synchronous communication and collaboration with other media forms. According to Heldman et al. (2013), social media conversations need to be listened to, and influencers engaged with. Furthermore, Freeman et al. (2015) observes that though the social media are unlikely to be the sole solution to changing behaviour, they can play a valuable role in contributing to campaign objectives. Similarly, Korda and Itani (2013) argue that with the rapid and innovative advances in participative Internet communication, social media offer opportunities for modifying health behaviour. Sufficient evidence about social media's impact on health knowledge, behaviour and outcomes show that it can be effective in meeting individual and population health needs (Neiger et al. 2013; Valkenburg et al. 2016).

Much as social media has been proven to be viable for setting health agenda even in the face of an epidemic, the two theories, HBM and agenda setting, suggest that substantial focus should be on the message. While information alone is not sufficient to change behaviour (Teutsch and Fielding 2013), it does help to set the right agenda and promote the desired health behaviour. Notwithstanding the deluge of information about COVID-19, what is required are messages that will break through the clutter, contents that are novel, creative, well-executed, comprehensively developed, culture-centric and mindful of the demographic and psychographic variables of the target audience. The message strategy is key; it is not just about knowing what to say but how best to say it. Loss of message control and proliferation of junk science and fake news have to be eliminated.

According to Farmer (2019), there are three fundamental components of communication for effective health advocacy: use of appropriate language to ensure messages are understood, incorporation of several forms of media to increase acceptance of the message being conveyed, and lastly, and perhaps the most important, careful consideration of social and cultural determinants of health. Messages delivered in a manner that meets the needs of the target audience and includes the perspectives of those who will benefit from health services can have a powerful impact. This is important because individuals and communities can play an important role in determining their health. In other words, message development should account for user characteristics, information preference and mode or type of social media.

As Korda and Itani (2013) affirm, priorities for all health promotion initiatives include the following: understanding target audiences and their information preferences, developing tailored messages for different audience segment, basing programme design and evaluation on theories of social behavioural change and defining process and outcome measures to access intervention impacts, intermediate outcome, and health status outcomes. These are priorities for all health promotion initiatives. The most powerful messages are communicated in a short period of time and must be culture and age-appropriate. This has been proved by the effectiveness of HIV/AIDS prevention behaviour messages designed for the masses and disseminated through edutainment programmes which had a wide reach and had a prolonged impact (Babrow and Mattson 2003).

Like Obregon and Airhihenbuwa (2000) argued, messages which are tailored, based on the cultural traits of the audience increase the likelihood that the messages will have optimal reach, impact and recall. There is so much about health messages that is culture-bound and the success or failure of the message may be because of the application of adequate or inadequate knowledge of the culture in message development. These cultural values are embedded in and influenced by notions of community rules, traditions, beliefs, socioeconomic ability, power structures, education, religion, spirituality, gender roles, exposures and pathways to negotiate health issues—individually and collectively. When messages are culture-centric, they reflect a within-culture view, portraying valid cultural essence by drawing directly from narratives of cultural members in naturalistic interactions. Thus, culturally consistent messages factor in the values, traditions, roles, rules and power structure of the target audience and thus yield result.

In order to ensure the appropriate use of culture-centric messages, scholars have reported that the use of narratives is an effective means of conveying messages because they are a natural form of communication which people can comprehend easily, and which can be easily adapted to motivate and support health behaviour change. Being a representation of connected events and characters within an identifiable structure, bound in space and time and containing implicit or explicit messages about the health topic being discussed, they can transmit culturally grounded health messages with underlying cultural values and norms consistent with cultural practices (Kreuter et al. 2007; Larkey and Hecht 2010). So, they move from story to the world of interaction as story elements and norms embedding cultural identity are woven into discussion to create a sense of resonance with the audience (Larkey and Hecht 2010).

The socially shared symbols and systems that express group membership make these personal stories, exemplars, anecdotes and testimonials have the unique ability to involve audiences mentally by transporting them into the world being talked about and arousing emotional reactions through integrative melding of attention, imagery and feelings and becoming meaningful to listeners by providing "good reason" that justify actions based on the dominant stories with the group (Shen et al. 2015). They replace arguments for readers to judge and invite readers into story actions and immerse them in the real or plausible life experiences of others that are often difficult either to disagree with or dispute. The additional use of audio or video messages for such narratives enables them to contain more vivid information and make them more effective than print-based information (Green 2006; Larkey and Hecht 2010).

Methodology

More than two hundred COVID-19 messages were collated and previewed from various social media and online platforms. The data was collected over a period of three months: June, July and August 2020. The search words included but were not limited to COVID-19 video clips, COVID-19 messages, COVID-19 jingles, health messages on COVID-19, and sensitisation messages. Thereafter, 40 videos and 20 posters were selected for analysis. The selection favoured comprehensively developed, well-executed and publicly available samples only. The inclusion criteria were that the message must be on COVID-19 and must be locally generated. Further exclusion was done if the message appeared too similar to others or lacked originality. Two experienced and qualified research assistants were trained to code independently, using an instrument that was designed by the researchers. Inter-coder reliability was calculated based on percentage of agreement between two coders, and the result (0.88) indicated that reliability was attained. Analysis of each video or poster was recorded on a content coding sheet. The findings were then cumulated and represented using simple percentages to delineate frequency of occurrence. Qualitative reports were also made from findings using descriptive discourse.

Results

Figure 19.1 Breakdown of the videos according to type.

Figure 19.2 presents the types of messages used in the selected videos. The commonest forms were drama (45%) followed by straight announcements (40%). Song and music constituted 12.5% of the videos, while 2.5% were documentaries. Thus, 85% of the messages were in the form of drama and straight announcements.

Figure 19.3 shows the percentile distribution of identified sponsors. Federal and state governments sponsored close to a third of all the selected messages while public-spirited individuals and various companies together sponsored more than half of the messages. Non-governmental

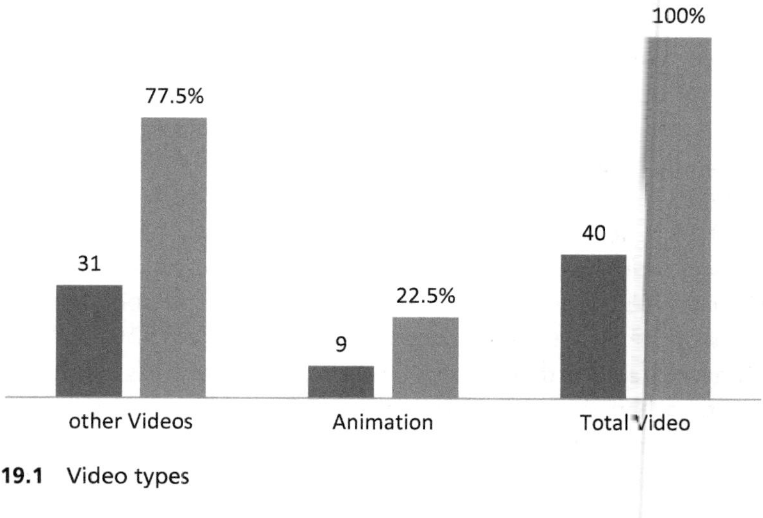

Fig. 19.1 Video types

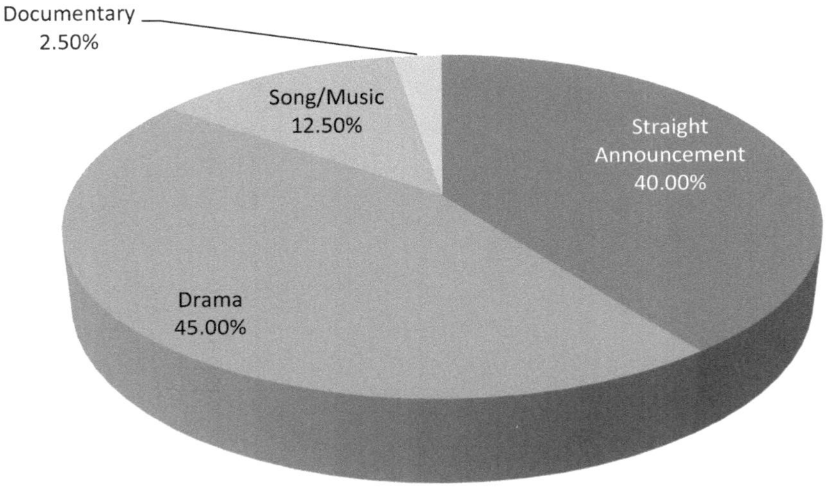

Fig. 19.2 Type of message

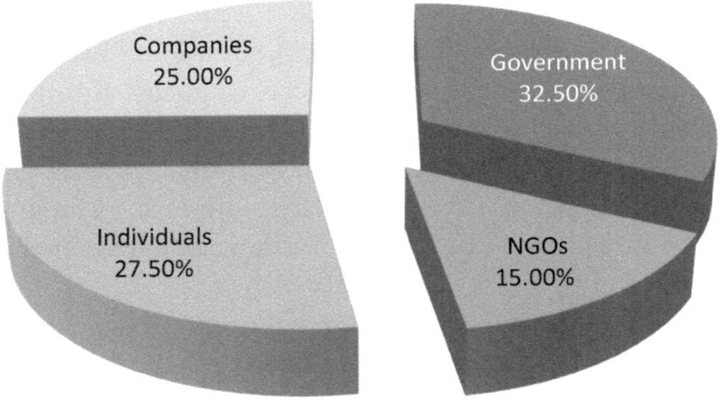

Fig. 19.3 Identified sponsors

organisations, including Faith-Based Organisations, sponsored the remaining 15%. Given the public health dimension of the epidemic, it is understandable that most of the sensitisation messages would come from government.

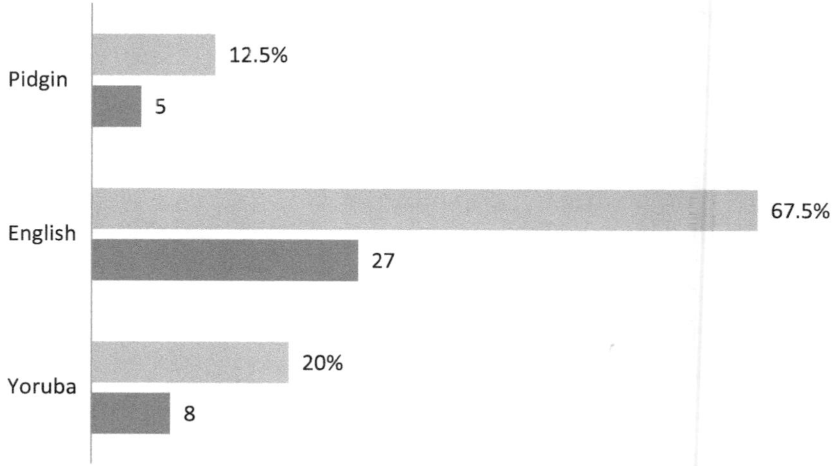

Fig. 19.4 Languages used

Figure 19.4 shows that 67.5% of the messages were crafted in English; 20% of the messages were in Yoruba while 12.5% of the messages were in Pidgin. It is not surprising that the most commonly used language of engagement was English, Nigeria's official language, through which a wider audience across indigenous language groups can be reached.

Most of the selected adverts combined emotional appeals, in the form of fear arousal, hope, positive or negative appeals. Humour featured prominently in some of the appeals as the qualitative analysis shows (Fig. 19.5).

Figure 19.6 shows elements of different aspects of Nigerian culture like the use of indigenous music, language, dressing, beliefs and religion.

Analysis

A total of 40 video and 20 e-posters were analysed for the study. The content coding sheet was divided into sections: A, B and C. In Section A, the coders recorded the message title, social media platform, number of views and the date released. In Section B, the coders identified name of the sponsor, language used, factors of cultural and religious resonance,

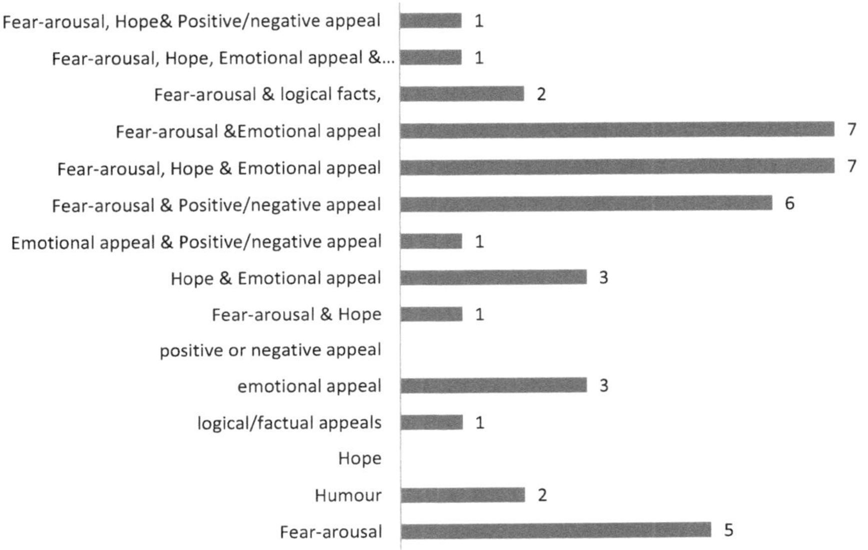

Fig. 19.5 Types of appeal

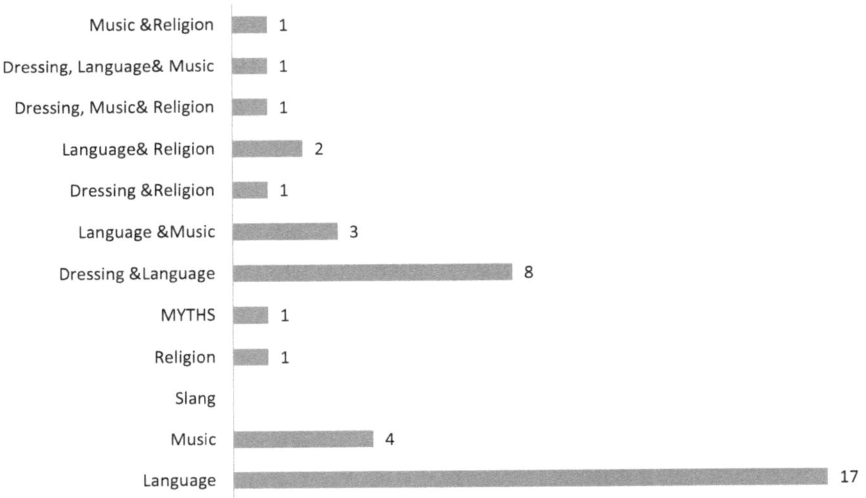

Fig. 19.6 Cultural resonance

target audience, message type, appeal, message presenter, description of the video, duration, unique features of the mention of preventive measures and call to action. In Section C, the coders analysed each message to show if and how encoders demonstrated the threat and severity posed by the pandemic, the benefits and barriers of taking action, message accuracy and agency of the audience. Section A shows that majority of the messages appeared across various social media—Facebook, Instagram, WhatsApp and Twitter with the highest frequency being on Facebook.

Research Question 1: To What Extent Do the Selected Messages Present Salient Issues on COVID-19, Drawn from the Health Belief Model and Agenda Setting Theory?

To answer the first research question, concepts were drawn from the template presented by the Health Belief Theory and Agenda Setting theory. The messages to a great extent covered salient issues relating to COVID-19. The message sponsors, as identified in the credits, belong to four major categories; government agencies sponsored more messages (32.5%) than any other group as shown in Fig. 19.3. These were the Federal Ministries of Health, Information, Youth and Sports and State Ministries of Health (especially Lagos State, the disease epicentre in Nigeria). Non-governmental agencies sponsored 15% of the messages. Some other sponsors included WHO, UNICEF, UKAID and the Nigeria Medical Association. A quarter of the messages (25%) were sponsored by private companies (e.g. the oil company, Oando). Other sponsors included media organisations (i.e. News Agency of Nigeria), television stations and media houses (i.e. Africa Independent Television, Television Commercial, Nigeria Television Authority, Guardian Newspapers). Equally represented (15%) were Faith-Based Organisations such as churches and church groups (Redeemed Christian Church of God, Methodist Church, Boys' Brigade), volunteer groups, celebrities, and public-spirited individuals.

The messages were relayed using facts, logic, statistics and medical evidence. Topics covered encompassed managing or curtailing the spread of the virus, especially social or physical distancing, curtailing movement, isolation and quarantine, handwashing, avoidance of touch or contact with eyes, mouth and nose. More of the messages (67.3%) focused more on the benefits of taking action than on the threats and severity of the pandemic. Seventy-one percent of the messages touched on the agency of the audience. A total of 96.7% of the messages gave accurate information about COVID-19. However, there were a few inaccuracies such as the distance to maintain in social distancing, coughing into elbow or covering the mouth, the duration of handwashing, the avoidance of eating game and stockpiling of food and medicine. Emphasis on the benefit of taking action was minimal (30%), just as the barriers to taking action were also not given priority attention (10%). Seventy-three percent (73%) of the messages made clear calls to action, with a notable one being cast in Yoruba, *Gbe ile ki o ba gbaye* ("Stay at home to stay alive"). This tagline would resonate with many native speakers of Yoruba, (one of the three major Nigerian ethnic groups) and the play on words "Gbe ile" and "Gbaye" makes for memorability.

The messages did not adequately reflect all the factors examined in the Health Belief Theory. Demonstration of the severity and threat of the epidemic was low (20%), probably because the message developers did not want to generate more fear and panic, as people were already scared. Translation of some technical terms (hand sanitizer, social distance, virus) from English into the indigenous language was not accurate or adequate. One particular fact-laden message, devoid of entertainment, garnered over half a million views (577,073) on Facebook alone(https://www.youtube.com/watch?v=G-wB_IANUzw). Another video titled "VSO NIGERIA raises awareness on COVID-19" was targeted at hearing impaired persons, a category of people usually, inadvertently sidelined in communication campaigns in Nigeria.

Examples of specific calls to action can be categorised as follows:

- Avoiding large gatherings: "Stay away from people in public places; Stay away from weddings, *owanmbe* (large, crowded parties; Use technology to worship)."

- Checking the media and NCDC updates: "Stay tuned to this TV channel to receive more updates on the corona virus; Take responsibility and call NCDC for information."
- Observing the health protocols: "Use hand sanitizer, no shaking hands with neighbours and friends; Stay away from cough droplets; Wash hands regularly for at least 20 seconds; Cough into elbows, avoid touching your mouth and sick people, cover mouth when sneezing; Wear facemask."
- Avoiding rumour mongering: "Don't spread rumours; Spread this message, not the virus."
- Providing information on treatment procedure: "Self-isolate if you feel sick; Do not self-medicate; Don't panic; Do not buy fake drugs for cure; Call helpline if you feel or notice any of these symptoms."
- Being socially responsible: "Be a superhero; Don't discriminate against people who test positive."

Research Question 2: What Appeals Are Used in the Selected Messages for the Study?

The nature of information people consume can influence both the extent and the form of their opinions (Valkenburg et al. 2016), the probability of the individuals' response to threats to personal or community health and self-agency (Commodari 2017). This section shows samples of creative elements in the selected messages, notably the attempt to domesticate or indigenise the campaign through music, people's mode of dressing, location, language (especially the use of slang) and some transliterations. The videos featured drama, music, animation, straight announcement and documentary. The most common format for the messages was drama (40%). Some elements of fear concerning disease, epidemic and death were introduced into the video messages. In line with The Health Belief Model, some of the messages focused on the pandemic's deadliness, danger and fatality. These were reinforced by naming dead Nigerian elites, portraying health officials decked in Personal Protective Equipment (PPE) and images of hospitalised victims. The Anthill Corona PSA animation, which had garnered about 24,000 views at the time of data collection for this research played up the fear of families being separated. It featured young children with the warning, "Your parents will be taken by the government."

The videos and posters also featured Nigerian celebrities (Toyin Abraham, Oga Bello), religious leaders (Pastor Enoch Adeboye, General Overseer Redeemed Christian Church of God), sportsmen and women (past medallists like Mary Onyeali), musicians (e.g. Cobham, Don Jazzy, KWAM One and Ebenezer Obey), health professionals (Dr. Jafiya Abubakar, Head of Epidemiology, NCDC, a group of health professionals across disciplines from a teaching hospital), CEOs of companies (e.g. Aliko Dangote), town/community groups, among others. These notable personalities and institutions were featured to enhance the credibility of the messages, thus increasing the possibility of gaining the attention of the target audience. This corroborates the argument of Iyengar and Kinder (2010) that health promotion thrives when opinion leaders and existing communal structures own the message and audiences can hear their own voices in the communication.

The messages from the Faith-Based Organisations focused on hope, love, belonging, unity, togetherness, encouragement and a call for prayers. The pronoun "we" was more commonly used than the pronoun "you" or "I." The song, "We Go Win," by Cobham Asuquo (https://www.youtube.com/watch?v=G-wB_IANUzw) is an example of a message replete with a call to unify efforts at fighting Corona: *we go fight am, we fit beat am, we fit stop am, we get power, no let panic finish us, we go win o*. The song was a repeated call to fight Corona as one people. The copy of some of the other selected advertisements featured messages like "Let's save ourselves, let's save the world," "Take responsibility, do it for yourself and the rest of us." "You are the superhero Nigeria is waiting for, will you answer their call? Corona, alejo lo je; tete k'eru re malo" ("Corona, you are a stranger, pack and leave here quickly"). In the last message, Corona is personified as an unwanted guest. All of these were attempts to make the audience own the message and act as a cohesive group.

One rich and prominent element in the messages is the use of humour which, according to Obadare (2009: 245), ordinary Nigerians use as a potent weapon to "deconstruct and construct meaning out of a reality that is decidedly surreal." The categorisation of humour styles by Martin et al. (2003) was particularly relevant. These are the affiliative, which is a benign style used to improve one's relationship with others; the self-enhancing, which is wholesome and favourable to oneself and others; the aggressive that is detrimental to others while enhancing oneself; and the self-defeating type which derides oneself while promoting one's relationships with others. Buttressing the Yoruba folk saying, *Oro euruku, toun terin* ("A grievous situation accompanied by laughter"), these humorous messages serve as coping mechanisms to limit the anxiety occasioned by the pandemic (Kuiper et al. 2004)

The Redeemed Christian Church of God (RCCG) for its 58th Annual Convention featured a video which employed self-enhancing humour to discourage members from attending the convention which normally attracts thousands of members and would have constituted a super-spreader event. An argument in Ijesa dialect of Yoruba, between a mother who is a diehard member and her sceptical daughter, provides accurate information on the efficacy of social/physical distancing and deploys the authority of a credible encoder, the General Overseer. Self-denigrating humour is employed in a video, "Palliative, Episode 8" produced by *20Mouth House of Humour* which highlights the deep distrust displayed by Nigerians about the government and its efforts to alleviate the effects of the pandemic on the citizens. The video dramatized the greed displayed by a couple who were intent on outwitting each other in ways that fractured the fidelity of the marriage, all in a bid to collect the cash subsidy promised by the government. This clip contains neither COVID-19 guidelines nor call to action and could undermine people's agency.

Despite the grim reality of COVID 19, Nigerians' zest for life and humour appears undiminished as is reflected in thirteen of the posters which attempt to mitigate the severity of the pandemic and laugh in the face of fear (Nabi 2016; Hendriks and Janssen 2018). In Nigeria, "jokes serve a double function as a tool for subordinate classes to deride the state (including its agents) and themselves" (Obadare 2009, 241).

Poster 19.1 derides a policeman, a state agent, who appears to enforce the use of face mask while greedily staring at a man eating a whole chicken. Poster 19.2 similarly derides the Inspector General of Police's announcement banning the Special Anti-Robbery Squad and police checkpoints by proposing alternative means of extortion of the public.

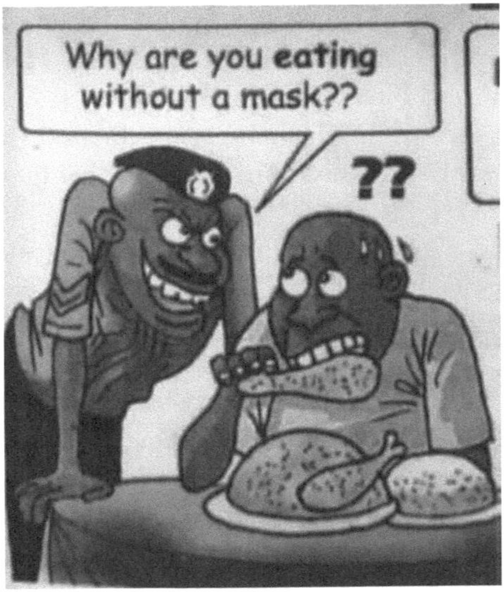
Why are you eating without a mask??
??

Poster 19.1

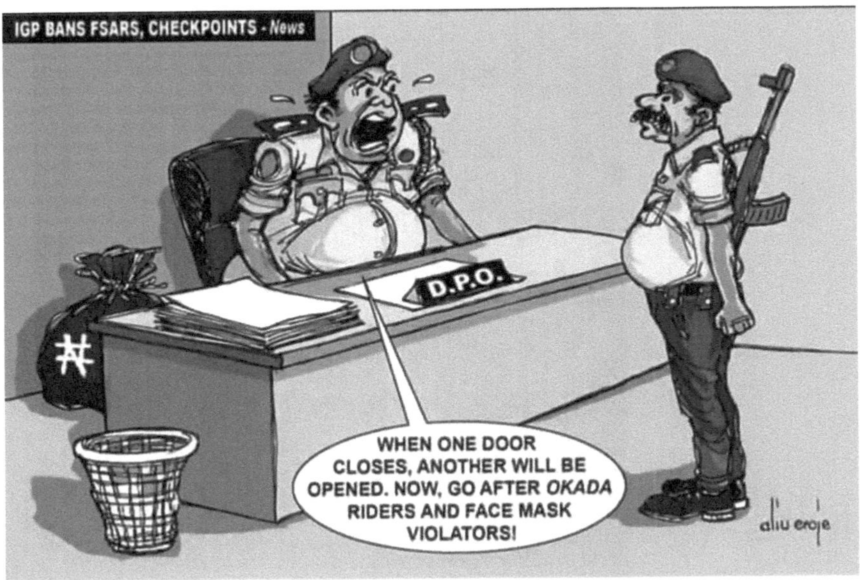
IGP BANS FSARS, CHECKPOINTS - News
D.P.O.
₦
WHEN ONE DOOR CLOSES, ANOTHER WILL BE OPENED. NOW, GO AFTER OKADA RIDERS AND FACE MASK VIOLATORS!
aliu eroje

Poster 19.2

Poster 19.3 creates humour from the famous last statement about Corona virus credited to Ibrahim Magu, the suspended Head of the much-dreaded Economic and Financial Crimes Commission (EFCC).

In Poster 19.4, there is linguistic inversion in a pun with the acronym of the World Health Organisation (WHO), being used as the pronoun "Who."

Posters 19.5 and 19.6 adopt comic incongruities to draw attention to the guideline on social distancing while the green frog in Poster 19.7, rather irreverently, compares breathlessness, a symptom of COVID 19, to the discomfort of wearing tight pants.

Poster 19.8, "Don't let them take your temperature on your forehead," ridicules the guideline on monitoring people's temperature before they are permitted to enter public places by inferring that it distorts a person's cognition. This self-defeating humour style in Posters 19.5, 19.6, 19.7,

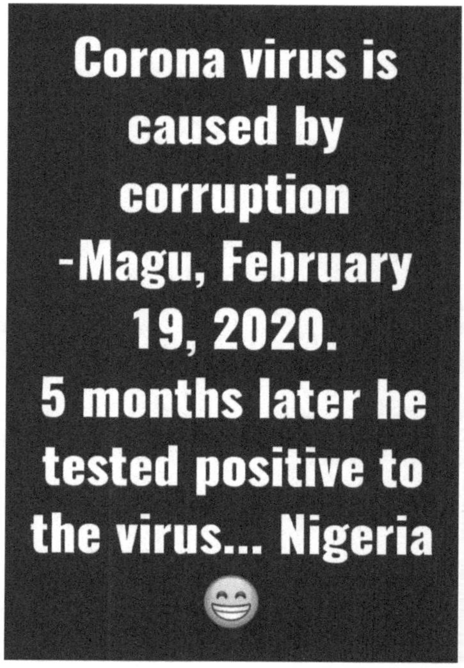

Poster 19.3

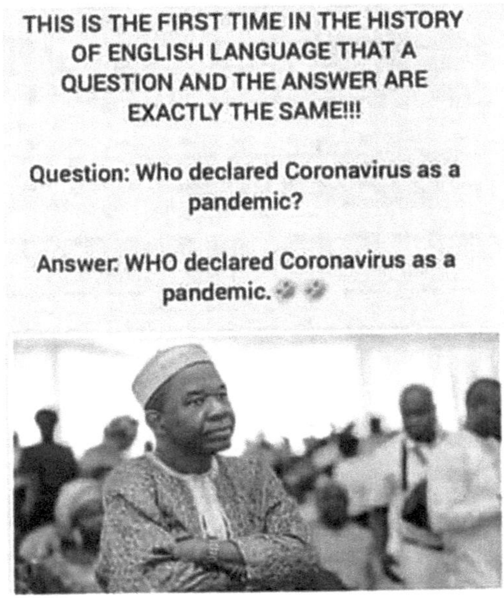

Poster 19.4

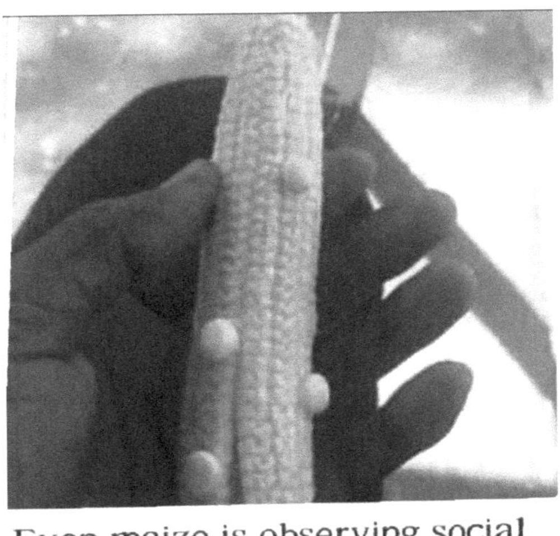

Poster 19.5

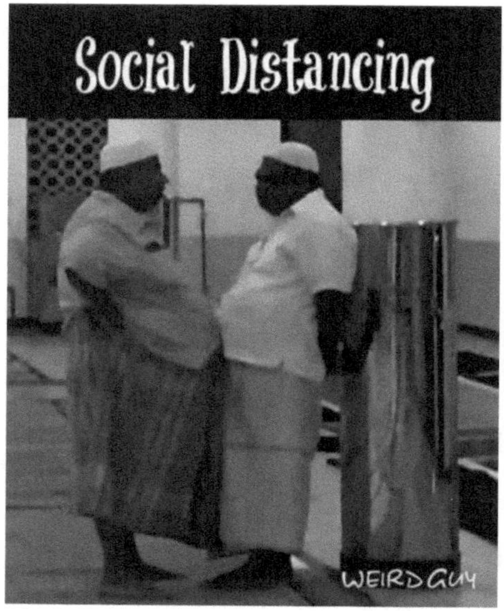

Poster 19.6

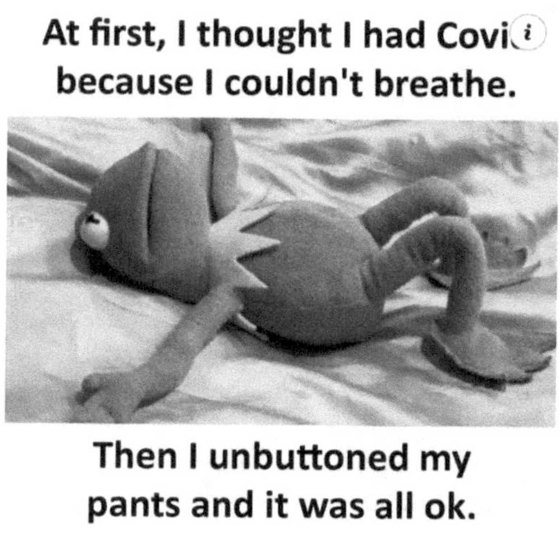

Poster 19.7

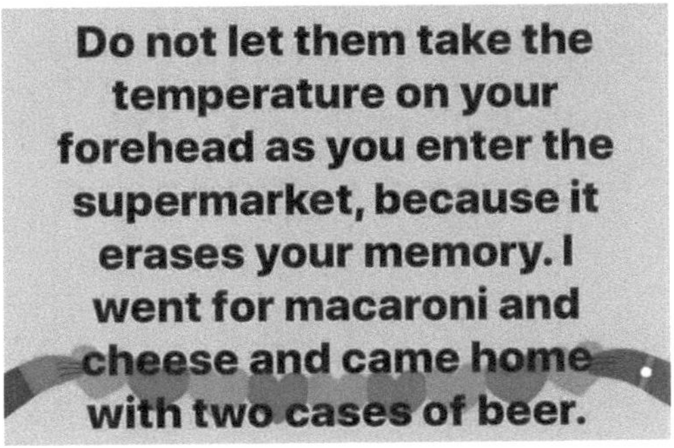

Poster 19.8

and 19.8, while ostensibly countermanding the protocols, uses counter-intuitive humour to sustain morale in the face of the stress of the pandemic.

Similarly, Poster 19.9 titled "God Abeg" ("Please God"), will resonate with the average Nigerian's belief in the existence of everyone's "destiny helper." This joke becomes more hilarious when juxtaposed with another one which had earlier celebrated the idea of face masks providing a debtor, a cover against being recognised by the creditor.

Poster 19.10 ridicules societal materialism exhibited in the ostentatious Nigerian *Owanmbe* tradition in which party attendees make outfits with the same material and incorporate matching face masks introduced by Nigerian fashion designers. However, this poster depicts an overkill where the face mask not only matches the wearer's attire but the entire décor, including the container of hand sanitizer. Even though this use of humour does not support the Health Belief Theory which requires that beyond rhetoric and humour, people need to know how to prevent COVID-19 (Kissler et al. 2020); it still attracts attention.

Posters 19.11 and 19.12 contrast sharply in the level of the compliance with COVID protocols. Poster 19.11 contains a striking and potentially damaging infodemic purported to be derived from opinions of medical practitioners. The message in the poster makes a call to "everyone in the world" to take part in inhalation of steam for one week and COVID-19 would be "eradicated." Compared to the message in Poster 19.12

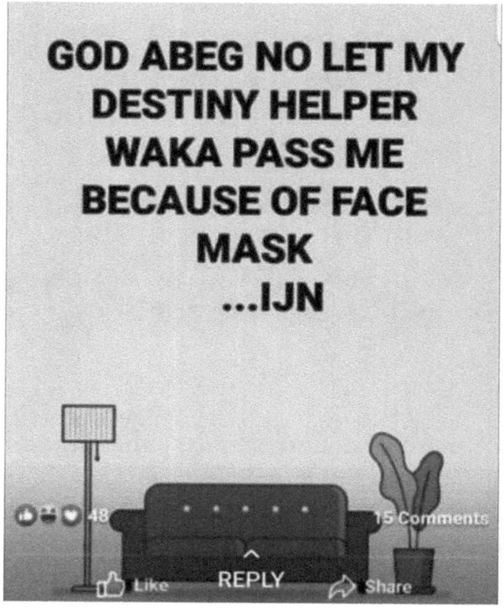
GOD ABEG NO LET MY
DESTINY HELPER
WAKA PASS ME
BECAUSE OF FACE
MASK
...IJN
48
15 Comments
Like
REPLY
Share

Poster 19.9

sponsored by the Oyo State Government, this claim of eradication by inhalation, though laughable, may be embraced by a gullible public, thus constituting an abuse of the principle of agency by the community. This kind of falsehood underscores the need for the media to set the right agenda and push information that will generate healthy choices and influence positive actions.

According to Olubodun (2018), to a large extent, to be African is to be religious. Therefore, factoring religion into message development is important because it is a locus of control and an integral part of the life of the African. Thus, Posters 19.13 and 19.14, while extending greetings to Muslims on the occasions of Eid Kabir and Eid Mubarak combine the COVID-19-compliant guideline by masking the Islamic symbol of the crescent and the sacrificial lamb for the Eid-el-Kabir or the Eid-al-Adha. The messages simply reiterate the need to celebrate the Eid with family and friends while observing the safety precautions for COVID-19. Similarly, Poster 19.15 adds an eleventh commandment to the existing

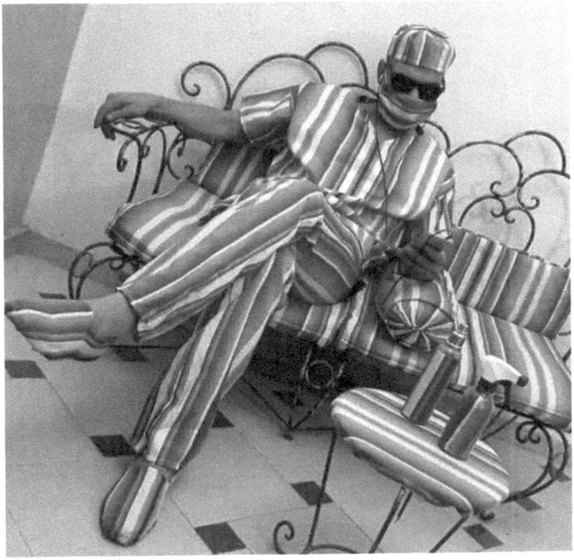

Poster 19.10

Dear All,
As per doctors view, COVID-19 is killed in nostril itself by steam inhalation and it costs very little or can say negligible.
To act upon above initiation, we request all everyone around the world to come togather and start this process of inhalation of steam for one week starting from 19th july to 25th july twice a day i.e one in morning between 7:00 AM -8:00 AM and at night between 7:00 PM -8:00 PM.By adopting this practice for a week we are sure that deadly COVID-19 will be eradicated
Please forward these message to all your groups,relatives,friends and neighbors so that we all come togather and kill this Corona virus and walk freely in this beautiful world
Thanks
09:17

Poster 19.11

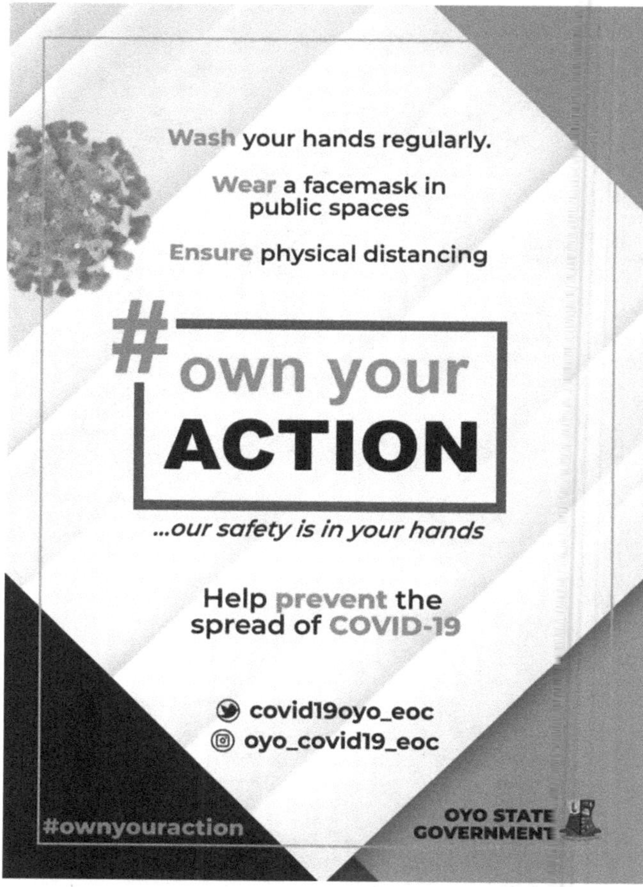

Poster 19.12

ten in the Bible by replacing the word "covet" in the tenth commandment with "COVID." Such use of humour is potentially attractive and makes a message memorable, fostering attitudinal change and knowledge acquisition (Cline and Kellaris 2007, Percy and Rossiter 1997), promoting interpersonal sharing and stimulating positive emotions (Greatbatch and Clark 2002). In the context of the new media, it can act as conversation starter/topic and an important determinant of information sharing (Dobele et al. 2007). This way, the media can assume an agenda setting role by telling people what to talk about.

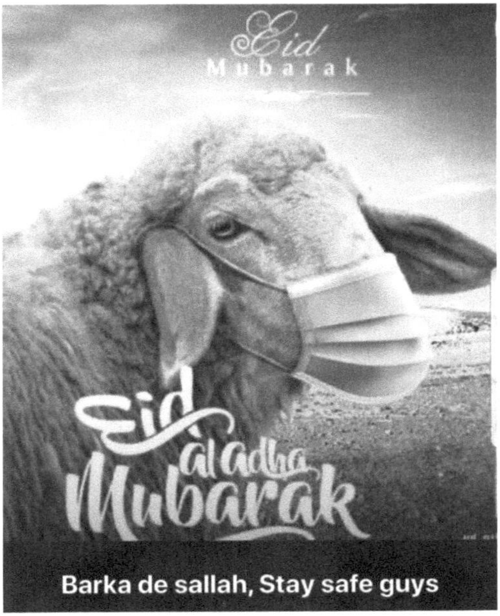
Eid
Mubarak
Eid al adha Mubarak
Barka de sallah, Stay safe guys

Poster 19.13

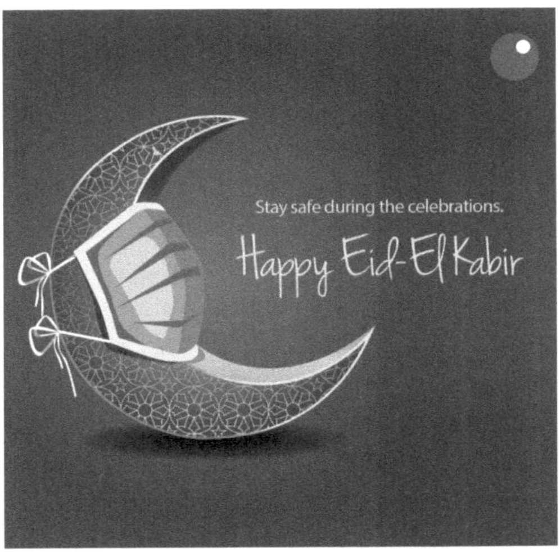
Stay safe during the celebrations.
Happy Eid-El Kabir

Poster 19.14

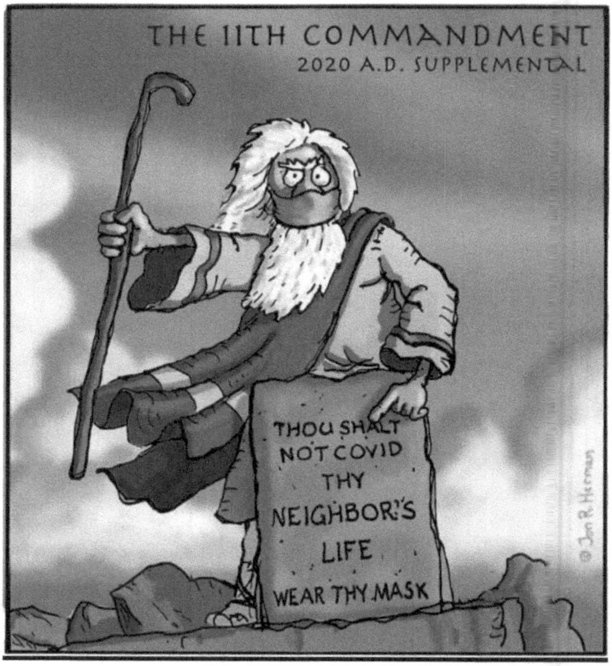
THE 11TH COMMANDMENT
2020 A.D. SUPPLEMENTAL
THOU SHALT NOT COVID THY NEIGHBOR'S LIFE
WEAR THY MASK

Poster 19.15

Conclusion

From the assessment of the selected COVID-19 messages, one could identify the salient issues addressed in the messages and the extent to which the messages leaned on the constructs of the Health Belief Model and Agenda Setting Theory. The literature shows that social media are relevant and highly potent for disseminating information on health campaign to support behaviour change. While humour served to provide relevant information, it was used to ridicule state agents and for self-critique, to sustain morale and cohesion of the community in ways that lessen the fear of the pandemic. The encoders, public health practitioners and social marketers utilised aspects of HBM variables and Agenda setting to package their campaigns to meet their communication objectives and reach the right target with the intended message. These health campaigns on COVID-19 shared on social media have the potential of receiving considerable attention, especially from literate young people. Consequently, due consideration should be given the pivots of health belief model in order to set the right agenda and directly increase the possibility that salient information on COVID-19 reaches the desired targets, and ultimately, impact health behaviour.

Recommendations Having examined closely the messages under study and their contents in line with the Health Belief Model and Agenda Setting Theory, we recommend that for health communication messages, especially on COVID-19, to fulfil the objective of improving the knowledge, attitude and practice of the target audience, message developers should incorporate receivers' cultural constructs, adopt and adapt traditional media of theatre, oratory and folk music. This should facilitate compliance with the health promotion interventions, especially in a country like Nigeria with its low literacy level, multi-ethnicity and religious affiliations and sensitivities. At the applied level, the results generated by this study underscore the popularity of humour in campaign development, the importance of encouraging sharing, and measuring potential impact as a component of health campaigns evaluation.

References

Arowolo, Olasunkanmi. 2017. Understanding Framing Theory. *Mass Communication Theory* 3 (6): 4.

Babrow, Austin S., and Marifran Mattson. 2003. Theorizing About Health Communication. In *The Routledge Handbook of Health Communication*, 49–76. London and New York: Routledge.

BBC News. 2021. https://www.bbc.co.uk/programmes/w3cszcmr. Accessed September 17.

Carpenter, Christopher J. 2010. A Meta-analysis of the Effectiveness of Health Belief Model Variables in Predicting Behavior. *Health Communication* 25 (8): 661–669.

Cline, Thomas W., and James J. Kellaris. 2007. The Influence of Humor Strength and Humor—Message Relatedness on Ad Memorability: A Dual Process Model. *Journal of Advertising* 36 (1): 55–67.

Commodari, Elena. 2017. The Role of Sociodemographic and Psychological Variables on Risk Perception of the Flu. *SAGE Open* 7 (3): 2158244017718890.

Dobele, A., A. Lindgreen, M.B. Beverland, J. Vanhamme, and R. van Wijk. 2007. Why Pass on Viral Messages? Because They Connect Emotionally. *Business Horizons* 50 (4): 291–304.

Farmer, Mychelle. 2019. Advocacy in Action for Improved Health Outcomes. In *Promoting Health Equity Among Racially and Ethnically Diverse Adolescents*, ed. Lisa Barkley, Maria Veronica Svetaz, and Veenod L. Chulani, 99–111. Springer.

Fitzpatrick, M.A., L. Vance, and H. Witteman. 1984. Autonomy and Interdependence Reflected in Informal Interaction Between Mates. *Journal of Language and Social Psychology* 3 (2): 81–95.

Freeman, Becky, Sofia Potente, Vanessa Rock, and Jacqueline McIver. 2015. Social Media Campaigns that Make a Difference: What Can Public Health Learn from the Corporate Sector and Other Social Change Marketers. *Public Health Research and Practice* 25 (2): e2521517.

Glanz, K., and B.K. Rimer. 2005. *Theory at a Glance: A Guide for Health Promotion Practice. National Cancer Institute, NIH*. Public Health Service. Washington, DC: US Government Printing Office.

Greatbatch, David, and Timothy Adrian Robert Clark. 2002. Laughing with the Gurus. *Business Strategy Review* 13 (3): 10.

Green, Melanie C. 2006. Narratives and Cancer Communication. *Journal of Communication* 56: S163–S183.

Hacker, Jacob. 1996. National Health Care Reform: An Idea Whose Time Came and Went. *Journal of Health Politics, Policy and Law* 21 (4): 647–696.

Heldman, Amy Burnett, Jessica Schindelar, and James B. Weaver. 2013. Social Media Engagement and Public Health Communication: Implications for Public Health Organizations Being Truly "Social". *Public Health Reviews* 35 (1): 13.

Hendriks, Hanneke, and Loes Janssen. 2018. Frightfully Funny: Combining Threat and Humour in Health Messages for Men and Women. *Psychology and Health* 33 (5): 594–613.

Huynh, Toan Luu. 2020. The COVID-19 Risk Perception: A Survey on Socioeconomics and Media Attention. *Economics Bulletin* 40 (1): 758–764.

Iyengar, Shanto, and Donald R. Kinder. 2010. *News that Matters: Television and American Opinion*. Chicago: University of Chicago Press.

Kissler, Stephen M., Christine Tedijanto, Edward Goldstein, Yonatan H. Grad, and Marc Lipsitch. 2020. Projecting the Transmission Dynamics of SARS-CoV-2 Through the Post Pandemic Period. *Science* 368 (6493): 860–868.

Korda, Holly, and Zena Itani. 2013. Harnessing Social Media for Health Promotion and Behavior Change. *Health Promotion Practice* 14 (1): 15–23.

Kreuter, Matthew W., Melanie C. Green, Joseph N. Cappella, Michael D. Slater, Meg E. Wise, and Doug Storey. 2007. Narrative Communication in Cancer Prevention and Control: A Framework to Guide Research and Application. *Annals of Behavioral Medicine* 33 (3): 221–235.

Kuiper, Nicholas A., Melissa Grimshaw, Catherine Leite, and Gillian Kirsh. 2004. Humor Is Not Always the Best Medicine: Specific Components of Sense of Humor and Psychological Well-being. *Humor* 17: 135–168.

Larkey, Linda K., and Michael Hecht. 2010. A Model of Effects of Narrative as Culture-centric Health Promotion. *Journal of Health Communication* 15 (2): 114–135.

Lennart, Sjoberg. 2000. Factors in Risk Perception. *Risk Analysis* 20 (1): 1–11.

Maiman, Lois A., and Marshall H. Becker. 1974. The Health Belief Model: Origins and Correlates in Psychological Theory. *Health Education Monographs* 2 (4): 336–353.

Martin, Rod A., Patricia Puhlik-Doris, Gwen Larsen, Jeanette Gray, and Kelly Weir. 2003. Individual Differences in Uses of Humor and Their Relation to Psychological Well-being: Development of the Humor Styles Questionnaire. *Journal of Research in Personality* 37 (1): 48–75.

Matsaganis, M.D., and J.G. Payne. 2005. Agenda Setting in a Culture of Fear: The Lasting Effects of September 11 on American Politics and Journalism. *American Behavioral Scientist 49* (3): 379–392.

McQuail, Denis. 2010. *McQuail's Mass Communication Theory*. London: Sage publications.

Msughter, Aondover Eric, and Deborah Phillips. 2020. Media Framing of COVID-19 Pandemic: A Study of Daily Trust and Vanguard Newspapers in Nigeria. *International Journal of Health, Safety and Environment (IJHSE)* 6 (5): 588–596.

Nabi, Robin L. 2016. Laughing in the Face of Fear (of Disease Detection): Using Humor to Promote Cancer Self-examination Behavior. *Health Communication* 31 (7): 873–883.

Neiger, Brad L., Rosemary Thackeray, Sarah A. Van Wagenen, Carl L. Hanson, Joshua H. West, Michael D. Barnes, and Michael C. Fagen. 2012. Use of Social Media in Health Promotion: Purposes, Key Performance Indicators, and Evaluation Metrics. *Health Promotion Practice* 13 (2): 159–164.

Neiger, Brad L., Rosemary Thackeray, Scott H. Burton, Christophe G. Giraud-Carrier, and Michael C. Fagen. 2013. Evaluating Social Media's Capacity to Develop Engaged Audiences in Health Promotion Settings: Use of Twitter Metrics as a Case Study. *Health Promotion Practice* 14 (2): 157–162.

Obadare, Ebenezer. 2009. The Uses of Ridicule: Humour, 'Infrapolitics' and Civil Society in Nigeria. *African Affairs* 108 (431): 241–261.

Obregon, Collins O., and Rafael Airhihenbuwa. 2000. A Critical Assessment of Theories/Models Used in Health Communication for HIV/AIDS. *Journal of Health Communication* 5 (Suppl. 1): 5–15.

Ohia, Chinenyenwa, Adeleye S. Bakarey, and Tauseef Ahmad. 2020. COVID-19 and Nigeria: Putting the Realities in Context. *International Journal of Infectious Diseases* 95: 279–281.

Olubodun, Feyisola Solomon. 2018. *The Villager*. South Africa: Tracey McDonald Publishers.

Orji, Rita, Julita Vassileva, and Regan Mandryk. 2012. Towards an Effective Health Interventions Design: An Extension of the Health Belief Model. *Online Journal of Public Health Informatics* 4 (3).

Percy, Larry, and John R. Rossiter. 1997. "A theory-based approach to pretesting advertising." Measuring advertising effectiveness. 267–281.

Pierce, John P., Terence Dwyer, Anne Chamberlain, Rosemary N. Aldrich, and Julia M. Shelley. 1987. "Targeting the smoker in an anti-smoking campaign." Preventive medicine 16, no. 6 : 816–824.

Reuben, Rine Christopher, Margaret M.A. Danladi, Dauda Akwai Saleh, and Patricia Ene Ejembi. 2021. Knowledge, Attitudes and Practices Towards COVID-19: An Epidemiological Survey in North-Central Nigeria. *Journal of Community Health* 46 (3): 457–470.

Scheufele, Dietram A. 1999. Framing as a Theory of Media Effects. *Journal of Communication* 49 (1): 103–122.

Schultz, Rosemary. 2005. The Agenda Setting Function of Mass Media, Tampa, John Howard, Print Media and Public Opinion: How It All Came Together in Melbourne. *Independent Study Project (ISP)*. digitalcollections.sit.edu 482.

Shen, Fuyuan, Vivian C. Sheer, and Ruobing Li. 2015. Impact of Narratives on Persuasion in Health Communication: A Meta-analysis. *Journal of Advertising* 44 (2): 105–113.

Sijbesma Christine. 2010. Coming into its own: Hygiene promotion for development in : WaterAid, IRC and CWR, Sharing Experiences:effective hygiene promotion in South East Asia and the Pacific. http://www.wateraidcommunity.org.au/hygienebook

Sleator, Roy D., Steven Darby, Alan Giltinan, and Niall Smith. 2020. COVID 19 in the Absence of Vaccination- 'Mask the Nation'. *Future Microbiology* 15 (11): 963–966.

Sunjaya, Anthony Paulo, and Christine Jenkins. 2020. Rationale for Universal Face Masks in Public Against COVID-19. *Respirology (Carlton, Vic.)*, April 30: 1–9. https://doi.org/10.1111/resp.13834.

Tatyana, S., and L. Jim. 2015. Health Belief Model. In *Health Encyclopedia of Public Relations*, ed. L. Robert, vol. 1. Thousand Oaks: Sage Publication.

Teutsch, Steven M., and Jonathan E. Fielding. 2013. Rediscovering the Core of Public Health. *Annual Review of Public Health* 34: 287–299.

Valkenburg, Patti M., Jochen Peter, and Joseph B. Walther. 2016. Media Effects: Theory and Research. *Annual Review of Psychology* 67: 315–338.

Wakefield, Melanie A., Barbara Loken, and Robert C. Hornik. 2010. Use of Mass Media Campaigns to Change Health Behaviour. *The Lancet* 376 (9748): 1261–1271.

World Health Organization. 2009. *A Guide to the Implementation of the WHO Multimodal Hand Hygiene Improvement Strategy*. Geneva: World Health Organization.

———. 2020. *COVID 19 Public Health Emergency of International Concern (PHEIC). Global Research and Innovation Forum: Towards a Research Roadmap*. 12 February. https://www.who.int/.

Yoo, Woohyun, Min-Woo Kwon, and Linda J. Pfeiffer. 2013. Influence of Communication on Colorectal Cancer Screening: Revisiting the Health Belief Model. *Journal of Communication in Healthcare* 6 (1): 35–43.

Zain, N.R.M. 2014. Agenda Setting Theory. *International Islamic University Malaysia*: 1–11. Accessed on researchgate.net.

Zhang, Yiyan. 2020. When Politics Intervene in Non-political News Flow. *The Agenda Setting Journal* 4 (2): 173–119.

20

COVID-19 (Post)Proverbials: Twisting the Word Against the Virus

Aderemi Raji-Oyelade

Already we are familiar with the concern generated by "nervous diseases," and the awareness that man becomes more delicate in proportion as he perfects himself. As the century advanced, the concern became more pressing, the warnings more solemn. Already Raulin had observed that "since the birth of medicine…these illnesses have multiplied, have become more dangerous, more complicated, more problematical and difficult to cure.
—Michel Foucault, *Madness and Civilization (1989: 211)*

Preamble: Tracing the Virus

COVID-19 stands for "Coronavirus Disease 2019," a transmissible respiratory disease caused by a novel coronavirus, which first broke out in the city of Wuhan, Hubei Province, China, on November 17, 2019.[1]

[1] https://www.livescience.com/first-case-coronavirus-found.html.

A. Raji-Oyelade (✉)
Department of English, University of Ibadan, Ibadan, Nigeria

F. Egbokhare, A. Afolayan (eds.), *Global Health, Humanity and the COVID-19 Pandemic*, https://doi.org/10.1007/978-3-031-17429-2_20

COVID-19, caused by the SARS-CoV2, is a new strain of SARS-CoV, i.e., severe acute respiratory syndrome-coronavirus. It was identified as an epidemic in 2002 in the city of Guangdong, China, affecting 26 countries with 8000 documented cases.[2] Unlike SARS-CoV, COVID-19 (SARS-CoV2) has attained the status of a pandemic, barely 150 days after its outbreak, with over 6.5m cases in 210 countries across the world.[3]

As researches on the origin, nature, and volatility rate of the contagion continued, there have also been concerted, international efforts to contain its spread, with the race for the vaccine to conquer the virus. While medical responses have been the most obvious to contain the pandemic, there have also been other responses to the ravaging illness, ranging from trado-medicinal, homeopathic, and the religious to conspiracy theorems including the scare of the biblical Armageddon, the end of days, the interrelation of the scourge with 5G wavelength radiation, and the counter-accusations of bio-terrorism, which suggest an economic third-world war between the USA and China. Thus, the responses to COVID-19 have been notably medical, spiritual, philosophical, economic, political, sociological, and sociolinguistic. Across the African continent, following healthcare instructions, most national governments introduced a combination of testing, contact tracing, social distancing, face-masking, sanitization, handwashing, and total or partial lockdown of the citizenry as measures to mitigate the pandemic.[4] According to a United Nations Habitat report, the control measures of most African countries to curtail the spread of COVID-19 included "restrictions on inter-regional movements to total lockdowns at the local, provincial or national level" (2020: 20).

[2] https://www.who.int/ith/diseases/sars/en/.

[3] https://www.worldometers.info/coronavirus/.

[4] The first confirmed case of COVID-19 in Africa was in Egypt on February 14, 2020. Nigeria had its first case on February 27, 2020. The first case in South Africa was announced on March 5, 2020, and in Ghana, the first two cases were reported on March 12, 2020.

Breaking the Outbreak

In the ascendancy of COVID-19, different categories of creative materials including memes, video and audio skits, GIFs, quips, and proverbs are produced on social media as part of the larger sociological and psychological (motivational) responses to the disease. Particularly, some inventive turns have been served on a number of proverbs that they can be categorized as novel creations of the postproverbial imagination, given the strains noticeable in the breaking and re-composition of the words. Amidst the challenge and containment of the affliction, the strains of invented proverbs are phenomenal reactions of the people to the outbreak, deserving of attention and analysis. The radical imagination of the users of the proverb text within particular language communities are evident of their philosophy of engagement with the pandemic. The postproverbial text itself is a cultural-linguistic "outbreak," an *outgrowth* of the conventional text, and, thus, symbolically, a response to the viral outbreak.

In Search of the Deviant Text

The focus of this chapter is to draw on the available range of postproverbial response to COVID-19, that is, the manner in which reactions to the scourge have been reconfigured in particular proverbial utterances in some African communities. An open call for contributions (OCC) was shared on March 15, 2020, on social media, including WhatsApp, Twitter, and Facebook.[5] Respondents were not limited to the number of entries that they could supply. In selecting the entries for this study, consideration was given to appropriateness, logic, and translation. In some cases where clarifications were needed, direct correspondence with particular respondents was initiated for follow-up. The proverbs were collected within the time range of 4 weeks (March 16–April 15, 2020) by means of question and sampling from respondents. In addition to the

[5] All the respondents who supplied examples of coronavirus-related proverbs did so freely and approved of the use of the illustrations. The interpretations of the postproverbials are without any prejudice to the respondents' own comments and suggestions.

open call, other examples or illustrations of coronavirus-related proverbs were drawn from available sources in news reports, Twitter, and other platforms. Furthermore, permission was sought to cite all the collated entries only for academic purpose and publication.

This study contains 23 postproverbials related to COVID-19 in six African languages, including Hausa, Ibibio, Igede, Igbo, Yoruba, and Zulu. As it will be evident in the interpretation section of this chapter, the collected samples are radicalized sayings (in the season of anomie), emerging as decidedly playful but instructive fabrications out of the welter of traditional African proverbs. Also, given the ethnic background of most of the respondents, examples from Yoruba language are more predominating, representing up to three-quarter of the total number of the proverbs collected. The preliminary observation is that the collected responses are admonitions, which draw attention and awareness to the dangers of the pandemic, and in other cases, they are verbal jousts against the virus itself. In relation to the basic principles of rift, suture, and super(im)position of the theory of postproverbials, these are absolute creations of the radical imagination, with new values, new functions, and different significations.

The Postproverbial Order

Transgressive paremiology is the study of innovations and transformations in contemporary proverb scholarship. Its crucial interest is to deal with significant structural violence done to traditional or conventional proverbs, the deconstruction of the idiomatic pathogen of the conventional utterance which invariably affects its meaning, knowledge transmission, and the overarching philosophy of life.

To be sure, conventional proverbs have never been dismissed as jaded, outworn, or clichés in spite of their ubiquitous and repetitive use. Yet, the human penchant for creativity, modernist, or iconoclastic energies, coupled with a critical detachment from the heritage of traditional wisdom, have questioned the sacrosanct status of the proverbial text in culture. The term "antisprichwort" (German for "anti-proverb") was first used by

Wolfgang Mieder in 1983.[6] Mieder would collaborate later with Anna Litovkina, the Hungarian sociolinguist, to publish the first major work on the tradition of innovation in the use and making of proverbs titled *Twisted Wisdom: Modern Anti-Proverbs* (1999). In European and Anglo-American studies, proverb scholars have drawn on the label "anti-proverb" for alterations, transgressions, and transformations: *anti(-)proverb* (French), *антипословица* (Russian), and *anti(-)proverbium* (Hungarian). In African proverb scholarship, the term "postproverbial" was first coined in 1995 by Aderemi Raji-Oyelade in an essay that would be published later in *Research in African Literatures* in 1999.[7]

COVID-19 Postproverbials: Interpreting the Twisted Word

The set of COVID-19 postproverbials collected so far are verbal reflections on the reality of the pandemic, the experience of lockdown, social distancing, hygiene, as well as the invocation and reification of the morbid potential and presence of the virus in the community. The interpretive minimum, which runs through all but one of these radicalized texts, is the personification of the coronavirus as subject and agency. As organized, each pair of proverb text for analysis contains the conventional proverb and the postproverbial engendered by the disease; thus, the commentary that follows serves as contextual explication of the interrelation of the given proverbemes. In the basic structural pattern of the postproverbial act, a part of the conventional proverb—clausal, phrasal or

[6] Mieder, W. *Antisprichwörter*. Band I. Wiesbaden: Verlag für deutsche Sprache, 1983.

[7] Relevant publications on postproverbials or anti-proverbs include the following: Raji-Oyelade, A. "Posting the African Proverb: A Grammar of Yoruba Postproverbials, or Logophagia, Logorrhea and the Grammar of Yoruba Postproverbials." *Proverbium: Yearbook of International Proverb Scholarship* 21 (2004): 299–314; T. Litovkina, A. and Mieder, W. *Old Proverbs Never Die, They Just Diversify: A Collection of Anti-Proverbs*. Burlington & Veszprém: The University of Vermont & The Pannonian University of Veszprém, 2006; Mieder, W. "Anti-Proverbs and Mass Communication: The Interplay of Traditional and Innovative Folklore". *Acta Ethnographica Hungarica* 52.1 (2007): 17–46; Aleksa, M. and Hrisztova-Gotthardt, H. & T. Litovkina, A. "The Reception of Anti-Proverbs in the German Language Area", in Soares, R. & Lauhagankas, O. (eds.), *Actas ICP08 Proceedings*. Tavira: Tipografia Tavirense, 2009. pp. 83–98; and Raji-Oyelade, A. *Playful Blasphemies: Postproverbials as Archetypes of Modernity in Yoruba Culture*. Trier: Wissenchaftlicher Verlag, 2012.

lexical—is suspended and replaced by a newly extracted clause, phrase, or lexis, which is directly related to coronavirus as agency. In other cases, the conventional proverb remains intact but supplemented by a postproverbial retort. The double act of suspension and superimposition which takes place is a structural fissure, albeit, a locking down or twinning of the old with a new artifice which thus gives birth to a hybrid or rogue text.

On Lockdown

The first set of proverbial retorts to the pandemic are devoted to the people's reaction toward the sudden change of lifestyle caused by the official declaration of lockdowns in most countries around the world. The lockdown was the first major regulatory act of governments, and attendant upon it were other restrictions including self-isolation, quarantine, face masking, and social/physical distancing. Medical tourism, the practice of travelling for therapeutic treatment, became downgraded, and in its place was medical curfew, the restriction of movement of persons across state borders, in control of the acute contagion.

1.
p1: Ibi orí dá'ni sí làá gbé.
A man's home is where he should reside.

p2: Ibi orí dá'ni sí làá gbé, níí gba'ni l'ọ́wọ́ọ àtànkálẹ̀ kòró.[8]
A man's home is where he should reside. Thus, one is saved from the spread of coronavirus.

Comment: The conventional saying is a philosophical reference to the destiny as well as the contentment of humans who must submit to the natural order of birth. In troping on this, the postproverbial retort directly points at the need for human to remain within her location (locus) in order to be saved from the uncharted rout of the virus. The sense of the spiritual (fate) in the first proverb is replaced by the sense of the physical

[8] Supplied by a respondent, @Olushola-Excel Oyadiji (Yoruba).

(home) in the prosthetic proverb. This truly is a lockdown postproverbial.

2.
p1: Akpa sangha isang isi diagha se mbon ufok edia.
The one who walks about does not eat what those at home eat.

p2: Akpa sangha isang abi m^m COVID-19.[9]
It is the one who walks about that will contract COVID-19.

Comment: This is an apt example of a postproverbial that is induced by the sense of precaution. Whereas the conventional proverb points at the adventurous nature of humans, the radical response in COVID-19 addresses the danger of indiscriminate wandering.

3.
p1: Ukwu n'aga wam wam wam marakwa na anya n'aga wam wam wam na eleya.
The leg that walks about should know that the eye that looks around is watching it.

p2: Ukwu n'aga wam wam wam mara kwa na COVID-19 na eche ya.[10]
The leg that walks about should know that COVID-19 is waiting for it.

Comment: In this example of a lockdown postproverbial, a person is admonished against aimless wandering and transgression that could lead to infection. The restrictive tone of the original proverb is retained in the new proverb; the warning is not about extra vigilance ("of the eye that looks around") as it is about the presence of the virus (COVID-19) that lurks around the corner for the wanderer.

[9] Supplied by a respondent, @Hanson Utibe-Abasi (Ibibio).
[10] Supplied by a respondent @Miracle Francis (Igbo).

On Social Distancing

The act of lockdown, with the creation of physical and social boundaries, was the direct cause of the condition of isolation and dissociation. The popular term for the practice of regulated spacing and dissociation is called social distancing. Social distancing is the accepted measure of remoteness between persons and groups of people with a view to reducing or canceling any act of intimacy especially for the purpose of medical (psychological or psychiatric) healing. It is noteworthy that most of the postproverbial creations in the season of the coronavirus reflect directly or indirectly on the logic and necessity of safe distancing.

4.
p1: Ká rìn ká pọ̀, yíyẹ níí yẹni.
Moving together in unison brings honour and respect.

p2: Ká rìn ká pọ̀, pípa níí pani.[11]
Moving together in unison brings death.

Comment: The original proverb here reflects on the joy of communal relations and association, but the postproverbial admonishes against the danger of crowding, which increases the rate of viral infection in COVID-19 time. The radicalized proverb is already used as part of a musical composition entitled "Koro" which was released on April 16, by Jubal Music (2020). The song is itself a persuasive melody drawing on the lesson of good hygiene, social distancing, counsel against overcrowding in the home and in public places, as well as an invocation of spiritual protection and hope for the future.[12]

[11] Composed in a special song released by Jubal Music, entitled "Koro"; https://www.youtube.com/watch?v=kqYnB9T9rUU.

[12] In popular imagination, coronavirus is shortened as "koro," being the colloquial form of corona/korona.

5.
p1: Ara kìí sá f'ára, bíí ti kúrúnà kọ́.
Bodies do not run from bodies, not with scabies infection.

p2: Ara kìí sá f'ára, bíí ti kófìdì kọ́.[13]
Bodies do not run from bodies, not with the outbreak of COVID-19.

p2: Ara kìí sá f'ára, bíí ti *kórónà* kọ́.
Bodies do not run from bodies, not with coronavirus infection.

Comment: In the conventional proverb, a bacterial skin disease is the referent effect of non-cautionary physical interrelations; in the postproverbial creation, the discomfort of scabies is replaced by the stigma of coronavirus. Thus, COVID-19 is figured as the symptomatic repercussion of bodily interactions. The other postproverbial variant here—Ara kìí sá f'ára, bíí ti *kórónà* kọ́—is a direct pun of the phonetic similarity of corona/korona (English) and kúrúnà (Yoruba).

6.
p1: Ìsúnmọ́ni, là á mọ̀ ṣe ẹni.
Close association brings understanding.

p2: Ìsúnmọ́ni, àrùn níí dá sára.[14]
Close association breeds illness.

Comment: This is a proverb on the virtue of close interpersonal relations and how affiliations make understanding and awareness of a person's character possible. But the postproverbial creation becomes a warning, a counsel about social distancing as crucial mitigation of the danger of infection and spread. Therefore, as in the previous example, close physical association is a veritable source of illness and death.

[13] Supplied by a respondent, @Tolulope Akinrinde (Yoruba).
[14] Supplied by a respondent, @Ope Oyetunji (Yoruba).

7.
p.1: Òde kìí yá aláṣọ rè.
Partying never tires the dresser.

p2: Òde kìí yá aláṣọ rè, l'áyé kòró kọ́.[15]
Partying never tires the dresser, not in the time of coronavirus.

Comment: The conventional proverb is apparently a praise of the material possessions of someone with a chest of clothes and who is therefore never tired of going to parties. A general stereotype of the Yoruba is that of a people given to hedonism and lavish celebrations. One of the effects of the lockdown is the absolute absence of social gathering. The supplement of the postproverbial text is predictably cautionary, inferring that interaction or partying is no longer a fanciful or virtuous in the age of the coronavirus.

8.
p1: Igi gogoro má gùn míi lójú, àtòkèrè la tí ǹ'wó.
That we may not be blinded by the tall, pointed tree, one must watch it from afar.

p2: Igi kòró má gùn míi lójú, àtòkèrè la tí ń'júbà.[16]
That we may not be blinded by the tall, corona tree, it takes a salute from a distance.

Comment: While the original proverb expresses the need for extra caution and prudence in all proposals and actions, the postproverbial discourages socialization and encourages extra care. In the new proverb, there is an attribution, the qualification of the presence of the virus in a material object of nature—"igi kòrónà" (corona tree).

[15] Supplied by a respondent, @Wale Oyedeji (Yoruba).

[16] Supplied by a respondent, @Adeshewa Adekoya (Yoruba).

On Spread and Awareness

By the context of their creation and use, some postproverbials have served as disseminators of the existence of the pandemic in the society. They also serve as verbal evidence, admonitions, or confirmation of the aggressive virus with its morbid power of fear and death among the people.

9.
p1: Ó jọ ate, kò jọ gàté, ó fi ẹsẹ̀ méjì lé lẹ̀ ate-gàte!
So steadily, so unsteadily, the matter plants its feet wobbly in the land!

P2: Ó jọ ate, kò jọ gàté, kòró má ǹ'fi ẹsẹ̀ mú lẹ̀![17]
So steadily, so unsteadily, the coronavirus is planting its feet solidly in the land!

Comment: In this example, both proverb and postproverbial call attention to the awareness of a crucial matter or event within the community with the potential of becoming permissive and endemic. In the conventional proverb, reference is to an unnamed matter or situation; in the radical proverb however, the situation becomes known and named. Also, its presence is described as potentially grounded in the community.

10.
p.1: Oun tó wà l'ẹ́yìn *Ọfà*, ó ju *Ọ̀jé* lọ.
What is after the border of *Ofa* is more than the encampment of *Oje*.

p.2: Oun tó wà l'ẹ́yìn kòró, ó ju ikọ́ lọ.[18]
What comes after the coronavirus is more than coughing.

Comment: The traditional proverb here is usually uttered as a caution on an action that has repercussion, should the warning be ignored. In its historical context, *Ọfà* was a Yoruba settlement in the northern border of

[17] Supplied by a respondent, @Lanre Oladoyinbo (Yoruba).
[18] Supplied by a respondent, @Remi Akinpelu (Yoruba).

old Oyo Empire; it used to be a major garrison of the warriors before the Fulani Jihad of 1804; beyond the old garrison was *Òjé*, another settlement which later developed into a huge encampment for warriors on strategic missions. It is therefore said, in military sense, that when a battle rages and ends in *Ọ̀fà*, there is a greater one with greater repercussion waiting in *Oje*. Thus, in the postproverbial turn of the conventional saying, the infection of the coronavirus is the initial battle, but the minimum symptom of cough is itself the euphemism for death.

11.
p1: Ong ole kojuwa hwume gen gen ka gba chu gbei.
Whatever is making the bush to shake must come to the road by and by.

p2: Okumu nyi koro ole kowe hume gen gen aka dai lo gba chu gbei ka.[19]
The corona masquerade that is shaking the bush must eventually appear on the road.

Comment: The conventional proverb here notes that whatever is hidden even for a long time will eventually be revealed. But the postproverbial turns the general ("whatever") into the specific presence of the pandemic which is personified as a masquerade ("okumu nyi koro"). This is a radical proverb not only about the awareness of the virus but more about its impending outbreak and danger.

12.
p1: "Mai zan yi da abinda ya gagare wuta," inji kishiyar konania.
"I have no business with a fire fighter," says the co-wife of a burnt woman.

p2: "Mai zan yi da abinda ya gagare wuta," inji kishiyar mai korona.[20]
"I have no business with a fire fighter," says the co-wife of a corona patient.

p2: "Ba ruwana da asibiti," inji kishiyar mai korona.
"I have no business with the hospital," says the co-wife of a corona patient.

[19] Supplied by a respondent, @Maria Ajima (Igede).
[20] Supplied by a respondent, @Rahila Luka (Hausa).

Comment: "'Mai zan yi da abinda ya gagare wuta,' inji kishiyar konania" is a proverb that is generally used to address negligence and indifference. Its postproverbial other ("Mai zan yi da abinda ya gagare wuta, inji kishiyar mai korona") addresses the negligence of the Kano state people toward the outbreak of COVID-19. Whereas the original proverb dwells on the negligence, as well as the complicity, of the wife in the misfortune of the co-wife, the postproverbial is used to focus on the reported cases of negligence and even denial of a cross-section of Kano state youths. In the third week of April 2020, there was a spike of mystery deaths in Kano, the main hub of the economy of Northern Nigeria. A record number of over 150 mortalities were reported within 3 days, followed by counter-statements about the cause of the death, especially of the elderly and high-profile individuals in the city.[21] Weeks before the outbreak of deaths, scenes of crowds in different parts of the city defying the stay-at-home order were familiar and displayed in online sites and in conventional news channels. A virus-defying song was even composed by the predominantly youthful population: "Malam ya ce babu korona, muma mun ce babu korona"—"Malam says there is no corona, we also say there is no corona."

13.
p1: Girman kai rawanin tsiya.
Pride is the turban of trouble.

p2: Girman kai rawanin mai karyata korona.
Pride is the turban of a corona denier.[22]

Comment: In the symbolic use of an abstract characteristic as a sign for another condition, the original proverb is as metonymic as its postproverbial other. The attribute of pride (girman) in both proverb and

---

[21] https://www.theguardian.com/world/2020/apr/28/nigerian-authorities-deny-wave-of-deaths-is-due-to-covid-19.

[22] Supplied by a respondent, @Rahila Luka (Hausa).

postproverbial is employed as agency and cause. In the conventional proverb, pride is the crown (rawanin) of trouble; but in the postproverbial, pride becomes the handle, the carriage for the denial of the existence of the coronavirus.[23]

On Invocation

With its confirmation as qualifier of the new normal in societies, the coronavirus becomes the reference in daily dialogues and conversations that it becomes easily invoked and named in place of other material elements. Thus, a number of the postproverbials supplied by respondents sound like invocation or qualification of the embodiment of coronavirus as disease, as an infective, drug-defying pandemic which is open to awe or derision according to the perspective of the particular speaker. The invocation of the virus itself points at its agency, volatility, and morbidity.

14.
p1: Òkùnkùn kò m'ẹni ọ̀wọ̀.
Darkness does not recognize the noble person.

p2: Òkùnkùn kò m'ẹni ọ̀wọ̀, kòró lẹ̀ ń'ké sí.[24]
Darkness does not recognize the noble person, the praise-name of coronavirus.

Comment: This is another classic example of a postproverbial text composed with a supplement. The conventional proverb is used to qualify the state or area of darkness as a place of anonymity which does not respect an individual's importance or class. In the postproverbial, the quality of darkness is invoked as the power or praise-name of the coronavirus. As it were, the disease is thus infused with the epithetic and descriptive agency of "darkness" over humans, irrespective of standing, stature, or status.

---

[23] "Rawanin" is the Hausa word for the emir's turban, which has the connotation of "crown"; "karya" means lie, so the word used for denial in Hausa is karyata, i.e., claiming that something is not true.

[24] Statement made by an unidentified speaker on a live call in a radio program (Yoruba).

15.
p1: Uwar kishiya, kwadon kulle mai yawon banza.
The mother (matriarch) of co-wives is a padlock for the restless wanderer.

p2: Korona, kwadon kulle ma yawon banza.
Corona, the padlock that keeps the restless wanderer at home.

Comment: Like the example before this, the postproverbial here is created as an invocation of the power of the coronavirus. In the conventional proverb, the "mother of co-wives" is actually the matriarch of the home, literally the senior wife who controls the home, and is therefore described as "the padlock" to the restlessness of the co-wives. In the postproverbial, the power of the matriarch is attributed to the coronavirus, signified as the padlock which restricts and confines the restless wanderer at home.

16.
p1: Nala kungheko iquhude liyasa.
Even when the rooster is not present, the day breaks.

p2: Nala Ukorona ekhona, usuku liyasa.[25]
Even when the corona is present, the day breaks.

Comment: The conventional proverb reflects on the eternity and constancy of nature, in spite of other condition, opportunity, or challenge. The postproverbial is itself no less different in the philosophy of the natural law of existence, that in spite of the invocative morbidity of the coronavirus, day will still break. In other words, the pair of proverbs here deflates the power of the disease, with an underlying sense of optimism that in spite of the darkness, the day will break.

[25] Supplied by a respondent, @Bernice Badal (Zulu).

17.
p1: Ẹni éégún ńlé, kó máa r'ọ́jú; bó ti ń'rẹ ará ayé náà ló ń'rẹ ará ọ̀run.
He who is pursued by the masquerade should endure; as the human tires so does the spirit tire.

p2: Ẹni éégún kòró ńlé, kó máa r'ọ́jú, bó ti ń'rẹ ará ayé náà ló ń'rẹ ará ọ̀run.[26]
He who is pursued by the corona masquerade should endure; as the human tires so does the spirit tire.

Comment: In this example, the deflation of the power of the coronavirus is the subject of the postproverbial utterance. Both proverbs establish the importance and necessity of endurance in the face of adversity. The masquerade in the conventional proverb becomes the corona masquerade in the radical proverb, but the impermanence of trials is the constant trope of the (post)proverbial text.

On Hygiene

In the new normal, one of the precautions against the coronavirus is the hygiene of humans and their environment. In addition to social distancing and lockdown, the main measures of that precaution include the covering of the mouth and the nose with face masks and the regular washing and sanitization of the hands. The responsibility to prevent the transmission of the virus, which is tied to hygienic orientation, has also been a subject of postproverbial creativity.

18.
p1: Àgbájọ ọwọ́ la fi ń'sọ àyà.
With all hands together we beat the chest in solidarity.

[26] Supplied by a respondent, @Adetutu Olubummo (Yoruba).

p2: Àgbájọ ọwọ́ la fi ń'wẹ ọwọ́.[27]
With all hands together we wash (the hands) to cleanliness.

p2: Àgbájọ ọwọ́ la fi ń'sọ àyà; l'áyée kòró kọ̀ọ́.[28]
With all hands together we beat the chest in solidarity; not in the age of coronavirus.

Comment: In the conventional proverb, the focus is on solidarity and collective action; whereas the first postproverbial points at the indexical and individual action of hand hygiene, the second example of the postproverbial functions as a declamation against collective physical activity.

19.
p.1: F'ọ̀tún w'òsì, f'òsì w'ọ̀tún, lọwọ́ fi ńmọ́.
Washing the left with the right, washing the right with the left, makes the hand clean.

p.2: F'ọ̀tún w'òsì, f'òsì w'ọ̀tún, ló ń'lé kòró lọ.
Washing the left with the right, washing the right with the left, lays off the coronavirus.

Comment: This is a pair of proverbs that focuses on the physical activity of hand washing as manual process of hygiene. On the one hand, the conventional proverb is predictively embedded with the metaphor of solidarity and cooperation; on the other hand, the postproverbial directly affirms the necessity of hand hygiene as a crucial way of preventing coronavirus infection.

20.
p1: Tí ará ilé ẹni bá ń'jẹ kòkòrò burúkú, tí kò bá r'ẹ́ni sọ fun un, hùrùhẹrẹ rẹ̀ kò ní jẹ́ kí ará ilé gbádùn.
When one's relation feeds on a forbidden insect without warning, his restive reaction will not allow the neighbours to rest.

[27] Supplied by a respondent, @Charles Akinsete (Yoruba).
[28] Supplied by a respondent, @Morounfolu Akinpelu (Yoruba).

p2: Tí ará China bá ń'jẹ kòkòrò burúkú, tí kò bá r'ẹ́ni sọ fún un, kòró kò ní jẹ́ kí gbogbo àgbáyé gbádùn.[29]
When the Chinese feeds on forbidden animals without warning, the coronavirus will not allow the whole world to rest.

Comment: Literally speaking, this is a proverb that anticipates the symptomatic effect of harmful food intake; it also draws attention to how a strain of poisonous food/object consumed by one person can affect the well-being of other people around. In the postproverbial, the subject becomes specified as "the Chinese," apparently echoing the widespread insinuation that the coronavirus disease emanated from an exotic animal market in China. Thus, the radical proverb is as cautionary as much as it is accusatory.

On Morbidity

The very absolute repercussion of coronavirus infection and spread is death. This is an awareness that has been part of the scary reality of living with the pandemic. Therefore, through a number of postproverbials, the creative imagination is devoted to the fearful connotation of death and the sense of morbidity connected to the agency of the virus which is as yet unyielding to the science of vaccine production.

21.
p1: A kìí gbé'lé ẹni ká f'ọrùn rọ́.
One cannot stay at home and get injured.

p2: A kìí gbé'lé ẹni ká f'ọrùn rọ́, òwe kòró kọ́. F'ọwọ́ ẹ![30]
One cannot stay at home and get injured, no such proverb in corona time. Wash your hands!

Comment: The conventional proverb here is a terse figuration of the home as a place of comfort, security, and safety. It is a philosophical

[29] Supplied by a respondent, @El-Nasir Al-Amin (Yoruba).
[30] Supplied by a respondent, @Lanre Oladoyinbo (Yoruba).

assumption that no one gets involved in a ghastly accident while within the confines of his own residence. The accident is specified, that is, having a forced sprain to the neck ("f'ọrùn rọ́"). In the postproverbial utterance, the home is no longer given as safe or insulated from the scourge of the coronavirus. The original proverb is extended and doubly troped upon: first, there is the declamatory clause ("òwe kòrónà kọ"), followed by a full imperative statement which counsels physical hygiene ("F'ọwọ́ ẹ!"). In the postproverbial, the impact of injury (to the body or bones) is replaced with the trauma of infection that it is inherently implied in the radical utterance that the injury is not somatic but a viral one.

22.
p1: Àtẹ́lẹwọ́ ẹni kìí tan ni jẹ.
One's palm does not betray the bearer.

p2: Àtẹ́lẹwọ́ ẹni a má pa ni jẹ.
One's palm can become one's deathtrap.[31]

Comment: In the conventional proverb, the palm (àtẹ́lẹwọ́) is the symbol, the metonym, for a person's destiny; it is also the manual representation of the person's ability by which his industry is determined. Thus, it is said that a person's success or failure is dependent on the effort of her hand/palm. However, in the postproverbial text, the epistemic base of the original proverb is deflated such that the palm is no longer imagined as symbolic. Instead, the palm is taken literally as the inner surface of the hand between the wrist and fingers with the function of washing and cleansing. The palm is the site for physical hygiene and sanitization; if it is not duly taken care of, it may turn to the carrier of infection and death. In its brevity, the postproverbial utterance contains the dual resonance of counsel and threat: the palm can save, and the palm can kill.

23.
p1: Báòkú, ìṣe ò tán.
When there's life, activity does not cease.

[31] On Twitter, https://twitter.com/ajankoro/status/1250390293662380033?s=20 (April 15, 2020).

p2: Báòkú, ìṣekúṣe ò tán.[32]
When there's life, lustfulness does not end.

Comment: Here, the conventional proverb is otherwise rendered as "when there's life, there's hope." In its radical form, it is turned over, punned on, and infused with sexual undertones. Whereas the original proverb is motivational and positivist, the postproverbial stresses the possibility of promiscuity and the potential of lasciviousness *as long as there is life*. Contextually, being sexual or sensual is taken as an inevitable or primary human activity (even in corona times). This postproverbial creation was a direct inference from an unverified news item ascribed to a top official of the Ministry of Health in Uganda who reported that some quarantined coronavirus patients had been having sex with each other.[33] In spite of the possibility of being fake news, such seedy scenario is better left imagined as precarious and dangerously indulgent.

Values of the Postproverbials

The limitation of the study is that the data for analysis is highly topical: the postproverbials are volatile, and like the virus in its period of infection, incubation, and spread, the deployment and significance of COVID-19 postproverbials would probably be active and virtually meaningful within the marked period of invention, currency, and inscription. But ultimately, the values of COVID-19 postproverbials reside in the general attempt to create paramedical awareness against the pandemic, the expression of wisdom in social or physical distancing, of the danger of overcrowding, and of the importance of sanitization, tracing, self-isolation, self-preservation, and in community hygiene

[32] Shared by a Nigerian author, Tade Ipadeola (April 15, 2020).

[33] https://weetalknaija.com.ng/news/breaking-govt-raises-alarm-says-those-in-quarantine-have-started-having-sex-with-each-other.html.

Conclusion

Finally, I assert that these are inexhaustive samples of invented proverbs in the age of the coronavirus. There are four cardinal stems that may be added to conclude the interrogation of these strains of contemporary radical sayings, viz:

1. As a category of postproverbials, they are the eponymous type, in the sense that they are deliberately invented proverbs identified with their initial "authorship" or traceable to particular individuals as referenced in this chapter.
2. As formalized utterances, these entries are essentially retorts, reactions, or bluffs to extant African proverbial thoughts. Indeed, they are ingenious responses to the experience of medical affliction, through the artifice of proverb-making; thus, it can be said that the typical COVID-19 postproverbial is a verbal innovation in the age of illness.
3. As literary and cultural materials in the possession of their users, they undergo a form of "genetic manipulation," and they become chromosomal mutants, aesthetically speaking, in relation to the conventional proverbial text.
4. As sociolinguistic verbal acts, they bear the therapeutic functions of jest and relief, deployed as a coping or healing strategy against the choleric season with its attendant condition of trauma. Pragmatically so, these postproverbials are verbal communicative strategies of living with the life-threatening force of the respiratory virus.

In its creation, the typical COVID-19 postproverbial is invariably volatile, and like the virus in its virtual period of infection, incubation, and spread, the deployment and significance of the radical text will probably be active within the life span of its invention, currency, inscription, and usage.

References

Aleksa, M., H. Hrisztova-Gotthardt, and T. Litovkina Anna. 2009. The Reception of Anti-proverbs in the German Language Area. In *Actas ICP08 Proceedings*, ed. R. Soares and O. Lauhagankas, 83–98. Tipografia Tavirense: Tavira.

Foucault, Michel. 1989. *Madness and Civilization: A History of Insanity in the Age of Reason*. London & New York: Routledge.

Mieder, W. 2007. Anti-proverbs and Mass Communication: The Interplay of Traditional and Innovative Folklore. *Acta Ethnographica Hungarica* 52 (1): 17–46.

Mieder, W., and A. Tóthné Litovkina. 1999. *Twisted Wisdom: Modern Anti-Proverbs*. Burlington: The University of Vermont.

Raji-Oyelade, A. 1999. Postproverbials in Yoruba Culture: A Playful Blasphemy. *Research in African Literatures* 30 (1): 74–82.

———. 2004. Posting the African Proverb: A Grammar of Yoruba Postproverbials, or Logophagia, Logorrhea and the Grammar of Yoruba Postproverbials. *Proverbium: Yearbook of International Proverb Scholarship* 21: 299–314.

———. 2012. *Playful Blasphemies: Postproverbials as Archetypes of Modernity in Yoruba Culture*. Trier: Wissenchaftlicher Verlag.

Tóthné Litovkina, A., and W. Mieder. 2006. *Old Proverbs Never Die, They Just Diversify: A Collection of Anti-proverbs*. Burlington & Veszprém: The University of Vermont & The Pannonian University of Veszprém.

United Nations Habitat Report. 2020. *COVID-19 in African Cities: Impacts, Responses and Policies*. A United Nations Human Settlements Programme (UN-Habitat), 34pp.

Index[1]

NUMBERS AND SYMBOLS

#EndSARS, 44, 185, 185n1, 330, 333, 343, 360n4

A

Adeboye, Pastor Enoch Adejare, 273, 277, 443
Africa
  "diseases continent," 8, 124, 145
  sub-Saharan, 53, 55, 56, 63, 136, 230
African traditional religion, 319–321
Akin Fadeyi Foundation (Nigeria), 355, 359–363, 368–370
Aladura movement, 260
Almajiri, 200, 223–244, 340
Anamnesis, 23–26
Animal, 35, 100, 151–157, 163, 165, 172, 269, 288, 409, 478
AstraZeneca, 3, 37, 180, 283
Asukwo, Etim Bassey, 329–344, 343n7, 348, 349

B

Bakhtin, Mikhail, 304–306, 308, 309, 314, 316, 317, 321
Black Death, v, 314
Border, 106, 128, 141, 181, 197–220, 234, 240, 338, 356, 390, 392, 414, 466, 471
Boundary, 7, 25, 113, 197–220, 270, 370, 414, 468

[1] Note: Page numbers followed by 'n' refer to notes.

F. Egbokhare, A. Afolayan (eds.), *Global Health, Humanity and the COVID-19 Pandemic*, https://doi.org/10.1007/978-3-031-17429-2

C

Capitalism, 2, 7, 128, 229
Cartoon/cartooning, 329–349
Case Fatality Ratio (CFR), 173
Center for Disease Control and Prevention (US), 52, 81, 133, 134, 199, 201, 295, 374–376
Center for Infectious Diseases (Senegal), 125, 129
China, v, 36, 40, 79, 98–106, 109, 110, 112–117, 152, 154, 167, 173, 176, 180, 181, 199, 202, 206, 207, 215, 248, 283, 308–310, 315, 316, 319, 320, 353, 354, 429, 461, 462, 478
  Wuhan, 8, 36, 79, 97, 100–103, 154, 173, 199, 248, 272, 283, 308, 401, 461
Christianity, 250, 255, 272, 313, 390, 413–415, 419, 420
Citizen, 9, 42, 76–80, 79n7, 84–88, 90, 91, 101, 128, 134, 137, 179, 185, 198, 201, 207, 210, 211, 213, 215, 225, 232, 235, 241, 242, 250, 254, 309, 330, 331, 335, 336, 344–346, 349, 358–360, 364, 365, 367, 375, 392, 393, 402, 405, 444
Civilization, v, vi, 4n1, 46, 133, 218
Colonialism, 64, 86n15
"Combat Coronavirus" stamp (Senegal), 137, 138
Communication, 10, 129, 251, 252, 267, 295, 332, 354–362, 367–370, 382, 427–455
Communion, 35, 49, 99, 100, 109–113, 117, 159, 160, 166–168, 238
  ethic of, 99, 100, 109, 110, 112, 113, 117
Communitarian/communitarianism, 45, 415
Community
  epistemic, 183
  Pentecostal, 249, 250, 253, 262
  political, 211, 215–217
  scientific, 10, 187
Conspiracy theories, 10, 103, 106, 115, 167, 172, 173, 186, 187, 191, 319, 342, 429
Coronavirus/COVID-19, v, 2, 16, 33–49, 51–66, 75, 97, 123–146, 151–169, 171–195, 197, 199–208, 212–219, 223–244, 247–277, 283, 303–323, 329–349, 353, 373–394, 401–422, 427–455, 461–481
Culture/cultural, vi, 10, 24, 27, 29, 34, 42, 46, 48, 52, 53, 58, 59, 61, 62, 64, 66, 105, 128, 131–133, 135, 139, 157, 163–165, 184, 210–213, 216, 229, 230, 237–240, 248, 257, 258, 275, 285, 295, 330–336, 331n2, 340–346, 343n6, 348, 349, 355–359, 367, 377, 389, 406, 409, 428, 433–435, 438, 439, 455, 464, 481

D

Death, v, 3, 17, 37, 54, 98, 105, 107, 115, 124n1, 126, 132–134, 145, 160, 163, 166, 173, 175, 176, 184, 199, 200, 202–204, 248–251, 254, 260–262, 264, 271, 272, 283–285, 292, 293, 297, 306, 316, 338, 362n5, 364, 374, 392, 402, 405, 442, 468, 469, 471–473, 478, 479

Dehumanization, 2, 232, 239
Democracy, 40, 44, 86, 213, 256, 413
Diagnosis, 23–26, 31, 175, 181, 283
Dialogism, 303–323
Dickens, Charles, 1, 2
Disease, 1–11, 25, 33, 51, 75, 100, 123–146, 153, 172, 202, 224, 248, 283, 307, 354, 374, 401, 428, 461
  infectious, 51, 52, 54, 55, 59, 76, 78n5, 81–84, 90, 107, 108, 124, 128, 131, 284, 285, 287, 291, 428
Distrust, 9, 63, 79–81, 85, 86, 88–91, 115, 152, 168, 182, 187, 260, 430, 444

E

Eating, 151–169, 410, 441, 444
Ebola, 43, 51–66, 107, 124, 128, 129, 145, 180, 181, 207, 298
Economy
  attention, 331n2
  prayer, 240
Education, 7, 8, 26, 29, 31, 42, 63, 190, 203, 205, 214, 225, 230, 231, 237, 239, 241, 242, 256, 267, 295, 304, 339, 353, 356, 369, 378, 434
Engagement/disengagement, 9, 19, 28, 30, 43, 61–63, 66, 135, 151, 153, 154, 156, 159, 219, 237, 291, 332, 335, 340, 348, 355–361, 363, 367n6, 370, 374, 376, 379, 416, 427–455, 463
The enigma of health, 15–31
Enlightenment, 3, 203, 228, 231, 236, 404, 414
Ẹnulẹbọ, 151–169
Epidemic(s), 2, 51, 53, 54, 58, 59, 61–63, 98, 100, 102, 108, 180, 190, 248, 250, 260, 265, 273, 277, 292, 296, 308, 317, 319, 387, 391, 421, 427, 433, 437, 441, 442, 462
Epidemiology, 166, 171–193
Epistemology, 7n2, 40, 156, 176, 178, 179, 225, 227, 243, 248, 268
Equilibrium, 19–22, 24, 25, 27, 29, 30
Ethics/ethical, 17, 41, 43, 46, 51, 53, 61, 65, 66, 76n1, 97–117, 151–169, 171, 208, 212–219, 238, 268, 283, 284, 406
European Union (EU), 79, 215, 236, 286

F

Facebook, 252, 329–349, 375, 377, 379, 381, 384, 387, 440, 441, 463
Faith-based organisations, 251, 437, 440, 443
Fake news, 10, 329, 365, 393, 432, 433, 480
Fela Anikulapo-Kuti, 342, 393, 394
Food, 29, 82, 145, 151, 153, 154, 156–158, 162–166, 182, 225, 227, 229, 231, 233, 239, 248n2, 264, 271, 318, 339, 365, 401–422, 441, 478

Foucault, Michel, 226, 238, 239, 358
Freedom, 9, 31, 45, 53, 76–78, 212, 239, 250–252, 266, 268, 319, 381, 401–422
  of choice, 77, 78

G

Gadamer, Hans Georg, 17–31
Geographic information system (GIS), 124, 125
Gestaltkreis, 20–22, 24
Ghana, 63–65, 107, 124n1, 262, 462n4
God, 160, 162–165, 164n6, 227, 229, 238, 249, 251, 254, 262, 263, 268, 269, 273–277, 310, 314–318, 321, 362, 387, 403, 410, 413–416, 418, 419
Good
  collective, 83–85, 89–91
  public, 81, 87–89, 87n16, 101
Government, 15n1, 37, 39, 41, 43–45, 47, 48, 62, 75, 77, 79–82, 79n7, 84, 86, 89, 90, 98, 99, 102, 104–106, 108, 109, 114, 115, 126, 129, 145, 171, 172, 176, 182–185, 187, 189, 192, 193, 198, 202–204, 207, 212, 214, 250, 251, 253, 254, 265–267, 272, 275, 277, 287, 290–292, 299, 308–310, 312, 333, 334, 341–343, 345, 349, 354, 355, 357, 358, 360, 367–369, 374, 375, 379, 384, 390–393, 401–405, 407, 411, 415, 417–422, 428, 430, 436, 437, 440, 443, 444, 462, 466
Guinea, 62–64, 129, 298

H

Healing, 19–23, 29, 31, 163, 230, 239, 249, 252, 257–259, 268, 271, 276, 316, 320, 387, 403, 468, 481
Health
  global, vi, 6, 9–11, 51–66, 100, 116, 217, 223, 283, 354
  infrastructure, 58
  mental, 2, 37, 295, 296, 298, 374, 377
  promotion, 428, 429, 434, 443, 455
  public, 16, 17, 31, 61, 76, 76n1, 78, 80n8, 81, 99, 107, 108, 123–125, 136, 137, 165, 167, 172, 176, 178, 181, 186, 197, 201, 202, 205, 213, 217, 248, 250, 251, 259, 274, 275, 277, 284–287, 291, 294, 296, 297, 311, 369, 374, 376, 379, 382–386, 390–394, 427, 431, 432, 437, 454
  sciences, 16, 17, 20, 22, 23, 26–31
  spiritual, 16, 28
  workers, 103, 108, 124n1, 129, 138, 224, 292–295, 297–299, 312, 374, 375
Healthcare, 17, 22, 25–27, 31, 56, 58, 63, 98, 99, 102, 107–109, 203, 205, 207, 213, 254, 284, 291, 292, 294, 296–299, 311, 312, 337, 374, 376, 391, 392, 431, 462
HIV/AIDS, v, 55, 107, 175, 285, 314, 434
Holy Spirit, 247–277

Human, v, 2, 15, 33, 51, 76, 98, 132, 151, 172, 197, 224, 249, 284, 304, 373, 402, 428, 464
Humanity/humanities, v, vi, 1–11, 18, 25–30, 33–36, 38, 40–42, 44–49, 51, 52, 58, 61–66, 109, 132, 136, 155, 162, 211, 216, 223–225, 230, 237, 243, 249, 262, 263, 293, 311–316, 318, 319, 321, 370

I

Identity, 47, 110, 111, 113, 167, 197–220, 270, 332, 338, 406, 409, 435
Ifá, 157, 162, 169
Immunity, 37, 55, 78, 80, 82–84, 83n12, 85n14, 89, 190, 203, 353, 354, 388
  herd, 55, 80, 82–84, 83n12, 85n14, 190, 203
Immunization, 7n2, 59, 78n5, 82
Individual, 16, 22, 25, 26, 30, 36, 40, 45–48, 75–78, 80–91, 83n12, 85n14, 100, 110, 114, 124n1, 126, 131, 132, 136, 144, 159, 171, 172, 182, 184, 201, 204, 208, 209, 212, 213, 224, 238, 239, 241, 250, 254, 263, 293, 305, 316, 333, 334, 342, 344, 346, 356, 358, 359, 365, 376, 381, 382, 384, 389, 403, 407, 428, 431, 433, 436, 440, 442, 473, 474, 477, 481
  rights, 81, 83, 84, 89–91, 201
Inequality, 8, 9, 17, 47, 58, 144, 202, 203, 207, 209, 214, 215, 219, 220, 226, 232
Inferiorisation, 188, 189
Infodemic, 10, 167, 186, 364, 375, 430, 449
Information/misinformation, 10, 64, 79, 79n7, 80, 86–90, 87n16, 98, 103, 104, 106, 124, 129, 171, 179, 183, 185–187, 189, 191, 192, 199, 206, 240, 252, 286, 307, 308, 330, 332, 354, 355, 357, 361, 362, 364–365, 367, 369n7, 370, 374, 375, 379–383, 386, 393, 404, 421, 427–429, 431–435, 441, 442, 444, 450, 452, 454, 455
Islam, 135, 136, 139, 226, 235, 240, 313, 318, 319, 415, 419, 420
Isolation, 37, 49, 60, 104, 108, 182, 184, 198, 217, 263, 306, 377, 382, 391, 430, 441, 468

J

Joshua, Pastor T. B., 261, 262
Justice, 57, 58, 85–88, 91, 203–205, 210, 345, 348

K

Knowledge, vi, 3, 5–7, 7n2, 16, 19, 20, 27, 28, 31, 40, 42, 44–47, 51, 52, 55, 63, 64, 78n5, 87n16, 89, 123–146, 176, 178, 183, 185, 187, 225–232, 238, 239, 268, 283, 291, 297, 330, 333, 339, 349, 418, 428, 429, 431–434, 452, 455, 464
  indigenous, 428

L

Language/languaging, 3, 19, 22–24, 27, 28, 33, 52, 124, 210, 226, 238, 242, 257, 263, 304–314, 321, 322, 333, 348, 355–359, 367–369, 428, 433, 438, 441, 442, 463, 464
Leibniz, Gottfried, 189, 191, 192
Lockdown, 37, 41, 47, 52, 66, 75, 102, 124n1, 145, 172, 177, 181, 186, 188, 190, 198, 200, 203, 204, 206, 207, 213, 234, 250–259, 265, 267, 271, 273, 329n1, 336, 339, 364–366, 374, 376, 377, 380–382, 384, 394, 401–405, 416–422, 430, 462, 465–468, 470, 476

M

Magal pilgrimage, 139–141
Magufuli, John, 262, 310, 362n5
Meaning, 6, 23, 49, 208, 226, 238, 241, 249, 251, 270, 305–307, 309, 311, 313, 322, 332–334, 336, 338, 341, 342, 348, 356, 357, 360, 367, 368, 406, 412, 414, 443, 464
Medicine, 9, 16, 18, 19, 23, 31, 60, 62, 66, 85n14, 105, 287, 320, 392, 406, 429, 441
Metaphor, 21, 22, 153, 226, 308, 311, 312, 322, 477
Minority(ites), 56, 140, 200, 202, 204, 214, 241, 269, 346
Moderna, 3, 55, 180, 283
Monadology, 189–192
Moral/morality
  agent, 111, 409
  failure, 224
  theory, 100, 109–116
  value, 60, 61, 111, 112
Mouride Brotherhood, 139
Music, 376–384, 386–388, 390, 393, 394, 436, 438, 442, 455

N

Nationalism, 8, 207, 218, 224, 229, 344
Neurath, Otto, 3
Nigeria, 39, 64, 76, 98, 107–109, 159n4, 171–193, 200, 224, 252, 283–299, 329, 353, 373–396, 401–422, 427–455, 462n4
Nigeria Centre for Disease Control (NCDC), 114, 180, 181, 184, 186, 204, 284, 287, 290, 291, 299, 430, 442, 443
Nigerian Medical Association (NMA), 98, 105, 106
Nigerian National Pandemic Influenza Preparedness and Response Plan (NPIPRP), 284, 287–296, 298

O

Obadare, Ebenezer, 256, 330, 346, 413, 415, 416, 420, 443, 444
Oyakhilome, Pastor Chris, 186, 272, 273, 273n17, 365
Oyedepo, Bishop David, 272, 273, 276, 403, 404, 421

P

Pandemic
- diplomacy, 206
- discourse, 303–305, 307, 309, 313, 315, 317, 321, 322, 349
- Justinian, v
- management, 115, 125, 145, 198, 212
- philanthropy, 98–100, 102–106, 109–117
- planning, 283–299
- post-, vi, 36, 38, 41, 112, 208, 219, 291, 295

Pasteur Institute, 125, 129, 131
Pentecostal, 362, 363, 402, 404, 405, 412, 415, 416, 418–422
Pentecostalism, 249, 255–258, 263, 268, 271, 274–277, 362, 415, 416, 418, 420
Person, 4n1, 6, 16, 17, 22, 24–26, 30n2, 31, 35, 37–39, 41, 42, 46, 54, 57, 58, 78n5, 82, 83, 85, 85n14, 87, 111, 155, 156, 159, 163, 164, 173, 200, 211, 216, 217, 258, 263, 265, 273, 292, 293, 297, 363, 364, 384, 385, 389, 391, 405–407, 411, 429–431, 441, 446, 466–469, 474, 478, 479
Personal protective equipment (PPE), 25, 59, 98, 134, 185, 215, 271, 292, 293, 298, 442
Pfizer, 3, 55, 64, 283
Plague, v, 233, 235, 262, 268, 269, 285, 312, 313, 388, 389
Plato, 22, 23
Polio, 54, 59, 64, 80, 80n9, 129, 180
Politics, 25, 64, 97–117, 126, 205–207, 211, 215, 256, 307, 332, 334, 341, 342, 345, 346, 390, 408, 413, 415, 420, 421
Polyphony, 303–323
Population, vi, 3, 8, 15n1, 37, 52, 53, 55–66, 78, 107, 124–126, 132–136, 143–145, 173–175, 179, 180, 190, 200, 204, 207, 213, 215, 235, 239, 262, 265, 269, 284, 285, 291, 298, 342, 354, 356–358, 361, 367, 369, 417, 418, 433, 473
- elderly, 125, 134

Populism, 115, 205, 218
Positivism, 6, 7n2
Post-Covid, 10, 223–244, 277, 402
Power, 8, 20, 27, 28, 42, 45, 64, 76, 86, 113, 115, 123, 125, 132–134, 137, 167, 168, 183, 188, 201, 202, 206, 212, 214, 215, 218, 238, 239, 242, 249, 251, 254, 256–263, 266, 268, 270, 271, 274–276, 309, 316, 318, 320, 329–336, 331n2, 338–342, 344–346, 348, 349, 358, 362, 363, 403, 407, 408, 415, 419–421, 434, 443, 471, 474–476
Proverbs/postproverbials, 417, 461–481
Public sphere, 252, 332, 341, 344–346, 348, 412, 413, 416

Q

Quarantine, 277, 377, 394, 421, 441, 466
- arts, 377, 394

Quarantine Act (Nigeria), 76
Qur'an, 228, 229, 231, 239, 243

R

Ramadan, 239, 419, 420
Relationality, 100, 113, 114, 116
Religion/religious, 2, 86, 101, 131, 159n4, 184, 210, 230, 248, 304, 362, 378, 402, 429, 462
Rwanda, 124n1, 128

S

Salvation, 239, 270, 271
SARS-CoV, *see* Coronavirus/COVID-19
Science(s)
  natural, 27, 28
  social, 52, 379
Scientism, 5–7, 7n2, 10
Secular/secularism/secularity, 230, 405, 412–422
Self-determination, 78, 81, 83, 88, 90, 91
Sellars, Wilfred, 4–6, 4n1
Senegal, 123–146, 230
Sincerity, 76, 79, 84, 89, 90, 172, 192, 193
Social contract, 77, 84, 84n13, 88, 91
Social media, 79n7, 115, 172, 186, 251, 330–336, 331n2, 340, 342–349, 353, 373–394, 427–455, 463
  influencer, 331, 331n2
Social/physical distancing, 34, 37, 48, 52, 125, 131, 134, 136–139, 184, 188, 198, 199, 204, 212, 213, 250, 264, 265, 267, 273, 312, 339, 354, 361, 363–364, 367, 373, 374, 377, 383, 384, 401, 403, 404, 420, 428, 441, 444, 446, 462, 465, 466, 468–470, 476, 480
Society, 10, 18, 28, 39, 42, 44, 46, 47, 76, 80–82, 84, 85, 87, 89–91, 101, 110, 126, 132–136, 139, 141, 189, 197, 199, 200, 209–211, 218–220, 229, 232, 234, 235, 237–240, 248, 249n4, 250, 251, 254, 255, 257, 262, 269–271, 274n20, 275, 277, 285, 291, 293, 294, 305, 330, 335, 338, 343, 354, 359, 360, 370, 374, 378, 389, 406, 412, 416, 419, 471, 474
Socrates, 22–24, 38
Solidarity, 44, 53, 110, 111, 113, 116, 162, 165–167, 197–220, 343, 376, 377, 382, 386, 394, 477
South Africa, 36, 41, 107, 128, 143, 180, 207, 213, 214, 247n1, 252, 264, 266, 306, 342, 462n4
Spanish flu, v, 54–55, 285, 297
Spirit/spiritual, 8, 10, 16, 24, 28, 42, 45, 49, 52, 136, 186, 189, 229, 243, 254–259, 263, 267, 271, 275, 310, 313, 319, 320, 363, 377, 382, 386–390, 394, 403, 406, 416, 419, 462, 466, 468, 476
State, 9, 17, 38, 66, 75, 101, 123, 152, 172, 197, 201–205, 233, 250, 287, 309, 329, 353, 375, 403, 436, 466
Suffering, 24–26, 108, 109, 112, 116, 209, 228, 248, 249, 251, 255, 264–266, 274, 303, 312, 315, 316, 318, 417, 419

Sufficiency, 52, 53, 57–59, 239
approach/theory, 52, 53, 57–59
Sufi/Sufism, 135–137, 228, 237–239

T

A Tale of Two Cities, 2
Theology, 225–227, 249, 257, 275, 276, 409–412, 415, 416
Trump, Donald, 103, 128, 202, 212, 307–309, 364
Trust, 9, 57, 61, 65, 66, 100, 106, 109, 111, 114, 162, 168, 169, 172, 183, 192, 193, 209, 214, 251, 254, 265
Truth, 5, 9, 10, 16, 18, 19, 22, 24, 26, 31, 39, 40, 46, 89, 115, 140, 143, 172, 175–177, 187, 189, 191, 193, 239, 304–306, 308, 309, 313, 317, 322, 332, 345, 404, 412
Twitter, 252, 329, 330, 334–336, 377, 381, 440, 463, 464

U

Ubuntu, 33–49, 110
United States (US), 17, 54, 56, 64, 79, 81, 124, 128, 133, 134, 141, 152, 154, 167, 181, 200–206, 212, 214, 215, 248n2, 307–310, 316, 317, 320, 364, 376, 408, 429, 462
Universal Basic Education Commission (UBEC) Act (Nigeria), 241

V

Vaccination
advocates, 81, 82, 84, 85, 88, 89
debate, 75–91
moderationists, 81
Vaccine
anti-, 9, 59
hesitancy/hesitation, 9, 56, 60, 61, 65, 264, 276
nationalism, 8, 9, 56, 207, 224
Virus, v, 3, 16, 37, 52, 79n7, 97, 100–101, 128, 156, 172, 199, 225, 283, 303, 332, 353, 373, 403, 428, 461–481
Chinese, 8, 202, 307

W

World Health Organization (WHO), 3, 8, 8n3, 36, 37, 54, 55, 57, 62, 64, 79, 97, 107, 129, 130, 132, 144, 145, 152, 154, 167, 173, 181, 182, 186, 199, 201, 206, 215, 218, 223, 248n2, 258, 283, 285–289, 292, 295, 298, 299, 306, 307, 310–312, 353, 354n1, 355, 363, 366, 375, 392, 401, 427, 428, 433, 440, 446
Worship, 138, 141, 158, 184, 212, 214, 250, 319, 377, 401–422, 441

Y

Yoruba, 151–169, 240, 259, 438, 441, 444, 464, 469–471, 474n24
YouTube, 186, 252, 353, 361, 377, 379, 381

Z

Zimbabwe, 36, 261, 303–323

Kolibri 360 GmbH
Ferdinand-Jühlke-Straße 7
99095 Erfurt, Deutschland
produktsicherheit@kolibri360.de